MANAGERIAL

EPIDEMIOLOGY

MANAGERIAL
EPIDEMIOLOGY

Steven T. Fleming
F. Douglas Scutchfield
Thomas C. Tucker

Health Administration Press, Chicago, Illinois
AUPHA Press, Washington, D.C.

AUPHA
HAP

04   03   02   01   00   5   4   3   2   1

The paper used in this publication meets the minimum requirements of American National Standard for Information Sciences—Permanence of Paper for Printed Library Materials, ANSW Z39.48-1984.♾™

Library of Congress Cataloging-in-Publication Data

Fleming, Steven T., 1950–
  Managerial epidemiology / Steven T. Fleming, F. Douglas Scutchfield, Thomas C. Tucker.
     p.; cm.
  Includes bibliographical references and index.
  ISBN 1-567-93-129-4 (alk. paper)
  1. Health services administration.   2. Epidemiology—Methodology.   I. Scutchfield, F. Douglas.   II. Tucker, Thomas C., 1946–   III. Title.
  [DNLM: 1. Epidemiologic Studies.   2. Epidemiologic Research Design.
  3. Health Services Administration. WA 950 F598m 2000]
  RA971 .F54 2000
  614.4—dc21
                                                              00-039715

Health Administration Press
A division of the Foundation
  of the American College of
  Healthcare Executives
One North Franklin Street
Chicago, IL 60606
(312) 424-2800

Association of University Programs
  in Health Administration
1911 North Fort Meyer Drive
Suite 503
Arlington, VA 22209
(703) 524-5500

To our families, who never understood what managerial epidemiology is but were willing to allow us to blather on about it. Particularly our wives, Alayne, Phyllis and Nancy whose patience and support has sustained us through this publication, but also through the academy's little slings and arrows—research diversions, desperate students, and persnickity computers. There are also so many mentors to whom we owe a great deal of appreciation. These colleagues, friends, and teachers come along side to encourage, inspire, and enkindle. We also dedicate this book to them. They include Avedis Donabedian, Robin Blake, Kurt Deuschle, Alex Langmuir, Gilbert Friedell, and Victor Hawthorne.

CONTENTS

LIST OF FIGURES

Figure

LIST OF TABLES

Table

Acknowledgments

The editors wish to thank all of the authors who gave so generously of their time and talents to write chapters for this book. Their professionalism, responsiveness to criticism, and willingness to engage in this project are most appreciated. We also salute the staff of Health Administration Press for their encouragement, support, and for their wordsmithing prowess. Thank you for giving this book a distinct luster. The often hidden, but highly valued work of reviewers is a critical component of academic scholarship. Duncan, thank you for your helpful comments, suggestions, and advocacy.

FOREWORD

I magine that you are about to finish a degree and start a career in health management. You can view your career in either the traditional way, or a new, expanded way. In the traditional way, you can see yourself as a kind of highly specialized hotel manager for doctors and their patients. You are concerned that the electricity is on, the food hot, the laundry and floors clean, the equipment in working order, the staffing adequate, and the bills paid. Or you can see yourself as part of a team helping to organize the best possible care for a defined population within the budget limits imposed by capitation. In the traditional view, managerial epidemiology will have small appeal. In the expanded view, however, it will be essential and central.

You join the management team of a progressive healthcare organization that sees itself as providing best care (giving value for money) to the population it serves. One of your first assignments is to join the asthma care team. This team is charged with organizing the best asthma care for your population and consists of a primary care physician, an asthma specialist, a nurse educator, and a staff person from the information department. The board of your organization has said that all care here will be evidence based. The team has more questions than answers. What is good asthma care? To answer this question you have to be able to judge the quality of the evidence. That's why you need to evaluate the clinical literature using the tools of evidence described in Chapters 3, 4, 5, and 6 here. How many asthmatics are cared for? How many are mild, moderate, and severe cases? Although as many as 10 percent of American urban dwellers have asthma, it is only the much smaller number of severe cases that account for most of the costly hospital admissions. This kind of population-based perspective is at the heart of epidemiology. What is the total cost of asthma care for your health plan? You find out that asthma care is the most expensive category of care for your organization's Medicaid patients, largely due to emergency room visits and hospital admissions by 50 families with a severe asthmatic member out of 20,000 enrollees. Your specialist team member says that well-organized care could avoid nearly all these admissions, but it would require more nurse educators and community asthma coaches. How good is the evidence for this assertion? Can you help develop the plan and budget for such reorganized care? This is where management and the population-based thinking of epidemiology fit together. This is why you need the knowledge presented in Chapters 7 through 11.

Your team comes to realize that the skills of the manager are essential in order to reengineer your organization to achieve evidence-based, population-based best care, including measured outcomes and costs per enrollee.

How will the management information system be redesigned to meet these best-practice goals? Can your current information system track asthma hospital admissions in "real time"? How is the rate of severity-adjusted emergency room visits per 100 asthmatic enrollees compared across your organiztion's several group practices? Do you benchmark your performance measures with other world-class care systems?

The team believes that reorganized asthma care can improve quality and lower costs. The physicians and nurse team members now realize they can't do this without your help. The perspective of management and clinical epidemiology joined together could be the basis of providing best care for the people your organization serves.

If you think this is the future of healthcare, read on. However, if you think that health management is "all in potatoes and floor polish," (1913) you need read no further.

Duncan Neuhauser, Ph.D.
The Charles Elton Blanchard Professor of Health Management
Department of Epidemiology and Biostatistics, Medical School
Co-Director of the Health Systems Management Center
Case Western Reserve University

Managerial Epidemiology: Principles and Tools

AN INTRODUCTION TO MANAGERIAL EPIDEMIOLOGY

Thomas C. Tucker, Steven T. Fleming, and F. Douglas Scutchfield

Epidemiology has traditionally been defined as the study of the distribution and determinants of disease in human populations (Lilienfeld and Stolley 1994). As a discipline, epidemiology has developed the tools by which we (1) measure the burden of disease in specific populations, (2) determine differences in the burden of disease between populations, (3) explore the origins or causes for differences in disease burdens, and (4) determine the effect of treatments and interventions on reducing the burden of disease. In other words, we can think of epidemiology as the tools we use to determine everything we know about interventions, treatments, and healthcare services. This text examines ways to apply the principles and tools of epidemiology to the management of health services. Much like managerial accounting applies the principles of accounting to various management functions (Neumann, Suver, and Zelman 1988), this book applies the principles of epidemiology to the management of health services.

Many ways exist to define and describe health services management (Austin 1974; Hodgetts and Cascio 1983). One common way is to list the functions that managers perform, to describe them one by one, to elaborate on the descriptions, and to form connections. Rakich, Longest, and Darr (1992) list the functions as planning, staffing, organizing, directing, and controlling. With each of these functions, health services managers must make decisions. For example, in the planning function, they must decide which services they will provide and which ones they will not. As part of the staffing function, managers must determine the skills that are required to provide specified services and decide on the type and number of staff needed to provide them. The organizing function requires managers to decide how various parts of the organization will relate to each other in order to maximize positive impact on health outcomes. As part of the directing function managers provide vision and leadership intended to focus the organization on important goals. With the controlling function managers determine if the organization is effective and producing the desired results. Each of these managerial functions requires decisions, and the decisions made in one functional domain almost always have consequences in other functional areas. This functional definition of management is depicted in Figure 1.1.

Managerial epidemiology uses the principles and tools of epidemiology to help managers make better-informed decisions in each of these functional domains;

FIGURE 1.1
Managerial
Functions

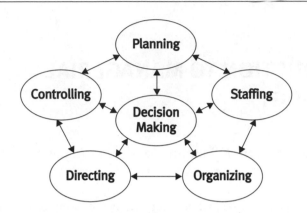

Source: Rakich, J. S., B. B. Longest, and K. Darr. 1992. *Managing Health Services Organizations, 3rd ed.* Baltimore, MD: Health Professions Press.

that is, **managerial epidemiology** is the application of the principles and tools of epidemiology to the decision-making process.

This text is organized into two parts. The principles and tools of epidemiology are presented in the first six chapters (Part I). Chapter 2 provides an overview of the concepts and principles of epidemiology. This includes the relationship between agent, host, and environment; concepts of disease transmission, incidence and prevalence rates; methods of standardizing rates; descriptive epidemiology across time, place, and people; levels of prevention; and test characteristics, such as sensitivity, specificity, and positive and negative predictive value.

Chapter 3 presents the basic statistical tools used in epidemiology and distinguishes between descriptive and inferential epidemiology, within the context of decision making for the healthcare manager. The chapter discusses the difference between continuous and categorical variables with measures of central tendency and variability for each type, and it describes various types of sampling methods. For inferential statistics, the authors discuss hypothesis testing, the concept of a p-value, and the distinction between type I (α) and type II (β) error.

Chapters 4, 5, and 6 relate to various types of epidemiologic study designs. Chapter 5 explores the case control design by describing selection of cases and controls; the concepts of exposure, relative risk, and confounding variables; attributable fraction; and various kinds of bias, with a focus on misclassification bias. Prospective and retrospective cohort studies are compared in Chapter 5. The authors discuss selection, exposure, and relative risk within the context of a cohort study, and the difference between attributable fraction and attributable risk, as well as the methods by which incidence is measured over time. Randomized clinical trials are the subject of Chapter 6, which includes the concepts of protocols, randomization, historical controls, crossover designs, and treatment effects. Moreover, the authors describe the importance of blinding, ethics, and integrity within the randomization process. The chapter also summarizes the concept of a hospital firm, the technique of meta-analysis, and the research design referred to as a community trial.

The application of these principles, tools, and study designs to the management of health services are discussed in Chapters 7 through 13 (Part II). The application of epidemiology to the planning function is the topic of chapter 7. Here the authors summarize the history of planning and distinguish among strategic, operational, institutional, and community planning. The chapter discusses community health planning, use of the Health People 2000 objectives, and ways in which epidemiology can be used to set priorities and objectives, obtain baseline information, and track progress toward meeting objectives.

The use of epidemiologic principles for making decisions related to the directing function is discussed in Chapter 8. Here the focus is on motivating, leading, and communicating. The authors articulate a theory of leadership, differentiate between managers and leaders, emphasize the importance of communication, and discuss the application of epidemiologic concepts and methods to each of these roles (i.e., how an understanding of epidemiology can become a source of power and credibility for the healthcare manager).

The application of epidemiology to the controlling function is discussed in Chapter 9, with a focus on quality assurance, measurement, and management. The author relates epidemiology to quality of care and discusses the various ways in which quality can be assessed using epidemiologic measures. This chapter explores the concepts of rates, surveillance, risk adjustment, and quality measurement using complication and mortality rates. Ambulatory care-sensitive conditions and avoidable hospitalization rates are discussed as measures of quality within the context of managed care. Finally, the chapter explores ways in which epidemiology can play a fundamental role in total quality management.

Chapter 10 explores the use of epidemiologic tools for making decisions about organizing and staffing. We discuss various types of organization design, the process of change over time, and ways for epidemiology to inform the decision-making process. Further, the chapter describes the process by which an organization can predict staffing needs using epidemiologic measures of morbidity or risk. This simple, and perhaps familiar, medical manpower model relates the assessment of need in the population served to the number of services that must be provided and to the number of medical professionals needed to provide those services.

Chapter 11 reviews the principles of epidemiology as they relate to financial management. Although financial management is considered a subset of activities related to the controlling function, it is of sufficient importance to health service managers to warrant a separate chapter. Here the authors thoroughly expostulate the concept of risk, differentiate between the kinds of risk (or exposure) facing the patient, and describe the capitation environment. In addition to a discussion on the basics of capitation and risk adjustment, the chapter suggests possible ways of using morbidity and risk factors to adjust capitation rates.

Clinical epidemiology is the focus of Chapter 12. The reason for including a chapter on medical decision making is to acquaint the reader with how physicians can use epidemiology to make clinical decisions. It would seem useful for healthcare managers to be at least somewhat familiar with how physicians think. In this chapter, the authors distinguish between tradition-based and evidence-based medical practice, where epidemiologic studies can inform the latter. The chapter describes the clinical encounter in terms of diagnosis, treatment, and prevention, and discusses how epidemiology should provide the evidence necessary for rational decisions.

Finally, Chapter 13 integrates the principles of epidemiology (Chapters 1–6) with their application to management (chapter 7–13) within the context of managerial decision making. The authors describe integrative decision making and problem solving within a healthcare setting by managers who embrace the concepts and principles of epidemiology. The case study originally presented in Chapter 1 is revisited in the last chapter in an attempt to describe the more effective decisions the epidemiologically informed healthcare manager might make.

The following case study presents a number of issues related to the various management functions. The case study should be carefully read. Think about how you would approach the problems identified in this case study. We will explore the relationship between the principles and tools of epidemiology and the variety of issues identified in the case study in Chapters 7–12. In the final chapter, this case study is revisited in an effort to show how the principles of epidemiology can be integrated into the decision-making process of health services managers.

Managerial Epidemiology: Case Study

Group Health East (GHE) is a 100,000-member HMO located in southern New England. It operates two large clinics in north and south Boston and five smaller satellite clinics in surrounding communities. GHE is a mixed-model HMO affiliated with two large multispecialty groups—Physicians Associates (PA) and Bayside Multispecialty Group (BMS)—in addition to 500 individual physicians in the community. PA provides in-house services in the north clinic; BMS provides services in the south. GHE is affiliated with two major metropolitan hospitals in the Boston area. The chief executive officer (CEO), Mr. Jones, is a 55-year-old hospital executive who crossed over into the managed care sector three years ago. Mr. Jones' autocratic style of management has caused no small amount of friction within and outside the organization since his arrival at GHE. GHE is going through a time of transition attributable to increased market competition, and it faces a number of important decisions that will affect its future. These decisions relate to organizational structure, staffing, incentives and performance appraisals, surveillance of adverse outcomes, strategic planning, and rate setting. Mr. Jones has alienated many of his senior staff as a result of his abrasive, dictatorial style, and he has virtually no rapport with the medical staff. Thus, his decisions tend to be made in a vacuum with very little decision support, including little epidemiologic input from key experts within the organization.

Each large GHE clinic maintains a functional organizational design with two main divisions (Support Services and Clinical Services) and separate departments in each division based on specific functions, such as housekeeping in Support Services and medicine in Clinical Services. An organization-wide medical staff, as well as separate medical staff organizations, practice at each of the two clinics. Based on his experience in large academic medical centers in the acute care sector and on the recommendation of the system's governing board, Mr. Jones is considering moving to a matrix model organizational design, with separate product lines that affiliate with, and draw services from, the functional departments (e.g., nursing). Mr. Jones is wrestling with a number of critical and fundamental questions at this juncture. What are the advantages and disadvantages of a matrix model for GHE in terms of direct and indirect costs, as well as benefits such as improved coordination? How many product lines should the organization identify? How should the organization determine which product lines ought to maintain separate identities as part of the matrix design? Mr. Smith has distanced himself from clinical issues and is totally unfamiliar with the disease burden of the enrolled population served by the HMO. What kind of data are needed to make him better informed?

The move to a matrix model is expected to affect staffing in a number of significant ways. Although the new model is expected to improve efficiency with regard to coordination of services, the effect of the new organizational structure is unclear in terms of the number of employees needed, both professional and otherwise, by the organization. More specifically, Mr. Jones is worried that the new structure will increase the total number of required physician generalists and specialists. His concern is founded, at least in part, on the uncertainty associated with the new structure and physician productivity. The focus on product lines may also break the market into segments in ways that would increase the demand for services. In addition to these staffing concerns, the nurse practitioners in two of the five satellite clinics have voiced concerns about workload and the amount of time they can spend with each patient. Mr. Jones is dealing with a number of critical staff questions at this point. How can he estimate the number of affiliated physicians that will be needed to support the north and south clinics when the matrix model of organization is in place? Will the new structure increase or decrease physician productivity? What kinds of data are necessary to determine staffing needs with regard to nurse practitioners at the satellite clinics?

A recommendation of the board has also moved GHE to consider restructuring of the incentive and performance appraisal system, specifically for physicians. Based on the experience of US Healthcare, GHE would like to link capitation payments to outcomes. Currently, GHE negotiates separate capitation contracts with both PA and BMS, wherein the two groups are paid monthly per-member-per-month payments based on the total number of enrolled members for which each group is responsible. Separate capitation contracts are negotiated with other affiliated physicians in the community as well. Currently, GHE withholds 20 percent of capitation payments until the end of the fiscal year and returns all or part of that amount based on expenses in three categories: hospitalization, emergency room use, and out-of-plan specialty services. GHE would like to provide incentives for physicians to deliver good quality care by linking capitation payments to patient outcomes. Although Mr. Jones has resisted this idea, the board has insisted that he develop a plan based on performance appraisal. Since Mr. Jones has eschewed contact with the medical staff in the past, he approaches this challenge with some degree of trepidation. His questions are many at this point. What aspects of performance, or quality of care, should be considered? Is it necessary to measure different outcomes for each type of physician specialist, or are there generic outcomes that can be assessed? How will the outcome measures incorporate risk? To what degree should capitation payments depend on performance appraisal? Will performance appraisal be the responsibility of GHE or the group practices or both? How will performance be assessed for the 500 individual physicians in the community?

For the last three years, GHE has retained most of the withhold payments as a result of substantial hospitalization expenses. The result has been an increase in friction between GHE and the two physician groups. The director for hospital services has alerted Mr. Jones and has presented him with a case-mix breakdown by diagnosis-related group (DRG). The concern seems to be that many of the hospital episodes are potentially avoidable. GHE does not currently have a surveillance program that would flag these specific episodes, nor does it have a system to identify those conditions that could result in hospital care if ambulatory care is deficient. The chief financial officer calculates the potentially avoidable cost to be 18.8 million dollars. Dr. Practice, medical director for BMS, urges Mr. Jones to reduce these episodes by developing a more sophisticated system for targeting those ambulatory care–sensitive conditions that are at risk for costly hospitalization. Mr. Jones faces a number of decisions at this point. Which ambulatory care-sensitive conditions need to be included in the surveillance system? How will these conditions be identified among the enrolled population? How will avoidable hospital episodes be monitored over time? How will GHE measure progress in this area?

GHE has contracts with several of the largest employers in the Boston area and with 50 mid-size businesses. Each employer contract is negotiated separately with past utilization primarily determining the capitation rates, although within companies the employees are assessed the same premium (i.e., they are community rated). The GHE board has urged Mr. Jones to become more proactive in setting capitation rates. More specifically, it has encouraged him to include not just the estimated disease burden of the enrolled population, based on past experience, but also the burden of risk factors to which enrollees are exposed (e.g., obesity, smoking, and alcoholism). Mr. Jones is puzzling over finding answers to a number of sensitive, but imperative, questions. How can the present and future disease burden of the enrollees be accurately measured or estimated? What are the significant risk factors of disease that can actually be measured? To what extent do they predict future morbidity? How should these risk factors be included in setting capitation rates? How feasible would such a rate-setting system be? To what extent would such a system affect profitability and market share?

In addition to all of these decisions that Mr. Jones needs to make, he is laboring over a five-year strategic plan. GHE has been well-positioned in the market but has recently suffered some decline in membership as a result of the entry of two new individual practice associations (IPAs) with very liberal point-of-service features: these IPAs allow their members to get services outside of the plan if they choose to, with little financial penalty. Moreover, the GHE plan has evolved to include a substantial number of elderly and poor members as the result of a decision five years ago to accept Medicare and Medicaid risk contracts. Mr. Jones is concerned that the membership profile has changed over the last several years, and he does not know the effect this will have on the kinds of services that are promised to enrollees. Because Mr. Jones would like to move to a matrix model of organization, he needs to identify specific product lines to meet the needs of GHE members, including a specific focus on the elderly and the poor. What kinds of data need to be collected by GHE to assess the needs of the members? How will GHE assess the risk factors that may lead to morbidity in the future? Which of these needs should be developed into specific product lines?

GHE obviously faces substantial, probably painful, changes outside and within the organization. The CEO has lost the respect of his senior staff, he has frustrated mid-level managers, and he has alienated the medical staff. He is being urged by others, including the governing board and affiliated medical groups, to make critical and significant decisions in organization, staffing, directing, planning, controlling, and finance. Mr. Jones will improve the efficiency and effectiveness with which he makes each of these decisions to the extent that he gathers the relevant epidemiologic measures and evaluates these data from an epidemiologic perspective. The purpose of this text is to convince the reader of the value of this approach.

References

Austin, C. J., 1974. "What Is Health Administration?" *Hospital Administration* 19 (27): 27–34.

Hodgetts, R. M., and D. M. Cascio. 1983. *Modern Health Care Administration.* New York: Academic Press.

Lilienfeld, D. E., and P. D. Stolley. 1994. *Foundations of Epidemiology, 3rd ed.* New York: Oxford University Press.

Neumann, B. R., J. D. Suver, and W. N. Zelman. 1988. *Financial Management: Concepts and Applications for Health Care Providers, 2nd ed.* Owings Wills, MD: National Publishing/AUPHA Press.

Rakich, J. S., B. B. Longest, and K. Darr. 1992. *Managing Health Services Organizations, 3rd ed.* Baltimore, MD: Health Professions Press.

PRINCIPLES AND CONCEPTS OF EPIDEMIOLOGY

F. Douglas Scutchfield and Steven T. Fleming

Many suggest that epidemiology is a relatively new discipline. They credit John Snow, a London anesthesiologist, with the creation of the modern notion of epidemiology as the scientific study and understanding of disease. Snow was able to demonstrate that water was the vehicle for the spread of the epidemics of cholera in the earlier half of the eighteenth century, a discovery that predated an understanding of the germ theory of disease. His efforts to use that information in controlling the epidemic of cholera also provide an excellent illustration of the use of epidemiology to control disease. However, others point to the fact that Hippocrates, the noted early Greek physician, studied and commented on issues such as the effects of environment on the occurrence and distribution of disease. They suggest that his description of the character of environmental influences on disease occurrence represents an earlier epidemiological approach to disease understanding and control. Certainly, we pay in tribute to the founding fathers of the field as we continue to call upon epidemiology for its vital role in advancing contemporary healthcare.

The latter point can be illustrated by examining one disease condition that we can follow to make various points about the importance of understanding epidemiologic principles. In 1981, Gottlieb published a brief report in the CDC's *Morbidity and Mortality Weekly Report* (*MMWR*) about the occurrence of a pneumonia caused by a rare organism, *Pneumocystis carinii*, in four homosexual males (Gottlieb 1981). An article soon followed in the prestigious *New England Journal of Medicine* (Gottlieb et al. 1981). In 1998, a total of 42,308 new cases of AIDS were diagnosed (*MMWR* 1999). The development of the epidemic we now know as AIDS (acquired immunodeficiency syndrome) is well chronicled in Stilt's book, *And The Band Played On* (Stilts 1987).

Since that initial case report, we have developed an effective understanding of the disease and its causative organism. However, until the virus responsible for AIDS (the human immunodeficiency virus, or HIV) was discovered, our only knowledge about the disease was what we were able to deduce from epidemiologic investigations. The early epidemiology of AIDS quickly suggested to researchers studying the disease that it was likely transmitted very much like hepatitis B. That led to an early understanding of AIDS risk factors and methods of prevention.

The Scope of Epidemiology

Webster's Collegiate Dictionary (10th Edition, 1995) defines **epidemiology** as "a branch of medical science that deals with the incidence, distribution and control of diseases in a population." Perhaps a more precise scientific definition is that in Last's *Dictionary of Epidemiology*, "the study of the distribution and determinants of health-related states or events in specified populations, and the application of this study to control of health problems" (Last 1995). This chapter sets out some basic principles for pursuing that study and some of the underlying concepts of epidemiology.

Epidemiology originated in efforts to describe and control the epidemics of infectious disease that swept the world during the nineteenth century. It is important to recognize, however, that one can apply the science of epidemiology in a number of ways. These include, for instance, the mobilization of researchers and clinicians to identify risk factors and to intervene in the epidemic of today's chronic diseases—cancer, heart disease, and stroke—that have replaced infectious diseases as the leading causes of death in most developed countries.

As we will discover, epidemiology can be used to examine agents of morbidity and mortality quite apart from specific disease states. The discipline has been used, for example, to examine the issues of violence and teen pregnancy in the population. It can also be effectively used to plan, implement, and evaluate the provision of health services, for example, using the prevalence of tuberculosis in planning and designing programs to control its occurrence and spread. These latter examples illustrate the use of epidemiology to study "health-related states or events," according to Last's definition.

Agent, Host, and the Environment

The development of disease requires the interplay of three major components. These three components are the **agent**, the **host**, and the **environment**. In the case of infectious disease, the agent is usually some microbiological organism such as a fungus, bacteria, or virus. In the case of AIDS, there are two kinds of agents: the virus, which destroys the immune system (HIV), and the microbiological agents that are responsible for the opportunistic infections that occur when the immune system is overwhelmed by HIV.

One typically thinks of agents as **pathogens**, or organisms that cause disease, and the course of disease development as **pathogenesis**. The agent can also be characterized in terms of **virulence** (or strength), **invasiveness** (ability to enter the host), and **communicability** (ease of the agent's spread from one host to the next). Note that communicability relates also to the characteristics of both environment and host.

As another illustration of agents, consider this example: in one's examinination of automobile injuries, the agent may well be the automobile or the energy transferred to the human body as the result of a collision. Or, for that matter, in the case of health services, the agent might be a program such as screening for breast cancer. In the case of evaluation of a new vaccine, the vaccine could well be the agent. Again, although the classic illustration of agent is the microbe, many particulars can comprise an agent in the context of epidemiology.

The host is the human body, and it can vary substantially in its reactions to agents of disease. For example, if the host has been vaccinated against measles ("immunized"), then exposure to measles will not result from exposure to a specific carrier of that specific disease. A variety of host factors, in addition to immunity, can contribute to the development of disease in response to exposure to a specific agent. In the case of AIDS, the development of the disease is influenced by host factors such as sexual behaviors on the part of the host who carries the virus and can transmit it. Host factors would also include genetic predisposition, exemplified by the female host that carries one of the genes linked to breast or other types of cancer. Age and gender are also factors that affect the incidence and course of disease as well as the response to treatment. Women have higher fatality rates than men from coronary artery bypass graft surgery because anatomically their coronary vessels are smaller. Age is related to the onset and progression of chronic disease. And, again, to return to the auto collision illustration, a child will have a response very different from that of an adult to the same energy release. Other illnesses, hereinafter referred to as **comorbidities**, may affect the incidence and course of illness in both positive and negative ways. Synergistic interactions may occur among diseases where the course of the illnesses interacting is greater than the sum of each disease in its separate progress. Some comorbidities may make a host less susceptible to infection, as happens in sickle cell anemia as a protection against malarial infection.

Hosts are **active carriers** if they are exposed to an infectious agent and harbor it. They are **incubatory carriers** in the early stages of illness, **convalescent carriers** while recovering, and **intermittent carriers** if they can spread the illness only occasionally. Many of us have fallen to the effects of the incubatory carriers of gastroenteritus (stomach flu) or the convalescent carriers of head colds. Some anguish over infection from the intermittent carriers of genital herpes. **Cases** are persons diagnosed with a particular disease. One can distinguish among the **primary case**, or first case in an epidemic; the **index case**, or the first case recognized by the epidemiologist; and the **secondary cases**, or those cases who got the disease from the primary case.

Finally, the environment in which exposure might take place also influences the development of disease. The epidemiologist takes a holistic view of the environment: its physical, social, and cultural components (as with AIDS, for example, whether or not use of a condom during sexual activity represents an environmental component). To further illustrate with our auto collision example, the severity of any collision might be influenced by the pre-crash condition of the auto and whether it contained air bags, the weather, seat belt use, and proper child restraints.

The environment has a substantial influence on the development of disease. The environment affects the survival of the agent as well as the route of entry.

For example, if individuals are confined to cramped quarters, airborne infections are increasingly likely to spread. Thus the communicability of airborne infection increases in cramped quarters. A decrease in crowding, therefore, lessens the occurrence of respiratory diseases. It has been suggested, for example, that the decline in the number of cases of tuberculosis since the mid-twentieth century is more a reflection of environmental influences than of the discovery of the tubercle bacillus or the development of antibiotics to kill the bacillus. The return of tuberculosis as a serious public health threat is related primarily to changes in host factors (the immunodeficiency of AIDS patients). Some evidence has emerged, however, that TB can be contracted during long overseas air travel—the modern day equivalent of the cramped living quarters of the early 1900s. The effect of physical environment on agent survival is perhaps exemplified best by the influenza virus, which lasts longer in the dry air of heated buildings in the winter.

Returning to our discussion of AIDS, epidemiologic evidence has suggested that the initial spread of the disease in Africa took place along the lines of major highways. Further examination has shown that the truck drivers using these routes were spreading HIV through contact with commercial sex workers along the road—an illustration of cultural environment as an influence on the spread of disease.

All three factors—agent, host, and environment—influence the development of disease. One's influence on at least one of these factors may be able to prevent the development of disease in human populations. A related phenomenon is the **web of causation**. The web of causation recognizes that a number of interrelated causes affect the development of disease, and that the relationship is not necessarily a simple, linear, cause-effect progression. For example, for a person to develop AIDS a number of antecedents are required: one must engage in risky behavior (which, as we know, can extend even—if seldom—to having surgery or working in the ER) and must have been exposed to infected blood, other body fluids, or tainted blood products. Some who are exposed do not develop the infection, for whatever reason. In all cases of developed disease, the virus lies dormant, with substantial variation in the period of time before overt AIDS develops. The ability to identify only one component in this web of causation allows the epidemiologist to intervene in the disease without necessarily knowing all of the specific relationships among the agent, host, and environment. Thus the concept of the web of causation represents an important opportunity for intervention in disease states. The web of causation for heart disease in a complex mesh of many factors, some of which promote heart disease (e.g., stress, obesity, diabetes, and hypertension), and some of which inhibit the disease (e.g., physical activity and a diet of polyunsaturated fats) (Timmreck 1998).

Concepts of Disease Transmission

Disease can be defined as an "abnormal" state during which time the host is incapable of normal functions. One can distinguish between **acute disease**

(typically of relative severity and short duration, and treatable) from **chronic disease**, which is usually less severe but of longer duration. The **spectrum of disease**, or **natural history**, refers to the typical sequence of events from exposure to the agent and death. These may include a **subclinical stage**, during which time the disease can be detected and characterized only by laboratory testing, and a **clinical stage**, when symptoms are more evident.

In the last section, we discussed the interaction of agent, host, and environment to facilitate the spread of disease. Within the environment there may also be **vectors**, which are living, nonhuman carriers of disease, such as insects (malaria transmitted by mosquitoes) or rodents (bubonic plague carried by fleas on rats). The environment may be the home of **reservoirs** of disease, which are living or inanimate objects in which infectious organisms multiply. Consider the quest in Africa for the reservoir of the deadly ebola virus. **Fomites** are inanimate objects within the environment—soiled linen or doorknobs, for example—that facilitate the spread of disease.

Outbreaks of disease may be attributable to a **common vehicle** such as water (with cholera) or tainted food (food poisoning), or a **serial transfer** may occur from one host to the next, for instance, with sexually transmitted diseases or influenza. An acute outbreak of disease that reaches levels greater than normal is referred to an **epidemic**; global or widespread outbreaks are **pandemics**. Some populations may have higher normal (or **endemic**) levels of disease, such as the nursing home population (pneumonia) or school-age children (head colds).

Rates and Ratios

Epidemiologists concern themselves with numbers. Epidemiology is based on examining the rates at which events occur. A **rate** must contain three parts: a numerator (the number of events), the denominator (the population in which the event occurs), and a multiplier (usually some power of 10). Rates are also expressed using a time dimension, as in the rate of occurrence of heart attacks (70 per 100,000 in 1998):

$$\text{Rate} = \frac{\text{occurrence of events in a specified population}}{\text{average population in which events occur}} \times 10^n$$

A rate is an expression of **probability**, as both affected and unaffected individuals are in the denominator. It expresses the risk that someone in a population has of the measured event occurring. The purpose of a multiplier is to convert an unwieldy fraction into a whole number for comparison purposes. For example, the rate of development of new cases of AIDS in the United States in 1998 was 17.6 per 100,000.

It is important to ensure that the numerator and denominator refer to a similar population; for example, if the numerator is white males only, then the denominator should also be white males only (the population at risk). In reporting the rate of cervical cancer one must have the denominator limited to females; with prostate cancer, the denominator should obviously include only men. It is important also to recognize that the population may not be a geographic population. If one were to examine the nosocomial infection rate—the rate of development of an infection in a hospital—the denominator should be all of those admitted to the hospital. Post-surgical infection rates may include in the denominator only persons at risk of a post-surgical infection, namely, those who underwent a surgical procedure (see the discussion of this concept in Chapter 8). Table 2.1 lists common rates used by epidemiologists.

Ratios are expressions of one number, events in a population with another number, and a multiplier. A ratio is distinguished from a rate in that the denominator is not the population at risk of the event: thus, a ratio is not a risk statement. The ratio is used when it is difficult to define the at-risk population. For example, it might be appropriate to express the stillbirth ratio as the number of stillbirths per 1,000 live births. Clearly, in this case, the numerator is not drawn from the denominator.

There is a specialized type of rate used in infectious disease epidemiology, the **attack rate**. The attack rate represents the total proportion of persons in an exposed population that develop a specific disease. There is also the notion of secondary attack rate that reflects the attack rate of those who are exposed to the new cases of the disease represented by the initial attack rate. For example, the attack rate of measles in a group of second grade students who were exposed to an index case (the initial child in the school who brought the infection to school) is the proportion of children in the class who develop the disease. The secondary attack rate is the proportion of the siblings of those second grade students who developed measles as the result of their exposure to the infected second grade students.

To illustrate the concept of rate, consider the various kinds of mortality rates that can be calculated for a reference population. In this case the event is

TABLE 2.1 Some Commonly Used Rates		
Crude mortality rate	Deaths among residents during a calendar year/midyear population × 100,000
Cause-specific mortality rate	Deaths assigned to a population in a given year/midyear population × 100,000
Age-specific mortality rate	Deaths in persons at a certain age range/midyear population in that same age range × 1,000
Case fatality rate	Number of deaths assigned to a cause/total number of cases occurring × 100
Infant mortality rate	Number of deaths of those less than one year of age/number of live births × 1,000
Perinatal mortality rate	Number of deaths less than 30 days old/number of live births × 1,000
Postneonatal mortality rate	Number of deaths age 30 days to one year of age/number of live births × 1,000
Maternal mortality rate	Number of deaths assigned to puerperal causes/live births × 1,000

death. The annual death rate would simply be the number of deaths that occur during a period of time, such as a year, divided by the population at risk of death (e.g., U.S. or state population) times the multiplier, in this case usually 100,000. The infant mortality rate would be the number of deaths that occur in infants less than a year old divided by the number of live births with a multiplier of 1,000. In 1990, for example, African Americans had more than double the infant mortality rate of whites: 18.0/1,000 compared with 7.9/1,000. Specific death rates and case fatality rates are two final examples. With specific death rates, the number of deaths are within certain age groups or disease categories, as in elderly mortality rates (for those ≥ 65) or rates for certain kinds of diseases (i.e., cardiovascular disease). Case fatality rates refer to the number of deaths from a specific disease divided by those diagnosed with the disease. Notice with the former that the at-risk population (the denominator) is all people in a population at risk of death, or in the case of age-specific deaths rates, a particular age group. With the latter, case fatality rates, the at-risk population includes only those diagnosed with a particular disease.

Prevalence and Incidence

The burden of illness in a population can be expressed by two different kinds of rates: prevalence and incidence. **Prevalence** is the number of events occurring in a population at a point in time or the presence of a state of disease in a population at a given point in time. For example, the number of individuals with asthma in Kentucky on July 1, 1999 is 250 per 100,000. This is referred to as **point prevalence**. **Annual prevalence**, sometimes called **period prevalence**, is the number of people who had the condition during the preceding year. The prevalence rate is complex and is rarely used because it contains notions of both prevalence and incidence; it also has more relevance for administrative issues than does the incidence rate since it allows for planning. Knowledge of the number of people with a certain condition or disease is most effective in planning for programs that deal specifically with the condition or disease in question.

Incidence, on the other hand, is the occurrence of a new event in a defined population over a period of time. Generally, the **reference population** is the midyear population in calculating annual incidence rates. Incidence is important in the examination of disease etiology and, although it has utility in health services, frequently it is of less use than prevalence rates. Because of the proximity of the development of the disease to the causes of that disease, the research epidemiologist prefers to use incidence rates as measures that are more likely to reflect causation. In making this distinction, consider the example of AIDS. In 1998, newly diagnosed cases numbered 48,269, but an estimated 271,115 people were living with AIDS. The first figure is used to calculate the incidence rate and the latter the prevalence rate. So with these numbers the incidence rate for 1998 was 17.6 per 100,000 and the prevalence rate was 98.9 per 100,000:

$$\frac{48,269}{274,000,000 \text{ (est. U.S. pop)}} \times 100,000 = 17.6/100,000$$

$$\frac{271,115}{274,000,000 \text{ (est. U.S. pop)}} \times 100,000 = 98.9/100,000$$

Clearly, incidence and prevalence are related. Figure 2.1 illustrates this relationship. The faucet dripping into the bowl represents the incidence. That is how the addition of new cases is accumulated in the prevalence rate. The volume in the bowl represents the prevalence. The faucet representing the outflow from the bowl reflects the fact that people with the illness either die or get well and no longer are in the prevalence bowl. Thus, prevalence and incidence are related by duration. The relationship is measured as:

$$\text{Prevalence} = \text{Incidence} \times \text{Duration}$$

This illustrates that an increase in prevalence may be the result of increases in incidence, duration, or both. Obviously, if you know two terms of the equation, it is possible to solve for the third term.

Adjusting Rates

Rates can occasionally appear confusing. For example, if the crude death rate for Miami, Florida is 250 per 100,000 and that for Lexington, Kentucky is 125 per 100,000, one might conclude that Miami is inherently less healthy than Lexington. However, an easy alternative explanation is that the people in Miami, on average, are older because many people retire to Florida. The mechanism for

FIGURE 2.1

Relationship Between Incidence and Prevalence

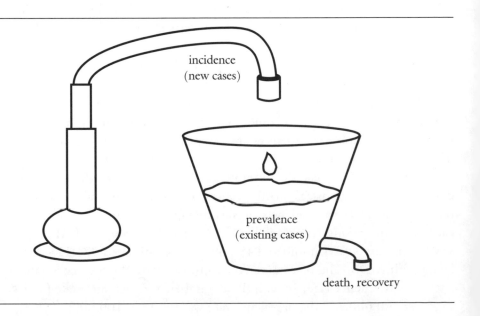

allowing comparisons among divergent groups is called **standardization.** The most common example is standardization for age, but other attributes, such as sex or race, may be the source of standardization, thus allowing for better comparisons of rate. In fact, rates may be adjusted for the risk of death associated with diagnosis, comorbidities, and other clinical factors (see the discussion of risk-adjusted mortality rates in Chapter 8).

Remember that the main purpose of standardization is to enable us to compare two or more population groups that may differ on the basis of age, sex, race, or other factors that influence mortality. In short, standardization "levels the playing field" in the interest of making valid comparisons. Two principle standardization methods are used to adjust mortality rates on the basis of age: direct and indirect standardization.

With the **direct method of standardization**, age-specific death rates from the two population groups to be compared are each applied to a third reference group, or standard population. This can be any population; however, for this example, we use the entire U.S. population for 1996. We calculate the expected number of deaths in the standard population using rates from each of the two comparison groups. For example, suppose we are comparing the mortality experience between Florida and Alaska. We want to take into consideration that Florida has more elderly citizens who are at an increased risk of dying. We take age-specific rates for both Florida and Alaska and apply these rates to a third reference population, say, the U.S. population. The number of expected deaths in the U.S. population is calculated for both Florida and Alaska. In other words, we calculate the number of the people in the United States who would be expected to die if the entire population of the country were dying at the rate of Florida and of Alaska, respectively. The expected deaths can easily be translated into expected death rates for both Florida and Alaska. Table 2.2 illustrates this concept and shows that Alaska has a somewhat lower age-adjusted mortality rate than Florida.

Through use of the **indirect method of standardization**, on the other hand, age-specific mortality rates from a standard population (e.g., the entire United States) are applied to the specific age groupings of the two comparison groups (e.g., Florida and Alaska). The numbers of expected deaths in each of the two comparison populations are calculated using the rates of the standard population. For example, here we estimate the number of people who would be expected to die in both Florida and Alaska as if they were dying at the same rate as people across the entire country. A Standard Mortality Ratio (SMR) is then calculated as the ratio of actual expected deaths in the two comparison populations times 100. If the ratio is more than 100 it means that actual deaths exceeded expected deaths, or that the comparison population was dying at rates in excess of the standard population. A ratio less than 100 implies that the comparison group had fewer deaths than expected, or that the rate was less than that of the standard population group. The SMRs for the two groups (Florida and Alaska) are directly comparable: the higher the SMR, the lower the mortality rate, taking age mix into consideration. Table 2.3 illustrates the indirect method

TABLE 2.2
Direct Method of Standardization Comparing Florida and Alaska, 1996

Age	Age-Specific Death Rate (Florida) per 100,000	Age-Specific Death Rate (Alaska) per 100,000	Reference Population (U.S., 1996)	Expected Deaths (Florida)	Expected Deaths (Alaska)
0–44	147	134	177,813,659	261,386	238,270
45–64	759	545	52,731,251	400,230	287,385
65+	4,415	4,242	33,860,882	1,494,958	1,436,379

Expected Death Rate (Florida)
$$\frac{(261,386 + 400,230 + 1,494,958)}{265,405,792 \ (\text{pop. U.S.})} \times 100,000 = 812/100,000$$

Expected Death Rate (Alaska)
$$\frac{(238,270 + 287,385 + 1,436,379)}{265,405,792 \ (\text{pop. U.S.})} \times 100,000 = 739/100,000$$

TABLE 2.3
Indirect Method of Standardization

Age Group	U.S. Mortality Rates per 100,000	Population (Florida)	Population (Alaska)	Expected Deaths (Florida)	Expected Deaths (Alaska)
0–44	125	8,790,255	452,315	10,988	565
45–64	717	2,958,761	122,019	21214	875
65+	5,061	2,672,719	30,952	135,266	1,566
Total expected deaths (summing columns)				167,468	3,006
Total observed deaths (to be given)				153,375	2,582
SMR (observed/expected × 100)				91.6	85.9

of standardization. Alaska has a somewhat lower SMR than Florida, although both states have lower mortality rates than the nation as a whole, as evidenced by SMRs less than 100.

Epidemiology Methods

There are three major domains of epidemiology: descriptive, analytic, and experimental. These types of epidemiologic inquiry are designed to follow a logical sequence to ascertain etiology and to design control measures for disease. While not always the case, the methods involve the following steps:

1. *Descriptive studies.* The disease distribution in various segments of the population is examined to ascertain variations in that distribution.

2. *Hypothesis generation.* Hypotheses are generated to explain the distribution of the disease.
3. *Analytic epidemiology.* The hypotheses undergo observation testing to ascertain the probability that one of them is correct.
4. *Experimental epidemiology.* The hypothesis is specifically tested.

Generally, the scientific evaluation of a disease or condition proceeds in this sequence—but not always. One may proceed to analytic studies without completing the descriptive work. A good illustration of the process began with the observation that individuals with mottled teeth had less tooth decay together with a descriptive examination of data. Following these steps, studies were designed to match communities that had high "naturally occurring" fluoride levels with those that had low fluoride levels. A substantial difference in decay rates was found between the two communities. The final step was to add fluoride to the water and to observe whether the fluoridated water resulted in fewer dental cavities. The latter is an example of experimental epidemiology that was used to test the hypothesis that fluoride added to the water prevented tooth decay.

Descriptive epidemiology focuses on answering questions about the distribution of disease across time, place, and person—the "who does and does not get what, when, and where" kinds of questions. Time can have a number of dimensions. Figure 2.2 illustrates the distribution of cancer deaths in men and women over time. The growth in the number of lung cancer deaths raises issues of identifying the agent responsible for that increase. It certainly could generate the hypothesis that smoking in women is on the increase and that smoking may be associated with lung cancer in women.

Similar examinations can be conducted by season. Figure 2.3 illustrates this point. This figure shows the cases of Lyme disease reported to the Centers for Disease Control and Prevention (CDC) from 1993 through 1997. Many of the infectious diseases follow a seasonal pattern. The season-disease connection is evidence of the effect of the environment on the spread of disease. This may include the physical environment, as is the case with Lyme disease, and the interaction of deer, mice, and ticks, and also the social environment, such as the school year.

A special time chart called the **epidemic curve** is frequently used in tracking acute infectious disease outbreaks. Figure 2.4 illustrates one such epidemic curve, in which the number of cases of a disease is plotted by day. This epidemic shows a sharp spike in the number of cases in a short period of time, characteristic of the **"common source" epidemic** that occurs when a large number of people are exposed to a common source of infection, such as contaminated potato salad consumed at a church social. In the case of an infectious disease outbreak, if you know the agent and the **incubation period** (the interval of time between agent contact and onset of illness or symptoms), you should be able to calculate the likely time of this common source exposure.

Place can be examined in a variety of ways to generate hypotheses for testing. Figure 2.5 illustrates a map of the United States showing the distribution of heart

FIGURE 2.2

Cancer Deaths in
Men and Women
over Time

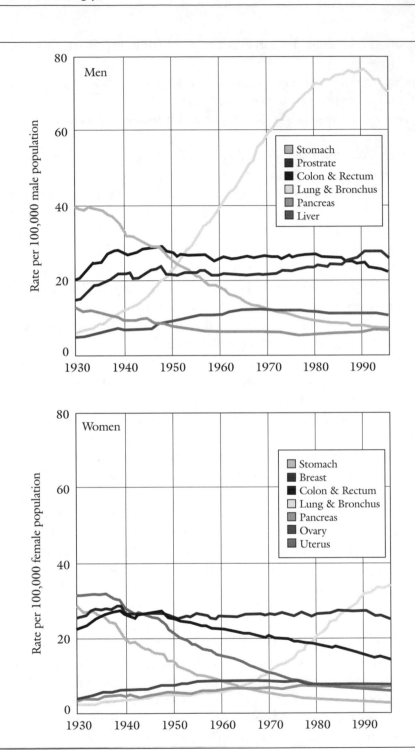

Source: Vital Statistics of the U.S., 1995.

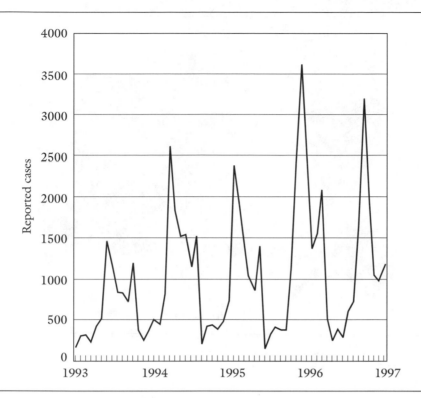

FIGURE 2.3
Seasonal Cycle of
Lyme Disease
Cases, 1993–1997

Source: Morbidity and Mortality Weekly Reports: 42 (53): 10/21/94; 43 (53): 10/6/95; 44 (53): 10/25/96; 45 (53): 10/31/97; 46 (54): 11/20/98.

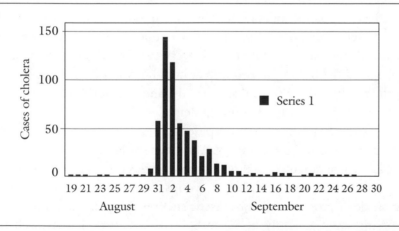

FIGURE 2.4
Epidemic Curve:
Cholera Cases at
Broad Street Pump,
London

Source: Timmreck, T.D. 1998. *An Introduction to Epidemiology, 2nd ed.* Sudbury, MA: Jones and Bartlett.

disease. The major occurrence in the Ohio and Mississippi Valley may suggest that heightened cardiovascular risk factors exist in this area, a testable hypothesis. In a similar way, the differences in urban and rural environments may be examined, or state/local maps may be analyzed for variations that occur.

FIGURE 2.5

Cardiovascular
Disease by State

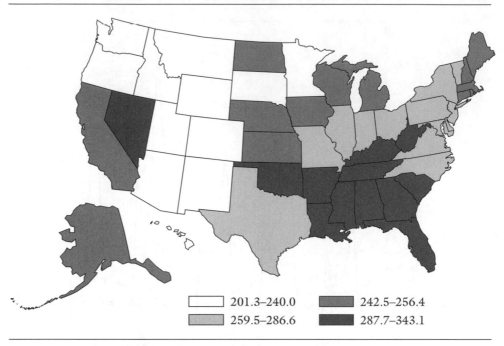

☐ 201.3–240.0	■ 242.5–256.4
▨ 259.5–286.6	■ 287.7–343.1

Source: http://www.cck.gov/nccdphp/cardiov.htm

A useful type of place examination is the **spot map** (Timmreck 1998). With
a spot map, a dot is placed on a map for every case. Snow (1936), in his examination
of cholera, effectively used spot maps to demonstrate a cluster of cases around the
Broad Street water pump in London. He also identified a number of cases outside
of the area usually served by the pump, and interviews with those patients showed
that they also used the Broad Street pump although it was not their closest water
supply. As the result of these place distributions, Snow removed the handle from
the Broad Street pump and stopped the epidemic.

Person is the final way to detect epidemiologic differences. The usual descriptors of a person are age, race, and sex. Almost all studies will report differences
in occurrence by these variables. In almost every case there will substantial variation
in the observed variable among different groups classified by age, race, and sex.
Other person descriptors can also be used, such as religious denomination. If
a disease occurs less frequently in Seventh Day Adventists, it may well relate
to their diet or low use of tobacco products. Socioeconomic status is likewise
a frequently examined person-related variable, as are such other attributes as
occupation, marital status, and education. Returning again to our AIDS example,
Table 2.4 shows the distribution of AIDS by sex and risk category, illustrating that
heterosexual sex is a substantially larger risk factor for women than men.

It is important to note that descriptive epidemiology is always grounded
in person, time, and place. It other words, it is not possible to calculate a rate
unless it refers to a specific type of individual (e.g., all, male, female), from a

	Males		Females	
	cases	percent	cases	percent
Men who have sex with men	27,316	51.8	—	
IV drug use	11,718	22.2	4,687	35.4
Men who have sex with men/IV drug use	3,044	5.8	—	—
Hemophilia/Coagulation disorder	300	0.6	21	0.2
Heterosexual	3,088	5.9	5,521	41.8
Sex with IV drug user	811	1.5	1,836	13.9
Transfusion	282	0.5	266	2.0
Undetermined	7,033	13.3	2,727	20.6
Total	52,781	100.0	13,222	100.0

TABLE 2.4

Distribution of AIDS Cases by Gender and Risk Category, 1996

Source: Centers for Disease Control and Prevention, National Center for HIV, STD, and TB Prevention, Division of HIV/AIDS Prevention.

specific geographic area (e.g., United States, state, county), or during a specific time period (e.g., 1999, 1990–1995).

Analytic epidemiology uses two major methodological approaches, both of which can be referred to as **observational studies**. These are the **case control** or **retrospective study** and the **prospective** or **cohort study**. These approaches will be discussed in more detail in subsequent chapters. This discussion is intended only to introduce these methods. The case control study starts with the disease and looks back to ascertain whether or not a potential etiologic factor existed. For example, descriptive studies may have suggested a relationship between tobacco and lung cancer. In the case control study, patients diagnosed with lung cancer are identified. These cases are "matched" with a control group made up of a similar group of individuals without lung cancer. Then each subject is asked about exposure to tobacco.

In the prospective study, a group of individuals—a cohort—is identified and classified by risk status, for example, whether or not they smoke. They are followed over time to ascertain whether or not they develop a particular outcome such as lung cancer. The case control study starts with subjects with and without a disease, and determines what happened in the past. The cohort study identifies the risk factor and follows the patient to ascertain whether the disease develops or not.

Prospective cohort studies have two major advantages. They allow for the direct estimation of risk, something that is more difficult to measure in case control studies. In addition, case control studies are subject to a phenomenon known as recall bias, in which a person with a disease is more likely than a person without the disease to remember a specific risk factor. Prospective cohort studies are large, expensive, and time-consuming. With even common study diseases that rarely occur, large groups of people must be followed for a prolonged period of time. Case control studies, on the other hand, are quicker, easier, and less expensive to conduct.

Experimental epidemiology involves specific experiments designed to test the hypothesis that flows from analytic studies. These studies typically involve large populations and the random assignment of subjects to either an experimental group (with the intervention) or a control group (without the intervention). Examples of experimental epidemiology exist for a number of different types of conditions. For example, vaccine trials are considered experimental, the initial experiments with fluoridation of water were experimental epidemiology, and the trials to ascertain the effect of lowering cholesterol on the occurrence of cardio-vascular disease also represent a type of experimental epidemiology. Occasionally, "natural experiments" arise (as in the case of fluoridation), when a hypothesis can be tested without a specific intervention. In this case the different levels of fluoride in the drinking water of various communities created an opportunity to study tooth decay and to correlate it with the occurrence of fluoride in the water.

Levels of Prevention

Because epidemiology is primarily concerned with the prevention of disease, it is appropriate to describe the various levels of prevention. Prevention is divided into primary, secondary, and tertiary prevention.

- **Primary prevention** involves the prevention of disease itself. The classic example of primary prevention is immunization: a person is immunized to avoid developing the disease even when exposed to the disease-causing agent. Similarly, chemoprophylaxis is a primary prevention activity. In this case an individual takes a drug, such as amantadine, to prevent the development of influenza.
- **Secondary prevention** involves early identification and treatment of a disease or risk factor, so that disease progression is stopped. Classic examples of such screening are breast cancer screening with mammography or screening for cervical cancer using the Pap smear. Screening for risk factors that can be treated, such as high blood pressure or elevated blood cholesterol, also represents cost-effective screening interventions. Screening of blood products for the HIV virus is another illustration of how screening, in this case, provides some primary benefits to those who do not receive an infected blood transfusion.
- **Tertiary prevention** involves attempts to ensure that disability does not increase after the disease has developed. For example, cardiac rehabilitation is a type of tertiary prevention designed to help a person avoid having another type of heart attack or developing heart failure. Using diet and exercise together with appropriate preventive medication often makes it possible to slow the progression of disability associated with heart disease.

The contemporary epidemiologist uses all of the strategies for prevention: primary, secondary, and tertiary. The appropriate use of primary prevention and secondary prevention, and the role of counseling in prevention, have been well laid out in the results of an examination of the appropriateness of these interventions in the *Guide to Clinical Preventive Services* (U.S. Preventive Services Task Force 1996).

Screening

Secondary prevention typically involves the use of screening tests to identify those individuals with a particular disease in the hope of finding the disease at an early and treatable stage. Any measure such as a screening test has both favorable and unfavorable characteristics. **Validity** refers to the accuracy with which a measure, such as a screening test, represents a particular phenomenon. For example, suppose a five-question screening test were developed for clinical depression: the test would have validity to the extent that the questions accurately characterized this mental disorder. As another example, the PSA screening test for prostate cancer has validity if a measurement of prostate-specific antigen accurately portrays prostate cancer. **Reliability** is a measure of consistency. Reliable screening tests yield the same results regardless of the number of times they are repeated. **Interrater reliability** measures the degree to which different reviewers get the same results with single or multiple applications of a test. **Intrarater reliability** refers to the consistency of test results found by the same reviewer. For example, one could assess the interrater reliability of a blood pressure screening test by determining the consistency of results with multiple tests by different nurses. The intrarater reliability of mammography could be assessed by measuring the consistency of test results when a single radiologist interprets a single film on multiple occasions.

Ideally, the screening test should distinguish between those individuals who have the disease (the true positives) from those who do not (the true negatives). The test should minimize the number of individuals who do not have the disease but test positive (the false positives) and those who have the disease but test negative (the false negatives). The logic of the screening test may involve the choice of a particular level (e.g., blood pressure level or level of prostate-specific antigen) as the critical juncture between the positive and negative test result in an effort to minimize false positives and negatives. Unfortunately, this represents a tradeoff. If one wants to be sure that the test identifies all true positives, then one must accept a higher level of false positives. By the same token, to ensure that those who test positive for the disease are in fact positive, one must accept more false negatives. These concepts are called sensitivity and specificity. **Sensitivity** measures the proportion of those who are actually diseased and test positive, whereas **specificity** measures the proportion of those who are actually not diseased and test negative. Thus, sensitivity is the ability of the test to identify those who are truly sick, whereas specificity is the ability of the test to correctly identify those who are well.

This relationship is illustrated mathematically in the two-by-two table of Figure 2.6. The columns represent those with and without the disease, herein labeled "reality," that is, "God only knows" whether or not the person really has the disease. The rows represent those who test positive and negative. Cell a represents the true positives, b represents false positives, c is the false negatives, and d is the true negatives. Assume that 2,000 people are tested, 1,000 with the disease and 1,000 without. Figure 2.7 is an example of what might be found when the test is done. The sensitivity is calculated by dividing a by $a+c$ and the specificity is calculated by dividing d by $b+d$. In our hypothetical case the sensitivity is 80 percent and the specificity is 90 percent. These represent not an ideal test, but one consistent with several commonly used laboratory tests.

Although the sensitivity and specificity of the test will remain the same, the number of false positives and false negatives will vary with the prevalence of the disease. The hypothetical example just presented assumed a prevalence of 50 percent, that is, of the 2,000 people tested, half had the disease. Figure 2.7 also illustrates the case with the same specificity and sensitivity in a group of 2,000 individuals where the prevalence is 10 percent. With a 50 percent prevalence, 100 people are incorrectly labeled as positive, whereas with a 10 percent prevalence the number rises to 180 of the 2,000 population. The circumstance worsens with a smaller prevalence rate, say, one percent. In order to identify 16 true positives, 198 people have been mislabeled as false positives.

The measure that examines the ability of a test to predict disease is called the predictive value. One can measure both the positive and the negative predictive value of a test. The **positive predictive value (PPV)** is the proportion of those who test positive and who actually have the disease. **The negative predictive value (NPV)** is the proportion of those who test negative and who actually do not have the disease. Again, returning to the two-by-two table of Figure 2.6, the positive predictive value is a divided by $a+b$ and the negative predictive value is d divided by $c+d$. Note the positive and negative predictive value in the circumstance where the prevalence of the disease is 50 percent, 10 percent, and one percent (Figure 2.7). The positive predictive value falls to less than 10 percent in the situation where the prevalence is one percent.

FIGURE 2.6
Screening for
Disease

		REALITY	
		YES	NO
TEST	YES	(a) True Positives	(b) False Positives
	NO	(c) False Negatives	(d) True negatives

	Disease (50%)		Disease (10%)		Disease (1%)	
	yes	no	yes	no	yes	no
Yes	800	100	160	180	16	198
No	200	900	40	1,620	4	1,782
Totals	1000	1000	200	1800	20	1980

(Test, row labels at left)

Disease (50%)	Disease (10%)	Disease (1%)
Sensitivity = 80%	Sensitivity = 80%	Sensitivity = 80%
Specificity = 90%	Specificity = 90%	Specificity = 90%
PPV = 0.88	PPV = 0.47	PPV = 0.07
NPV = 0.82	NPV = 0.98	NPV = 0.998

FIGURE 2.7
Sensitivity, Specificity, PPV, NPV by Disease Prevalence

The difference between sensitivity and positive predictive value, on the one hand, and specificity and negative predictive value, on the other, is not entirely intuitive. Sensitivity and specificity are intrinsic characteristics of the test itself and of the ability of that test to make a distinction—on the basis of some measureable characteristic, such as blood sugar or blood pressure levels—between those who are diseased and those who are not. Positive and negative predictive values are derived not only from characteristics of the test, but also from the prevalence of the disease in the population. As shown earlier, it can be demonstrated empirically that positive predictive value increases as disease prevalence does. The test itself has not changed, but one can place more trust in a positive test result from a screening test applied to a population wherein the disease is highly prevalent. Alternatively, negative predictive value falls as disease prevalence rises. One can trust a negative test result more with rare diseases than with common diseases.

In assessing the usefulness of a screening test, it is necessary to ensure that it is both sensitive and specific; however, it is also important to examine the predictive value of a test, as discussed earlier. A classic example of this issue is HIV testing. When the causative agent for AIDS was identified and a test was developed to screen for HIV, a great deal of pressure came into play to test various groups, frequently not of high risk. The obvious downside to testing a low-prevalence population for HIV is that many individuals would falsely test positive, given the low positive predictive value of a test with good sensitivity and specificity. This would result in labeling, incorrectly, many as having the virus. It would result in substantial time and energy to evaluate the extent to which the positive test was correct for a specific individual and would create a great deal of unnecessary anxiety in those who tested positive but did not have the virus. The better strategy was to use the test in high-risk populations, where the prevalence would be high enough to ensure a better positive predictive value.

Summary

Epidemiology has a long history of use in a variety of contexts. Traditionally it has been engaged to do disease detective work, originally to track infectious diseases. In the 1800s it was used to track the epidemics of major infections that swept across countries—the great pandemics, such as the cholera and yellow fever outbreaks. After the turn of the twentieth century, it was applied to individual infectious diseases, such as tuberculosis, in terms of tracking, etiology, and control. During the second half of the last century, epidemiologic research has focused on chronic diseases, with the elucidation of major risk factors for diseases such as cancer and heart disease. Finally, epidemiologic methods have recently been applied to the control of health problems that are neither acute infectious disease nor chronic disease, such as injury prevention.

Although epidemiology can boast of significant contributions in areas of disease etiology, prevention, and control, the contemporary epidemiologist can apply the tools and methods of this discipline to issues dealing more directly with the delivery of healthcare services. The use of epidemiology has much to recommend it to the student of health services management. The tools are easily and handily transferred from issues of disease to those that relate to the delivery of healthcare services. The ability to use epidemiologic tools in addressing the issues of access, cost, and quality of care is the hallmark of an effective practitioner of health services management.

Case Study 2.1

You are interested in comparing the treatment of cardiovascular disease in the states of New York and Alaska. Assume that the crude disease-specific mortality rate for cardiovascular disease is 314.9 (per 100,000) in New York and 152 (per 100,000) in Alaska. From these statistics alone, which state has the higher cardiovascular mortality rate? The population mix between Alaska and New York is quite different. In Alaska, 90 percent of the population is 55 years old or younger compared to 77 percent in New York. Assume a 1996 U.S. population of 210,183,450 (of which 55,222,342 persons are 55 and older). The age-specific cardiovascular mortality rates for the younger-than and older-than 55 age groups in Alaska are 22.7 and 1,316 per 100,000. For New York, these rates are 22.4 and 1,294 per 100,000. Calculate age-adjusted cardiovascular mortality rates using the direct age adjustment technique and the U.S. population as the standard. What are the age-adjusted cardiovascular mortality rates (per 100,000) for Alaska and New York? With the age-adjusted rates, which state has a higher mortality rate? Fifty-three percent of the population in Alaska are men compared with 47 percent in New York. Men have higher cardiovascular mortality rates than women. Perhaps one should adjust for both age and sex. Assume that 56.8 percent of the 55 and older U.S. population is female compared with 49.7 percent of the 54 and younger group. The age/sex–specific rates in Alaska are 33 per 100,000 (for males 54 and younger), 1,450 per 100,000 (for men 55 and older), 11 per 100,000 (for women 54 and younger), and 1,165 per 100,000 (for women 55 and older). These rates are 33 per 100,000, 1,400 per 100,000, 13 per 100,000, and 1,200 per 100,000 for the state of New York. Calculate age/sex–adjusted mortality rates from the data above. What are the age/sex–adjusted cardiovascular mortality rates (per 100,000) for Alaska and New York? With the age/sex–adjusted rates, which state has a higher mortality rate?

Case Study 2.2

Prostate-specific antigen (PSA) has become a common screening test for prostate cancer. In order to detect early-stage prostate cancer with a reasonable degree of success, a low serum level of PSA of 4.0 ng/ml is used as the cutoff point. Unfortunately, men with benign prostate hypertrophy (BPH) can also have elevated PSA levels. If 30 percent of men with BPH have PSA levels above 4.0 and 80 percent of men with prostate cancer have these elevated levels, can we calculate the sensitivity and specificity of the test with these data alone? What about the positive and negative predictive values? What are the positive and negative predictive values if the prevalence of prostate cancer are 10 percent? How do these values compare if the prevalence is 30 percent or 50 percent? Discuss the PSA test in terms of the costs of false positives and false negatives. How does our confidence in a positive or negative test result depend on the prevalence of prostate cancer in the population? Can the elderly with much higher rates of prostate cancer be more confident or less confident in a negative test result?

References

Gottlieb, M. S. 1981. "Pneumocystis Pneumonia—Los Angelos." *Morbidity and Mortality Weekly Report* 30 (1981): 250–252.

Gottlieb, M. S., R. Schroff, H. M. Schanker, J. D. Weisman, P. T. Fan, R. A. Wolf, and A. Saxon. 1981. "Pneumocystis Carinii Pneumonia and Mucosal Candidiasis in Previously Healthy Homosexual Men: Evidence of a New Acquired Cellular Immunodeficiency." *The New England Journal of Medicine* 305 (24): 1425–31.

Last, J. M. 1995. *Last's Dictionary of Epidemiology, 3rd ed.* New York: Oxford University Press.

Morbidity and Mortality Weekly Report. (48–49, 17 Dec. 1999): 1131–38.

Snow, J. 1936. *Snow on Cholera.* New York: The Commonwealth Fund.

Stilts, R. 1987. *And the Band Played on: Politics, People, and the AIDS Epidemic.* New York: St. Martin's.

Timmreck, T. D. 1998. *An Introduction to Epidemiology, 2nd ed.* Sudbury, MA: Jones and Bartlett.

U.S. Preventive Services Task Force. 1996. *Guide to Clinical Preventive Services, 2nd ed.* Baltimore: Williams & Wilkins.

STATISTICAL TOOLS USED IN APPLYING EPIDEMIOLOGICAL CONCEPTS TO THE MANAGEMENT OF HEALTHCARE RESOURCES

Mary Kay Rayens and Thomas C. Tucker

Introduction

Epidemiology can be viewed as utilization of the set of tools that measure the need for, and impact of, healthcare interventions. This chapter describes the basic statistical tools used by epidemiologists that health service managers can employ to guide the decision-making process. The sections that follow are intended to serve as an overview of these concepts; more detailed information may be found in the bibliography on p. 46 at the end of this chapter. The two basic sets of statistical tools are called **descriptive epidemiology** and **inferential epidemiology**.

Descriptive epidemiology is an attempt to describe a characteristic or characteristics of a defined population, including health needs, health events, and health outcomes. Thus, descriptive epidemiology typically summarizes the quantitative attributes either of a sample drawn from the population of observations (when the population is too large to assess completely) or of a known characteristic of the entire population of interest. For example, if you as a health manager need to assess the compliance of the hospital staff with the standard protocol for chart documentation, one way would be to review a randomly selected sample of charts to determine the number of sample charts that are in compliance (see Table A in the appendix at the end of this chapter for a table of random numbers). Another example of the use of descriptive statistics would be to record all of the reported cases of a particular disease in a registry and then to use this figure to summarize the incidence of this illness in the population during a specific time period. In other words, the tools of epidemiology can be used to describe characteristics of a population or to estimate these characteristics from a sample.

Inferential epidemiology is used to compare two or more populations for differences or similarities. An example of inference would be the use of statistical methods to ascertain whether or not males differ from females on the risk of developing hepatitis after exposure. In this situation, we can infer from the frequency of cases within the two gender groups the likelihood that the risk of disease is the same for both groups. Thus, the tools of epidemiology can also be used to compare differences between populations. This is possible because inferential methods allow one to generalize comparisons based on randomly-chosen samples and thus to reach conclusions about differences present in the underlying populations.

Levels of Measurement

The two basic classes of data used in epidemiologic statistical comparisons are the **continuous** and the **categorical**. Variables measured on an **interval scale**, which indicates that, for these variables, distance between points is meaningful and the variable can take any value within a continuous range, fall into the former class. Examples of continuous variables include age, height, weight, and systolic blood pressure. Categorical variables can take values only in a fixed number of categories. These types of variables may be either **ordinal**, which means that the categories can be ordered in some meaningful way, or **nominal**, which means that the categories are qualitative rather than quantitative. An example of an ordinal variable would be the assessment of patient satisfaction, graded on a four-point scale from "very satisfied" to "very dissatisfied," or of the extent of cancer invasiveness at diagnosis, coded as Stage I, II, III, or IV. Examples of nominal variables include race and gender.

Sampling

When it is not possible or practical to collect data from an entire population on the variable of interest, a subset of that population—a **sample**—is used to provide an estimate of the characteristic of interest. Although the purpose of sampling typically is to estimate population characteristics, it is likely that the sample will be drawn from a **sampling frame** rather than from the population itself. The sampling frame is a compilation of the members of the population who are available to be chosen in the sample, and it should include as many of the population members as possible. An example of a sampling frame is a telephone book. If the goal of a survey is to estimate the percentage of citizens in a certain town who wear seat belts, it may be impossible to have an exhaustive list of all citizens, but the phone book may be used as a reasonable sampling frame from which to randomly choose participants. Random-digit dialing techniques would increase the sampling frame to include citizens with unlisted numbers; this may improve the ability of the sample to provide a realistic estimate of the underlying population percentage of seat belt users.

The two basic ways to choose a set of elements from a sampling frame are **convenience sampling** and **probability sampling**. Convenience sampling is a nonrandom selection of elements from the population. An example of data collected using a convenience sampling scheme would be if the next n patients to enter a particular clinic were assessed on a relevant disease state, such as diabetic status.

A probability sample is drawn using the concept of randomness. The simplest example of a probability sample is a **simple random sample**, in which a random mechanism is used to select patients or records from an exhaustive list of the population. Using this sampling scheme, each member of the population is equally likely to be chosen. This type of sampling is considered the optimal type to use in planning an experiment, but it can be difficult to implement in practice. In the clinic patient example used earlier to illustrate convenience sampling, simple random sampling would involve randomly choosing a subset of patients from the entire list of patients who are seen at that clinic. Although simple random sampling may be a relatively straightforward task in this example (because the population is well defined and can be listed), it becomes difficult or even impossible to do in settings where the population defies enumeration.

Other types of probability sampling include **systematic sampling, cluster sampling,** and **stratified random sampling**. Each of these types of sampling involves schemes in which the sample of subjects is chosen in a more patterned way than by using simple random sampling. As an example of a systematic sampling scheme to derive data on the prevalence of diabetes, the entire list of the population of a clinic's patients would make it possible, first, to randomly choose one of the first 20 charts and then to pull for review every 20th chart from the entire population after that first selection. Thus, a 5 percent sample would be obtained using this scheme, and the sample information could be used to estimate the prevalence of diabetes in the clinic population.

The goal of probability sampling is to garner samples that are **representative** of the populations from which they come, so that conclusions can be extended from the sample comparisons to the populations. Convenience sampling, although easier to implement, may lead to estimates that are not representative, since the specific population that the sample members represent is not clear. If a convenience sample is drawn from a population of clinic patients seen during cold and flu season, for example, the sample may in fact represent the subpopulation of patients most likely to succumb to those two illnesses, rather than the larger population of all clinic patients.

Descriptive Statistics for Continuous Variables

Once the sample has been chosen and the relevant characteristics have been measured, the first step in describing a continuous variable is typically to assess the **mean** and **standard deviation** of that measure in the sample. The mean is the average value, while the standard deviation is a measure of the variability of the observations about the mean.

The formulas for the sample mean, $\bar{X}$ and sample standard deviation, s, are given below. With n subjects in the sample:

$$\bar{X} = \frac{\sum_{i=1}^{n} X_i}{n} \text{ and } s = \sqrt{\frac{\sum_{i=1}^{n}(X_i - \bar{X})^2}{n-1}} = \sqrt{\frac{n\sum_{i=1}^{n} X_i^2 - \left(\sum_{i=1}^{n} X_i\right)^2}{n(n-1)}}$$

Notice that the first formula given for the standard deviation illustrates how this statistic is a function of the distance of each of the sample values from the mean value, while the second formula provides a shortcut for computation. The **variance** is simply the square of the standard deviation, and thus also is a gauge of variability of the measurements. In the case of simple random sampling, the **standard error of the mean** is the sample standard deviation divided by the square root of the sample size. While the standard deviation is a measure of the variability of observations about the sample mean, the standard error of the mean is a measure of how accurate the sample mean is likely to be in estimating the true population mean. An additional summary measure for sample data is the **median**, or 50th percentile. This is the value wherein half of the observations lie above it and half below (in the case of an even number of observations, the median is the average of the middle two values). An additional method for describing the variability of the sample data would be to assess the **range**, or the difference between the highest and lowest observed value. The mean and median are both measures of **central tendency**, while the standard deviation, variance, and range are measures of **dispersion** or variation. A graphical method for summarizing continuous data is a **histogram**, which is a display of bars whose size is determined by the number or percent of the sample that fall into the range of values prescribed for that bar. Two distinguishing features of a histogram are that the bars touch and that the ranges for each bar are equally spaced. This graphical method allows one to discern patterns in the distribution of values, for instance, age of the population (Figure 3.1).

FIGURE 3.1

U.S. Resident Population by Age Group, 1997

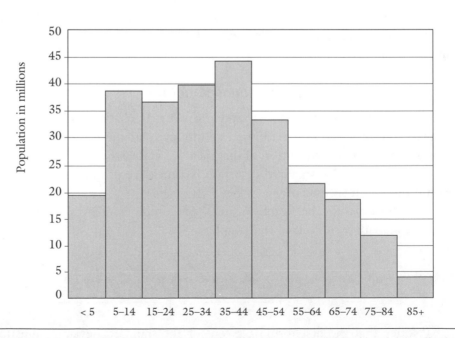

Source: National Center for Health Statistics. 1999. *Health, United States, 1999, with Health and Aging Chartbook.* Hyattsville, Maryland: NCHS.

Example 1

Here is an example to help illustrate how descriptive measures for continuous variables are calculated. As the manager of a health clinic, you want to describe the age of patients who come to your clinic on weekdays in the summer. Age is a continuous variable, so you decide to calculate the mean age, the median age, the standard deviation of ages observed, and the range of ages. You have selected a random sample of ten patients seen at the clinic between Monday and Friday during the first week in July. In practice your sample may be considerably larger. However, this limited sample size is used here to give examples of calculating the measures of central tendency and variability without being too computationally cumbersome. The presumption is that this sampling frame (i.e., the weekdays during the first week in July) has members who are representative of the population, namely, all patients who are seen in the clinic on summer weekdays. The ages of the ten patients in your sample are 9, 3, 11, 42, 81, 17, 59, 7, 26, and 32:

$$\text{The mean age is } \bar{X} = \frac{\sum_{i=1}^{10} X_i}{10} = \frac{(9 + 3 + 11 + 42 + 81 + 17 + 59 + 7 + 26 + 32)}{10} = 28.7 \text{ years}$$

In order to determine the median age of all patients seen at your clinic, it is useful to reorder the ten sample observations from lowest to highest: 3, 7, 9, 11, 17, 26, 32, 42, 59, 81. Because of the even number of observations in the sample, the median is the average of the two middle-ordered values; thus:

$$\text{Median age} = \frac{(17 + 26)}{2} = 21.5 \text{ years}$$

If the number of sample members had been odd, the median would simply have been the middle value from the ordered list of ages.

To determine the sample standard deviation using the shortcut formula, it is necessary to calculate both $\sum X_i$ and $\sum X_i^2$:

$$\sum_{i=1}^{10} X_i = 9 + 3 + 11 + 42 + 81 + 17 + 59 + 7 + 26 + 32 = 287$$

$$\sum_{i=1}^{10} X_i^2 = 9^2 + 3^2 + 11^2 + 42^2 + 81^2 + 17^2 + 59^2 + 7^2 + 26^2 + 32^2 = 14{,}055$$

Using the shortcut formula for the standard deviation:

$$s = \sqrt{\frac{n \sum_{i=1}^{n} X_i^2 - \left(\sum_{i=1}^{n} X_i\right)^2}{n(n-1)}} = \sqrt{\frac{(10 \times 14{,}055) - (287 \times 287)}{(10 \times 9)}} = 25.4 \text{ years}$$

The standard error of the mean for this sample is $25.4/\sqrt{10} = 8.0$ years. Finally, the age range of this sample of ten patients is the difference between the oldest and youngest patients, or 78 years.

Descriptive Statistics for Categorical Variables

The descriptive summary for categorical data usually consists of a **frequency distribution**, which summarizes in a table or graph the percentage or number of responses in each category. In its graphical form, the frequency distribution can be summarized in a **bar chart**. The bar chart is immediately differentiated from the histogram by the fact that the bars have spaces between them: this is to underscore the need to resist the temptation to look for trends by comparing bar heights or lengths, particularly in the case of nominal data (when the ordering of the bars is quite arbitrary) (Figure 3.2). Another summary measure that may be used for categorical data is the **mode**, the most commonly occurring value for the variable of interest. It is possible for sample data to have multiple modes or no mode.

It is common in epidemiology to study **binary variables**, categorical variables with only two outcomes. Examples of binary variables include survival status (alive or dead), disease status (present or absent), and gender (male or female). In this context, it is often useful to summarize binary data as either a **proportion** or a **rate**. A proportion is calculated by dividing the number of observations with an attribute (i.e., characteristic of interest) by the total number of observations.

FIGURE 3.2

Mothers Who Smoked Cigarettes During Pregnancy, 1997

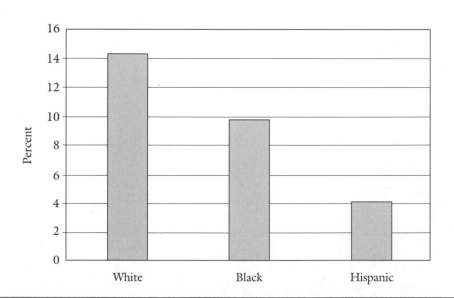

Source: National Center for Health Statistics. Health, United States, 1999 With Health and Aging Chartbook. Hyattsville, Maryland: 1999.

The **percentage** is the proportion multiplied by 100. A rate is a proportion that has been multiplied by a factor to make the order of magnitude of the proportion more meaningful. In the case of a rare health event, it is more meaningful to present incidence, prevalence, or mortality rates as per 1,000 or per 100,000 population rather than as a percent. For example, if the proportion of people in the United States who have a particular rare disease in the current year is equal to 0.000042, the rate of this disease in the U.S. population would then be 4.2 cases per 100,000 population. Rates are typically used to describe only populations, whereas proportions may be used to summarize populations or samples. The sample standard deviation in this context is $s_{\hat{p}} = \sqrt{[\hat{p}(1 - \hat{p})]/n}$, where $\hat{p}$ is the observed proportion with the attribute in the sample and n is the sample size. Thus for the case of binary data, the observed proportion $\hat{p}$ is the measure of central tendency while the standard deviation, $s_{\hat{p}}$, is the measure of variability.

Example 2

This example is provided to help illustrate the calculation of descriptive statistics for binary measures. When the previous sample of ten patient ages was collected, you also recorded whether each patient was male or female. Recall that this sample was taken from patients who visited your clinic on a weekday during the first week in July. Thus, this sample can also be used to provide an estimate of the proportion of females (or males) seen in the clinic during the weekdays in summer. The sample proportion is denoted $\hat{p}$; this statistic is an estimate of the population proportion, p. In your sample, seven patients were males and three were females. The proportion of the sample who are female is 3/10 or 0.3. The proportion of the sample who are male is 7/10 or 0.7. Thus 70 percent of the sample are males and 30 percent are females. The sample standard deviation is:

$$s_{\hat{p}} = \sqrt{\frac{\hat{p}(1 - \hat{p})}{n}} = \sqrt{\frac{(0.3) \times (1 - 0.3)}{10}} = \sqrt{0.021} = 0.14$$

Notice that because this is a binary variable, it does not matter if you calculate the standard deviation based on the male proportion or the female proportion, since the proportion of males is equal to one minus the proportion of females and vice versa.

Inferential Statistics: Overview

The statistical comparison of two or more samples that represent distinct underlying populations can be accomplished in a variety of ways depending on the goals of the study and on whether the variables are continuous or categorical. Many inferential techniques are designed to test specific **hypotheses**, or statements that compare the populations in a quantitative way. A simple example is the comparison of two population means. The **null hypothesis**, or the statement to be tested, is typically that the two populations have the same mean. The **alternative hypothesis**—assumed to be true if the null hypothesis is rejected—is typically that the two population means differ. This is an example of a **two-sided hypothesis**, since there is no presumption that one mean should necessarily be greater than the other one. As an example of a **one-sided hypothesis**, we may want to test whether a new drug is *more effective* than the current standard, and thus are interested only in obtaining a significant difference in mean response in a particular direction. In practice, two-sided hypothesis tests are more widely used. In the context of hypothesis testing, the **test statistic**, which is a function of the sample data, is used to reject the null hypothesis or fail to reject it. The conclusion in the former case is that the groups are not equal, while the conclusion in the latter case is that not enough evidence is present to suggest that the groups are significantly different.

A key element of hypothesis testing is the concept of the **p-value**. The p-value is the probability of observing a test statistic as extreme as the one obtained if the null hypothesis of equality is actually true. Stated another way, the p-value is the likelihood that the difference observed in the measures of central tendency between two groups relative to the variability of the observations is attributable to random chance. Intuitively, then, the smaller the p-value, the more evidence there is to suggest that the null hypothesis is false. In other words, the smaller the p-value, the less likely it is that the observed differences result from random chance. The general rule-of-thumb is that p-values less than .05 are considered **significant**, thus giving ample evidence to reject the null. P-values larger than .05 but less than .10 are typically considered **marginally significant**, perhaps indicative of a trend that did not quite reach strict statistical significance. A p-value below .01 or below .005 may be considered **highly significant**, depending on the context.

When conducting a hypothesis test, one of four possible outcomes will occur. Two positive outcomes would be either to reject the null hypothesis when, in fact, it is false or to fail to reject it when it is actually true. If the null hypothesis is rejected even though it is true, this is considered making a **Type I error**. Conversely, if the null hypothesis is not rejected even though it is false, a **Type II error** has been committed. The probability of making a Type I error is denoted α and the probability of making a Type II error is commonly referred to as β. Although it would be ideal to make both α and β as small as possible, so that the likelihood of reaching a wrong conclusion is minuscule, an inverse relationship exists between α and β, making it impossible to minimize one without increasing the other. The conventions for α and β are typically 0.05 and 0.20, respectively. That is, we are willing to wrongly reject the null hypothesis 5 percent of the time and to fail to reject the null when it is false 20 percent of the time.

The probability that we will *correctly* discern that the null hypothesis is false is the **power** of the test. The power and the Type II error rate sum to one, so that when a Type II error rate of 0.2 is specified, this is equivalent to a power of 80 percent. The convention of setting α to 0.05 is what drives the comparison of p-values to this level. The α level, also referred to as the **level of significance**, is a general guideline set in the planning stage of hypothesis testing, while the p-value is associated with a specific test statistic. If the p-value is less than the α level, the conclusion is that the test statistic is significant. In other words, if the p-value is less than the α level, we would reject the null hypothesis.

Two-sample t-Test

The most common type of hypothesis testing involves the comparison of the mean values for two groups on some continuous attribute. The null hypothesis in this situation is:

$$H_o : \mu_1 = \mu_2$$

The parameters μ_1 and μ_2 are the true population means for the continuous variable of interest. These population means are estimated using the sample means (i.e., $\bar{X}_1$ and $\bar{X}_2$) from each of the two groups. In order to test this hypothesis, a two-sample t-test can be used. The formula for the test statistic is:

$$t = \frac{\bar{X}_1 - \bar{X}_2}{\sqrt{(s_1^2/n_1) + (s_2^2/n_2)}}$$

The sample sizes from each group are n_1 and n_2, respectively. This is the general form of the t-test. For the special case in which the standard deviations of the two groups are not statistically different (which may be ascertained via another hypothesis test, this one for equality of variances; see below for details), the t-test formula simplifies to:

$$t = \frac{\bar{X}_1 - \bar{X}_2}{\sqrt{(s^2/n_1) + (s^2/n_2)}} \text{ with } s^2 = \frac{(n_1 - 1)\,s_1^2 + (n_2 - 1)\,s_2^2}{(n_1 - n_2 - 2)}$$

The formula given for s^2 in this equation provides a **pooled** estimate of the variance for this case, in which the two variances are not significantly different. The null hypothesis of no difference between the group means is rejected when the observed value of the t-test statistic is "large" in absolute value. To determine the significance level, the test statistic is compared to a t distribution, which has a bell-shaped form that is approximately normal, particularly for large sample sizes. Assuming a sample size of at least 30 per group and an alpha level of 0.05, the **critical value** for the test statistic is approximately 2. The critical value associated with a particular hypothesis test gives a cutoff beyond which the observed test statistic (in absolute value) is deemed to be significant. The interpretation is that, with this sample size, if the absolute value of the test statistic obtained is at least as large as the critical value, the null hypothesis is rejected since the p-value is at most 0.05. The critical value is a function of both the α level and the **degrees of freedom**. The sample size does play a role in determining the critical value since the degrees of freedom are a function of the sample size. In particular, the degrees of freedom (v) for the t-test based on pooled variances are equal to $n_1 + n_2 - 2$. For the t-test based on unpooled variances, the degrees of freedom are determined by:

$$v = \frac{\left\{ \dfrac{s_1^2}{n_1} + \dfrac{s_2^2}{n^2} \right\}^2}{\dfrac{s_1^4}{n_1^2\,(n_1 - 1)} + \dfrac{s_2^4}{n_2^2\,(n_2 - 1)}}$$

If this formula leads to a fractional value for the degrees of freedom, this value may be rounded to the nearest degree. Once the degrees of freedom are known and the test statistic has been calculated, the observed test statistic may be compared to the appropriate critical value displayed in Table B located in the appendix.

To determine which form of the t-test is appropriate, a test for the equality of variances is needed. The null and alternative hypotheses in this case are:

$$H_o : \sigma_1^2 = \sigma_2^2$$

$$H_A : \sigma_1^2 \neq \sigma_2^2$$

The population variance for each group, σ_1^2, is estimated using the sample variance, s_1^2, to test the null hypothesis. To test this hypothesis, label the larger sample variance as s_1^2 and the smaller as s_2^2. The corresponding sample sizes for each are labeled n_1 and n_2, respectively. The form of the test statistic is simply s_1^2/s_2^2. This observed test statistic is then compared to an F distribution with $v_1 = n_1 - 1$ numerator degrees of freedom and $v_2 = n_2 - 1$ denominator degrees of freedom. Table C in the appendix presents the critical values of the F distribution for one-sided tests with $\alpha = 0.05$ and 0.01. These tabled critical values are equivalent to the critical values for two-sided tests with significance levels of .10 and .02, respectively.

Example 3

The following is an example of the use of the t-test in comparing a continuous measure between two populations.

As the manager of a clinic you want to compare the average age of the previous sample of ten patients seen during weekdays in the summer with that of a sample of ten patients seen during weekdays in the winter. The hypothesis you would like to test is whether a significant age difference will be found between the two patient groups given the possibility that more injuries in summer may involve young patients and more viral infections in winter may involve older patients. Given this hypothesis, you would expect the average patient age in summer to be significantly different from the average age in winter. The null and alternative hypotheses are:

$$H_o : \mu_s = \mu_w$$

$$H_A : \mu_s \neq \mu_w$$

Example 1 already showed that the average age of the summer weekday patients (denoted $\bar{X}_1$) was 28.7 years with a standard deviation (s_2) of 25.4 years. In order to test the hypothesis of equal age in the two groups of patients, you select a random sample of ten patients treated at the clinic on a weekday during the first week of February. The average age of the second sample ($\bar{X}_2$) is 47.1 years with a standard deviation (s_2) of 21.0 years. We first test the null hypothesis of equality of variances using the sample standard deviations:

$$\frac{s_1^2}{s_2^2} = \frac{25.4^2}{21.0^2} = 1.5$$

Notice that the critical value for the two-sided test from appendix Table B, with $\alpha = 0.1$ and 9 degrees of freedom for both the numerator and the denominator, is equal to 3.18. Since our test statistic is less than the tabled value, the conclusion is that the p-value for this test exceeds 0.1 so that the null hypothesis is not rejected. Since the variances are not significantly different, the correct form of the t-test is:

$$t = \frac{\bar{X}_1 - \bar{X}_2}{\sqrt{(s^2/n_1) + (s^2/n_2)}} \text{ with } s^2 = \frac{(n_1 - 1)\, s_1^2 + (n_2 - 1)\, s_2^2}{(n_1 - n_2 - 2)}$$

In this case:

$$s^2 = \frac{(9 \times 25.4 \times 25.4) + (9 \times 21.0 \times 21.0)}{18} = 543.1$$

so that:

$$t = \frac{(28.7 - 47.1)}{\sqrt{(543.1/10) + (543.1/10)}} = 1.8 \text{ and } |t| = 1.8$$

The critical value for a two-sided test with $\alpha = 0.05$ and 18 degrees of freedom is 2.101 (see appendix Table B). Thus, we conclude that the p-value for this observed test statistic exceeds .05, so we fail to reject the null hypothesis and conclude that the evidence is not sufficient to suggest that the two patient groups differ significantly on age. This conclusion may seem counterintuitive given the apparent large difference in means between the two samples. However, the standard deviations are relatively large and the sample sizes are modest, and both of these affect the p-value of the test statistic.

z-Test for Differences in Proportions

The z-test for differences in proportions between two groups is similar in form to the t-test for two group means. The null and alternative hypotheses in this case are:

$$H_0 : \; p_1 = p_2$$

$$H_A : \; p_1 \neq p_2$$

The statistics $\hat{p}_1$ and $\hat{p}_2$ are the sample proportions of subjects with the attribute of interest from each of the groups. These are estimates of the population parameters, p_1 and p_2. As before, n_1 and n_2 are the sample sizes obtained from the two groups. The critical value for the z-test is determined using the standard normal distribution (also denoted the z distribution). A table of critical values from this distribution (Table D) is found in the appendix.

The z-test has the form:

$$z = \frac{\hat{p}_1 - \hat{p}_2}{\sqrt{[\hat{p}_1 (1 - \hat{p}_1) / n_1] + [\hat{p}_2 (1 - \hat{p}_2) / n_2]}}$$

In general, the z distribution provides accurate critical values for the z-test statistic. However, if the sample sizes are limited, the z-test tends to underestimate the true p-value, which may lead to an increased Type I error rate. To correct for this, a slight adjustment to the test statistic is suggested. The correction is referred to as the **Yates correction** and is a subtraction from the numerator of the test statistic; this modification decreases the test statistic, which in turn increases the p-value. As the sample sizes get large, the impact of the Yates correction is negligible. The form of the test statistic with this correction is:

$$z = \frac{|\hat{p}_1 - \hat{p}_2| - \frac{1}{2} (1/n_1 + 1/n_2)}{\sqrt{[\hat{p}_1 (1 - \hat{p}_1) / n_1] + [\hat{p}_2 (1 - \hat{p}_2) / n_2]}}$$

The observed test statistic is compared to the standard normal (z) distribution; critical values are displayed in Table D found in the appendix. The body of the table contains the probabilities, or area under the curve, for each possible value of the test statistic. For example, 95 percent of the z distribution is contained between -1.96 and 1.96, so that the choice of 1.96 as a critical value for a z-test would result in a test with an α level of 0.05.

Example 4

As the manager of a clinic, you want to know if there is a significant difference between the proportion of males or females seen during the summer compared with the gender distribution of patients seen in winter. You have already determined (in Example 2) that the proportion of males seen in summer is 0.7. If the sample of ten patients seen during the first week of February has four males, the test statistic for the comparison of these two proportions is:

$$z = \frac{(0.7 - 0.4) - \frac{1}{2} (1/10 + 1/10)}{\sqrt{[(0.7 \times 0.3) / 10] + [(0.4 \times 0.6) / 10]}} = 0.94$$

It is important to use the Yates correction in this case because the sample sizes are small. Comparing this observed value to Table D in the appendix reveals that the probability associated with observing 0.94 under the null hypothesis of equal proportions is equal to $(1 - [.3264 \times 2])$ or 0.34. This is the proportion of area under the standard normal curve that is in the two tails with a critical value of 0.94. With a p-value of 0.34, there is no evidence to reject the null hypothesis, so we conclude that the two proportions are not significantly different.

Confidence Intervals

The construction of a confidence interval around a sample estimate provides an alternative to the hypothesis test. The general form of the confidence interval is the test statistic plus or minus a particular quantity; this quantity is a function of the variability and the sample size. The motivation behind this method is to provide a range of values within which the true population parameter is likely to lie. Test statistics with relatively high variability or small sample sizes, or both, will have wider confidence intervals than those based either on smaller standard deviations or on more robust sample sizes, or both. Although confidence intervals can be constructed for virtually any test statistic, the confidence interval for the difference in means is:

$$\left(\bar{X}_1 - \bar{X}_2\right) - t_\alpha \times s < \mu_1 - \mu_2 < \left(\bar{X}_1 - \bar{X}_2\right) + t_\alpha \times s$$

The sample means $\bar{X}_1$ and $\bar{X}_2$ are used in this calculation as is the appropriate form of the sample standard deviation, s. This standard deviation is either the pooled or unpooled version discussed in the previous section on the two-sample t-test, depending on whether the variances are significantly different or not. The quantity t_α is a function of the alpha level and sample size and may be determined using Table B in the appendix. For example, if each group has 16 subjects, the significance level is chosen to be .05, and the two population variances are not different, the correct t_α would be 2.042 and s is the pooled standard deviation. If the α level is 0.05, the resulting confidence interval is referred to as a **95 percent confidence interval**. For alternative levels of significance, different t_α values would be specified to increase or decrease the width of the interval in line with the increase or decrease in the percent confidence. As the percent confidence increases, the size of t_α also increases so that the width of the interval is larger. Conversely, t_α is smaller for smaller levels of confidence so that the width of the confidence interval shrinks.

A 95 percent confidence interval means that we are 95 percent confident of the method used to generate it. In other words, we do not know with certainty that the obtained confidence interval contains the true population parameter of interest, but we do know that 95 percent of the time the obtained confidence interval will contain the population parameter. We summarize this interpretation by stating that we are 95 percent confident that the difference between the two population means is between a and b, where a and b are the lower and upper limits of the obtained 95 percent confidence interval.

The relationship between hypothesis testing and confidence intervals is direct. In the example of the confidence interval for the difference in means, if the obtained $(1 - \alpha)$ 100 percent confidence interval does not contain 0, this is analogous to the conclusion that the two means are significantly different at a significance level α. The appeal of the confidence interval over the hypothesis test is that it provides perhaps a more concrete representation of the "typical" range of values that the sample statistics are likely to take. The appeal of hypothesis testing when compared with confidence intervals is that the former provides a p-value that may be compared with various α levels to determine significance, while the latter is calculated for a preset α level.

Example 5

This example indicates the differences and similarities between hypothesis testing and confidence intervals. Recall in Example 3 the comparison of mean ages between summer and winter patients. The 95 percent confidence interval for the difference in mean ages is:

$$(47.1 - 28.7) - (2.1 \times 23.3) < \mu_1 - \mu_2 < (47.1 - 28.7) + (2.1 \times 23.3)$$

Thus, the 95 percent confidence interval for the difference in means is from -30.5 to 67.3. The zero contained in the interval confirms the fact that the two means are not statistically different at the $\alpha = 0.05$ level. Notice how the width of the interval is influenced both by the variability (i.e., the pooled standard deviation) as well as the sample size (through the degrees of freedom associated with the t-value, which determines the magnitude of the t-value used).

Conclusions

The material in this chapter and the examples provided offer a basic introduction to the statistical tools used in epidemiology. These are tools that can be invaluable to health services managers by providing objective ways for making decisions. In this chapter we have provided only a brief overview of the univariate (i.e., descriptive) and bivariate (i.e., inferential methods for two groups) statistics commonly used in epidemiology. Multivariate methods, such as multiple regression, multiple logistic regression, and analysis of variance, are beyond the scope of this overview. For more detailed information on the methods presented here or on multivariate analysis strategies, see the bibliography at the end of this chapter. Health services managers are encouraged to consult practicing statisticians or epidemiologists for assistance in planning the studies, making the important decisions, or answering the complex questions that may come up in the pursuit of epidemiologic problem-solving.

A Bibliography of Epidemiologic Tools for Healthcare Managers

Glantz, S. A. 1997. "Primer of Biostatistics." New York: McGraw-Hill.

Hamilton, L. C. 1990. *Modern Data Analysis: A First Course in Applied Statistics.* Pacific Grove, California: Brooks/Cole Publishing Company.

Kanji, G. K. 1999. *100 Statistical Tests.* London: Sage Publications.

Motulsky, H. 1995. *Intuitive Biostatistics.* New York: Oxford University Press.

National Center for Health Statistics. 1999. *Health, United States, 1999, with Health and Aging Chartbook.* Hyattsville, MD: NCHS.

Selvin, S. 1996. *Statistical Analysis of Epidemiologic Data.* New York: Oxford University Press.

Snedecor, G. W. and W. G. Cochran. 1967. *Statistical Methods, 6th ed.* Ames: The Iowa State University Press.

Vogt, W. P. 1999. *Dictionary of Statistics and Methodology: A Nontechnical Guide for the Social Sciences.* London: Sage Publications.

Appendix

	00–04	05–09	10–14	15–19	20–24	25–29	30–34	35–39	40–44	45–49
00	54463	22662	65905	70639	79365	67382	29085	69831	47058	08186
01	15389	85205	18850	39226	42249	90669	96325	23248	60933	26927
02	85941	40756	82414	02015	13858	78030	16269	65978	01385	15345
03	61149	69440	11286	88218	58925	03638	52862	62733	33451	77455
04	05219	81619	10651	67079	92511	59888	84502	72095	83463	75577
05	41417	98326	87719	92294	46614	50948	64886	20002	97365	30976
06	28357	94070	20652	35774	16249	75019	21145	05217	47286	76305
07	17783	00015	10806	83091	91530	36466	39981	62481	49177	75779
08	40950	84820	29881	85966	62800	70326	84740	62660	77379	90279
09	82995	64157	66164	41180	10089	41757	78258	96488	88629	37231
10	96754	17676	55659	44105	47361	34833	86679	23930	53249	27093
11	34357	88040	53364	71726	45690	66334	60332	22554	90600	71113
12	06318	37403	49927	57715	50423	67372	63116	48888	21505	80182
13	62111	52820	07243	79931	89292	84767	85693	73947	22278	11551
14	47534	09243	67879	00544	23410	12740	02540	54440	32949	13491
15	98614	75993	84460	62846	59844	14922	48730	73443	48167	34770
16	24856	03648	44898	09351	98795	18644	39765	71058	90368	44104
17	96887	12479	80621	66223	86085	78285	02432	53342	42846	94771
18	90801	21472	42815	77408	37390	76766	52615	32141	30268	18106
19	55165	77312	83666	36028	28420	70219	81369	41943	47366	41067
20	75884	12952	84318	95108	72305	64620	91318	89872	45375	85436
21	16777	37116	58550	42958	21460	43910	01175	87894	81378	10620
22	46230	43877	80207	88877	89380	32992	91380	03164	98656	59337
23	42902	66892	46134	01432	94710	23474	20423	60137	60609	13119
24	81007	00333	39693	28039	10154	95425	39220	19774	31782	49037
25	68089	01122	51111	72373	06902	74373	96199	97017	41273	21546
26	20411	67081	99950	16944	93054	87687	96693	87236	77054	33848
27	58212	13160	06468	15718	82627	76999	05999	58680	96739	63700
28	70577	42866	24969	61210	76046	67699	42054	12696	93758	03283
29	94522	74358	71659	62038	79643	79169	44741	05437	39038	13163
30	42626	86819	85651	88678	17401	03252	99547	32404	17918	62880
31	16051	33763	57194	16752	54450	19031	58580	47629	54132	60631
32	08244	27647	33851	44705	94211	46716	11738	55784	95374	72655
33	59497	04392	09419	99964	51211	04894	72882	17805	21896	83864
34	97155	13428	40293	09985	58434	01412	69124	82171	59058	82859
35	98409	66162	95763	47420	20792	61527	20441	39435	11859	41567
36	45476	84882	65109	96597	25930	66790	65706	61203	53634	22557
37	89300	69700	50741	30329	11658	23166	05400	66669	48708	03887
38	50051	95137	91631	66315	91428	12275	24816	68091	71710	33258
39	31753	85178	31310	89642	98364	02306	24617	09609	83942	22716
40	79152	53829	77250	20190	56535	18760	69942	77448	33278	48805
41	44560	38750	83635	56540	64900	42912	13953	79149	18710	68618
42	68328	83378	63369	71381	39564	05615	42451	64559	97501	65747
43	46939	38689	58625	08342	30459	85863	20781	09284	26333	91777
44	83544	86141	15707	96256	23068	13782	08467	89469	93942	55349
45	91621	00881	04900	54224	46177	55309	17852	27491	89415	23466
46	91896	67126	04151	03795	59077	11848	12630	98375	52068	60142
47	55751	62515	21108	80830	02263	29303	37204	96926	30506	09808
48	85156	87689	95493	88842	00664	55017	55539	17771	69448	87530
49	07521	56898	12236	60277	39102	62315	12239	07105	11844	01117

TABLE A
Ten Thousand
Randomly Assorted
Digits

TABLE A
(*Continued*)

	50–54	55–59	60–64	65–69	70–74	75–79	80–84	85–89	90–94	95–99
00	59391	58030	52098	82718	87024	82848	04190	96574	90464	29065
01	99567	76364	77204	04615	27062	96621	43918	01896	83991	51141
02	10363	97518	51400	25670	98342	61891	27101	37855	06235	33316
03	86859	19558	64432	16706	99612	59798	32803	67708	15297	28612
04	11258	24591	36863	55368	31721	94335	34936	02566	80972	08188
05	95068	88628	35911	14530	33020	80428	39936	31855	34334	64865
06	54463	47237	73800	91017	36239	71824	83671	39892	60518	37092
07	16874	62677	57412	13215	31389	62233	80827	73917	82802	84420
08	92494	63157	76593	91316	03505	72389	96363	52887	01087	66091
09	15669	56689	35682	40844	53256	81872	35213	09840	34471	74441
10	99116	75486	84989	23476	52967	67104	39495	39100	17217	74073
11	15696	10703	65178	90637	63110	17622	53988	71087	84148	11670
12	97720	15369	51269	69620	03388	13699	33423	67453	43269	56720
13	11666	13841	71681	98000	35979	39719	81899	07449	47985	46967
14	71628	73130	78783	75691	41632	09847	61547	18707	85489	69944
15	40501	51089	99943	91843	41995	88931	73631	69361	05375	15417
16	22518	55576	98215	82068	10798	86211	36584	67466	69373	40054
17	75112	30485	62173	02132	14878	92879	22281	16783	86352	00077
18	80327	02671	98191	84342	90813	49268	95441	15496	20168	09271
19	60251	45548	02146	05597	48228	81366	34598	72856	66762	17002
20	57430	82270	10421	00540	43648	75888	66049	21511	47676	33444
21	73528	39559	34434	88596	54086	71693	43132	14414	79949	85193
22	25991	65959	70769	64721	86413	33475	42740	06175	82758	66248
23	78388	16638	09134	59980	63806	48472	39318	35434	24057	74739
24	12477	09965	96657	57994	59439	76330	24596	77515	09577	91871
25	83266	32883	42451	15579	38155	29793	40914	65990	16255	17777
26	76970	80876	10237	39515	79152	74798	39357	09054	73579	92359
27	37074	65198	44785	68624	98336	84481	97610	78735	46703	98265
28	83712	06514	30101	78295	54656	85417	43189	60048	72781	72606
29	20287	56862	69727	94443	64936	08366	27227	05158	50326	59566
30	74261	32592	86538	27041	65172	85532	07571	80609	39285	65340
31	64081	49863	08478	96001	18888	14810	70545	89755	59064	07210
32	05617	75818	47750	67814	29575	10526	66192	44464	27058	40467
33	26793	74951	95466	74307	13330	42664	85515	20632	05497	33625
34	65988	72850	48737	54719	52056	01596	03845	35067	03134	70322
35	27366	42271	44300	73399	21105	03280	73457	43093	05192	48657
36	56760	10909	98147	34736	33863	95256	12731	66598	50771	83665
37	72880	43338	93643	58904	59543	23943	11231	83268	65938	81581
38	77888	38100	03062	58103	47961	83841	25878	23746	55903	44115
39	28440	07819	21580	51459	47971	29882	13990	29226	23608	15873
40	63525	94441	77033	12147	51054	49955	58312	76923	96071	05813
41	47606	93410	16359	89033	89696	47231	64498	31776	05383	39902
42	52669	45030	96279	14709	52372	87832	02735	50803	72744	88208
43	16738	60159	07425	62369	07515	82721	37875	71153	21315	00132
44	59348	11695	45751	15865	74739	05572	32688	20271	65128	14551
45	12900	71775	29845	60774	94924	21810	38636	33717	67598	82521
46	75086	23537	49939	33595	13484	97588	28617	17979	70749	35234
47	99495	51434	29181	09993	38190	42553	68922	52125	91077	40197
48	26075	31671	45386	36583	93459	48599	52022	41330	60651	91321
49	13636	93596	23377	51133	95126	61496	42474	45141	46660	42338

	00–04	05–09	10–14	15–19	20–24	25–29	30–34	35–39	40–44	45–49
50	64249	63664	39652	40646	97306	31741	07294	84149	46797	82487
51	26538	44249	04050	48174	65570	44072	40192	51153	11397	58212
52	05845	00512	78630	55328	18116	69296	91705	86224	29503	57071
53	74897	68373	67359	51014	33510	83048	17056	72506	82949	54600
54	20872	54570	35017	88132	25730	22626	86723	91691	13191	77212
55	31432	96156	89177	75541	81355	24480	77243	76690	42507	84362
56	66890	61505	01240	00660	05873	13568	76082	79172	57913	93448
57	41894	57790	79970	33106	86904	48119	52503	24130	72824	21627
58	11303	87118	81471	52936	08555	28420	49416	44448	04269	27029
59	54374	57325	16947	45356	78371	10563	97191	53798	12693	27928
60	64852	34421	61046	90849	13966	39810	42699	21753	76192	10508
61	16309	20384	09491	91588	97720	89846	30376	76970	23063	35894
62	42587	37065	24526	72602	57589	98131	37292	05967	26002	51945
63	40177	98590	97161	41682	84533	67588	62036	49967	01990	72308
64	82309	76128	93965	26743	24141	04838	40254	26065	07938	76236
65	79788	68243	59732	04257	27084	14743	17520	95401	55811	76099
66	40538	79000	89559	25026	42274	23489	34502	75508	06059	86682
67	64016	73598	18609	73150	62463	33102	45205	87440	96767	67042
68	49767	12691	17903	93871	99721	79109	09425	26904	07419	76013
69	76974	55108	29795	08404	82684	00497	51126	79935	57450	55671
70	23854	08480	85983	96025	50117	64610	99425	62291	86943	21541
71	68973	70551	25098	78033	98573	79848	31778	29555	61446	23037
72	36444	93600	65350	14971	25325	00427	52073	64280	18847	24768
73	03003	87800	07391	11594	21196	00781	32550	57158	58887	73041
74	17540	26188	36647	78386	04558	61463	57842	90382	77019	24210
75	38916	55809	47982	41968	69760	79422	80154	91486	19180	15100
76	64288	19843	69122	42502	48508	28820	59933	72998	99942	10515
77	86809	51564	38040	39418	49915	19000	58050	16899	79952	57849
78	99800	99566	14742	05028	30033	94889	53381	23656	75787	59223
79	92345	31890	95712	08279	91794	94068	49337	88674	35355	12267
80	90363	65162	32245	82279	79256	80834	06088	99462	56705	06118
81	64437	32242	48431	04835	39070	59702	31508	60935	22390	52246
82	91714	53662	28373	34333	55791	74758	51144	18827	10704	76803
83	20902	17646	31391	31459	33315	03444	55743	74701	58851	27427
84	12217	86007	70371	52281	14510	76094	96579	54853	78339	20839
85	45177	02863	42307	53571	22532	74921	17735	42201	80540	54721
86	28325	90814	08804	52746	47913	54577	47525	77705	95330	21866
87	29019	28776	56116	54791	64604	08815	46049	71186	34650	14994
88	84979	81353	56219	67062	26146	82567	33122	14124	46240	92973
89	50371	26347	48513	63915	11158	25563	91915	18431	92978	11591
90	53422	06825	69711	67950	64716	18003	49581	45378	99878	61130
91	67453	35651	89316	41620	32048	70225	47597	33137	31443	51445
92	07294	85353	74819	23445	68237	07202	99515	62282	53809	26685
93	79544	00302	45338	16015	66613	88968	14595	63836	77716	79596
94	64144	85442	82060	46471	24162	39500	87351	36637	42833	71875
95	90919	11883	58318	00042	52402	28210	34075	33272	00840	73268
96	06670	57353	86275	92276	77591	46924	60839	55437	03183	13191
97	36634	93976	52062	83678	41256	60948	18685	48992	19462	96062
98	75101	72891	85745	67106	26010	62107	60885	37503	55461	71213
99	05112	71222	72654	51583	05228	62056	57390	42746	39272	96659

TABLE A
(*Continued*)

TABLE A
(*Continued*)

	50–54	55–59	60–64	65–69	70–74	75–79	80–84	85–89	90–94	95–99
50	32847	31282	03345	89593	69214	70381	78285	20054	91018	16742
51	16916	00041	30236	55023	14253	76582	12092	86533	92426	37655
52	66176	34037	21005	27137	03193	48970	64625	22394	39622	79085
53	46299	13335	12180	16861	38043	59292	62675	63631	37020	78195
54	22847	47839	45385	23289	47526	54098	45683	55849	51575	64689
55	41851	54160	92320	69936	34803	92479	33399	71160	64777	83378
56	28444	59497	91586	95917	68553	28639	06455	34174	11130	91994
57	47520	62378	98855	83174	13088	16561	68559	26679	06238	51254
58	34978	63271	13142	82681	05271	08822	06490	44984	49307	61717
59	37404	80416	69035	92980	49486	74378	75610	74976	70056	15478
60	32400	65482	52099	53676	74648	94148	65095	69597	52771	71551
61	89262	86332	51718	70663	11623	29834	79820	73002	84886	03591
62	86866	09127	98021	03871	27789	58444	44832	36505	40672	30180
63	90814	14833	08759	74645	05046	94056	99094	65091	32663	73040
64	19192	82756	20553	58446	55376	88914	75096	26119	83898	43816
65	77585	52593	56612	95766	10019	29531	73064	20953	53523	58136
66	23757	16364	05096	03192	62386	45389	85332	18877	55710	96459
67	45989	96257	23850	26216	23309	21526	07425	50254	19455	29315
68	92970	94243	07316	41467	64837	52406	25225	51553	31220	14032
69	74346	59596	40088	98176	17896	86900	20249	77753	19099	48885
70	87646	41309	27636	45153	29988	94770	07255	70908	05340	99751
71	50099	71038	45146	06146	55211	99429	43169	66259	97786	59180
72	10127	46900	64984	75348	04115	33624	68774	60013	35515	62556
73	67995	81977	18984	64091	02785	27762	42529	97144	80407	64524
74	26304	80217	84934	82657	69291	35397	98714	35104	08187	48109
75	81994	41070	56642	64091	31229	02595	13513	45148	78722	30144
76	59537	34662	79631	89403	65212	09975	06118	86197	58208	16162
77	51228	10937	62396	81460	47331	91403	95007	06047	16846	64809
78	31089	37995	29577	07828	42272	54016	21950	86192	99046	84864
79	38207	97938	93459	75174	79460	55436	57206	87644	21296	43393
80	88666	31142	09474	89712	63153	62333	42212	06140	42594	43671
81	53365	56134	67582	92557	89520	33452	05134	70628	27612	33738
82	89807	74530	38004	90102	11693	90257	05500	79920	62700	43325
83	18682	81038	85662	90915	91631	22223	91588	80774	07716	12548
84	63571	32579	63942	25371	09234	94592	98475	76884	37635	33608
85	68927	56492	67799	95398	77642	54913	91583	08421	81450	76229
86	56401	63186	39389	88798	31356	89235	97036	32341	33292	73757
87	24333	95603	02359	72942	46287	95382	08452	62862	97869	71775
88	17025	84202	95199	62272	06366	16175	97577	99304	41587	03686
89	02804	08253	52133	20224	68034	50865	57868	22343	55111	03607
90	08298	03879	20995	19850	73090	13191	18963	82244	78479	99121
91	59883	01785	82403	96062	03785	03488	12970	64896	38336	30030
92	46982	06682	62864	91837	74021	89094	39952	64158	79614	78235
93	31121	47266	07661	02051	67599	24471	69843	83696	71402	76287
94	97867	56641	63416	17577	30161	87320	37752	73276	48969	41915
95	57364	86746	08415	14621	49430	22311	15836	72492	49372	44103
96	09559	26263	69511	28064	75999	44540	13337	10918	79846	54809
97	53873	55571	00608	42661	91332	63956	74087	59008	47493	99581
98	35531	19162	86406	05299	77511	24311	57257	22826	77555	05941
99	28229	88629	25695	94932	30721	16197	78742	34974	97528	45447

Source: Snedecor, G. W. and W. G. Cochran. 1967. *Statistical Methods, 6th ed.* Ames: The Iowa State University Press.

TABLE B
The Distribution of t (Two-Tailed Tests)

Degrees of Freedom	Probability of a Larger Value, Sign Ignored								
	0.500	0.400	0.200	0.100	0.050	0.025	0.010	0.005	0.001
1	1.000	1.376	3.078	6.314	12.706	25.452	63.657		
2	0.816	1.061	1.886	2.920	4.303	6.205	9.925	14.089	31.598
3	.765	0.978	1.638	2.353	3.182	4.176	5.841	7.453	12.941
4	.741	.941	1.533	2.132	2.776	3.495	4.604	5.598	8.610
5	.727	.920	1.476	2.015	2.571	3.163	4.032	4.773	6.859
6	.718	.906	1.440	1.943	2.447	2.969	3.707	4.317	5.959
7	.711	.896	1.415	1.895	2.365	2.841	3.499	4.029	5.405
8	.706	.889	1.397	1.860	2.306	2.752	3.355	3.832	5.041
9	.703	.883	1.383	1.833	2.262	2.685	3.250	3.690	4.781
10	.700	.879	1.372	1.812	2.228	2.634	3.169	3.581	4.587
11	.697	.876	1.363	1.796	2.201	2.593	3.106	3.497	4.437
12	.695	.873	1.356	1.782	2.179	2.560	3.055	3.428	4.318
13	.694	.870	1.350	1.771	2.160	2.533	3.012	3.372	4.221
14	.692	.868	1.345	1.761	2.145	2.510	2.977	3.326	4.140
15	.691	.866	1.341	1.753	2.131	2.490	2.947	3.286	4.073
16	.690	.865	1.337	1.746	2.120	2.473	2.921	3.252	4.015
17	.689	.863	1.333	1.740	2.110	2.458	2.898	3.222	3.965
18	.688	.862	1.330	1.734	2.101	2.445	2.878	3.197	3.922
19	.688	.861	1.328	1.729	2.093	2.433	2.861	3.174	3.883
20	.687	.860	1.325	1.725	2.086	2.423	2.845	3.153	3.850
21	.686	.859	1.323	1.721	2.080	2.414	2.831	3.135	3.819
22	.686	.858	1.321	1.717	2.074	2.406	2.819	3.119	3.792
23	.685	.858	1.319	1.714	2.069	2.398	2.807	3.104	3.767
24	.685	.857	1.318	1.711	2.064	2.391	2.797	3.090	3.745
25	.684	.856	1.316	1.708	2.060	2.385	2.787	3.078	3.725
26	.684	.856	1.315	1.706	2.056	2.379	2.779	3.067	3.707
27	.684	.855	1.314	1.703	2.052	2.373	2.771	3.056	3.690
28	.683	.855	1.313	1.701	2.048	2.368	2.763	3.047	3.674
29	.683	.854	1.311	1.699	2.045	2.364	2.756	3.038	3.659
30	.683	.854	1.310	1.697	2.042	2.360	2.750	3.030	3.646
35	.682	.852	1.306	1.690	2.030	2.342	2.724	2.996	3.591
40	.681	.851	1.303	1.684	2.021	2.329	2.704	2.971	3.551
45	.680	.850	1.301	1.680	2.014	2.319	2.690	2.952	3.520
50	.680	.849	1.299	1.676	2.008	2.310	2.678	2.937	3.496
55	.679	.849	1.297	1.673	2.004	2.304	2.669	2.925	3.476
60	.679	.848	1.296	1.671	2.000	2.299	2.660	2.915	3.460
70	.678	.847	1.294	1.667	1.994	2.290	2.648	2.899	3.435
80	.678	.847	1.293	1.665	1.989	2.284	2.638	2.887	3.416
90	.678	.846	1.291	1.662	1.986	2.279	2.631	2.878	3.402
100	.677	.846	1.290	1.661	1.982	2.276	2.625	2.871	3.390
120	.677	.845	1.289	1.658	1.980	2.270	2.617	2.860	3.373
∞	.6745	.8416	1.2816	1.6448	1.9600	2.2414	2.5758	2.8070	3.2905

Parts of this table are reprinted by permission from R. A. Fisher's Statistical Methods for Research Workers, published by Oliver and Boyd, Edinburgh (1925–1950); from Maxine Merrington's "Table of Percentage Points of the t-Distribution," Biometrika, 32:300 (1942); and from Bernard Ostle's Statistics in Research, Iowa State Univeristy Press (1954).
Source: Snedecor, G. W. and W. G. Cochran. 1967. *Statistical Methods, 6th ed.* Ames: The Iowa State University Press.

TABLE C—PART I
5% and 1% (Bold) Points for the Distribution of F

f_1 Degrees of Freedom (for greater mean square)

f_2	1	2	3	4	5	6	7	8	9	10	11	12	14	16	20	24	30	40	50	75	100	200	500	∞
1	161 **4,052**	200 **4,999**	216 **5,403**	225 **5,625**	230 **5,764**	234 **5,859**	237 **5,928**	239 **5,981**	241 **6,022**	242 **6,056**	243 **6,082**	244 **6,106**	245 **6,142**	246 **6,169**	248 **6,208**	249 **6,234**	250 **6,261**	251 **6,286**	252 **6,302**	253 **6,323**	253 **6,334**	254 **6,352**	254 **6,361**	254 **6,366**
2	18.51 **98.49**	19.00 **99.00**	19.16 **99.17**	19.25 **99.25**	19.30 **99.30**	19.33 **99.33**	19.36 **99.36**	19.37 **99.37**	19.38 **99.39**	19.39 **99.40**	19.40 **99.41**	19.41 **99.42**	19.42 **99.43**	19.43 **99.44**	19.44 **99.45**	19.45 **99.46**	19.46 **99.47**	19.47 **99.48**	19.47 **99.48**	19.48 **99.49**	19.49 **99.49**	19.49 **99.49**	19.50 **99.50**	19.50 **99.50**
3	10.13 **34.12**	9.55 **30.82**	9.28 **29.46**	9.12 **28.71**	9.01 **28.24**	8.94 **27.91**	8.88 **27.67**	8.84 **27.49**	8.81 **27.34**	8.78 **27.23**	8.76 **27.13**	8.74 **27.05**	8.71 **26.92**	8.69 **26.83**	8.66 **26.69**	8.64 **26.60**	8.62 **26.50**	8.60 **26.41**	8.58 **26.35**	8.57 **26.27**	8.56 **26.23**	8.54 **26.18**	8.54 **26.14**	8.53 **26.12**
4	7.71 **21.20**	6.94 **18.00**	6.59 **16.69**	6.39 **15.98**	6.26 **15.52**	6.16 **15.21**	6.09 **14.98**	6.04 **14.80**	6.00 **14.66**	5.96 **14.54**	5.93 **14.45**	5.91 **14.37**	5.87 **14.24**	5.84 **14.15**	5.80 **14.02**	5.77 **13.93**	5.74 **13.83**	5.71 **13.74**	5.70 **13.69**	5.68 **13.61**	5.66 **13.57**	5.65 **13.52**	5.64 **13.48**	5.63 **13.46**
5	6.61 **16.26**	5.79 **13.27**	5.41 **12.06**	5.19 **11.39**	5.05 **10.97**	4.95 **10.67**	4.88 **10.45**	4.82 **10.29**	4.78 **10.15**	4.74 **10.05**	4.70 **9.96**	4.68 **9.89**	4.64 **9.77**	4.60 **9.68**	4.56 **9.55**	4.53 **9.47**	4.50 **9.38**	4.46 **9.29**	4.44 **9.24**	4.42 **9.17**	4.40 **9.13**	4.38 **9.07**	4.37 **9.04**	4.36 **9.02**
6	5.99 **13.74**	5.14 **10.92**	4.76 **9.78**	4.53 **9.15**	4.39 **8.75**	4.28 **8.47**	4.21 **8.26**	4.15 **8.10**	4.10 **7.98**	4.06 **7.87**	4.03 **7.79**	4.00 **7.72**	3.96 **7.60**	3.92 **7.52**	3.87 **7.39**	3.84 **7.31**	3.81 **7.23**	3.77 **7.14**	3.75 **7.09**	3.72 **7.02**	3.71 **6.99**	3.69 **6.94**	3.68 **6.90**	3.67 **6.88**
7	5.59 **12.25**	4.74 **9.55**	4.35 **8.45**	4.12 **7.85**	3.97 **7.46**	3.87 **7.19**	3.79 **7.00**	3.73 **6.84**	3.68 **6.71**	3.63 **6.62**	3.60 **6.54**	3.57 **6.47**	3.52 **6.35**	3.49 **6.27**	3.44 **6.15**	3.41 **6.07**	3.38 **5.98**	3.34 **5.90**	3.32 **5.85**	3.29 **5.78**	3.28 **5.75**	3.25 **5.70**	3.24 **5.67**	3.23 **5.65**
8	5.32 **11.26**	4.46 **8.65**	4.07 **7.59**	3.84 **7.01**	3.69 **6.63**	3.58 **6.37**	3.50 **6.19**	3.44 **6.03**	3.39 **5.91**	3.34 **5.82**	3.31 **5.74**	3.28 **5.67**	3.23 **5.56**	3.20 **5.48**	3.15 **5.36**	3.12 **5.28**	3.08 **5.20**	3.05 **5.11**	3.03 **5.06**	3.00 **5.00**	2.98 **4.96**	2.96 **4.91**	2.94 **4.88**	2.93 **4.86**
9	5.12 **10.56**	4.26 **8.02**	3.86 **6.99**	3.63 **6.42**	3.48 **6.06**	3.37 **5.80**	3.29 **5.62**	3.23 **5.47**	3.18 **5.35**	3.13 **5.26**	3.10 **5.18**	3.07 **5.11**	3.02 **5.00**	2.98 **4.92**	2.93 **4.80**	2.90 **4.73**	2.86 **4.64**	2.82 **4.56**	2.80 **4.51**	2.77 **4.45**	2.76 **4.41**	2.73 **4.36**	2.72 **4.33**	2.71 **4.31**
10	4.96 **10.04**	4.10 **7.56**	3.71 **6.55**	3.48 **5.99**	3.33 **5.64**	3.22 **5.39**	3.14 **5.21**	3.07 **5.06**	3.02 **4.95**	2.97 **4.85**	2.94 **4.78**	2.91 **4.71**	2.86 **4.60**	2.82 **4.52**	2.77 **4.41**	2.74 **4.33**	2.70 **4.25**	2.67 **4.17**	2.64 **4.12**	2.61 **4.05**	2.59 **4.01**	2.56 **3.96**	2.55 **3.93**	2.54 **3.91**
11	4.84 **9.65**	3.98 **7.20**	3.59 **6.22**	3.36 **5.67**	3.20 **5.32**	3.09 **5.07**	3.01 **4.88**	2.95 **4.74**	2.90 **4.63**	2.86 **4.54**	2.82 **4.46**	2.79 **4.40**	2.74 **4.29**	2.70 **4.21**	2.65 **4.10**	2.61 **4.02**	2.57 **3.94**	2.53 **3.86**	2.50 **3.80**	2.47 **3.74**	2.45 **3.70**	2.42 **3.66**	2.41 **3.62**	2.40 **3.60**
12	4.75 **9.33**	3.88 **6.93**	3.49 **5.95**	3.26 **5.41**	3.11 **5.06**	3.00 **4.82**	2.92 **4.65**	2.85 **4.50**	2.80 **4.39**	2.76 **4.30**	2.72 **4.22**	2.69 **4.16**	2.64 **4.05**	2.60 **3.98**	2.54 **3.86**	2.50 **3.78**	2.46 **3.70**	2.42 **3.61**	2.40 **3.56**	2.36 **3.49**	2.35 **3.46**	2.32 **3.41**	2.31 **3.38**	2.30 **3.36**
13	4.67 **9.07**	3.80 **6.70**	3.41 **5.74**	3.18 **5.20**	3.02 **4.86**	2.92 **4.62**	2.84 **4.44**	2.77 **4.30**	2.72 **4.19**	2.67 **4.10**	2.63 **4.02**	2.60 **3.96**	2.55 **3.85**	2.51 **3.78**	2.46 **3.67**	2.42 **3.59**	2.38 **3.51**	2.34 **3.42**	2.32 **3.37**	2.28 **3.30**	2.26 **3.27**	2.24 **3.21**	2.22 **3.18**	2.21 **3.16**
14	4.60 **8.86**	3.74 **6.51**	3.34 **5.56**	3.11 **5.03**	2.96 **4.69**	2.85 **4.46**	2.77 **4.28**	2.70 **4.14**	2.65 **4.03**	2.60 **3.94**	2.56 **3.86**	2.53 **3.80**	2.48 **3.70**	2.44 **3.62**	2.39 **3.51**	2.35 **3.43**	2.31 **3.34**	2.27 **3.26**	2.24 **3.21**	2.21 **3.14**	2.19 **3.11**	2.16 **3.06**	2.14 **3.02**	2.13 **3.00**
15	4.54 **8.68**	3.68 **6.36**	3.29 **5.42**	3.06 **4.89**	2.90 **4.56**	2.79 **4.32**	2.70 **4.14**	2.64 **4.00**	2.59 **3.89**	2.55 **3.80**	2.51 **3.73**	2.48 **3.67**	2.43 **3.56**	2.39 **3.48**	2.33 **3.36**	2.29 **3.29**	2.25 **3.20**	2.21 **3.12**	2.18 **3.07**	2.15 **3.00**	2.12 **2.97**	2.10 **2.92**	2.08 **2.89**	2.07 **2.87**
16	4.49 **8.53**	3.63 **6.23**	3.24 **5.29**	3.01 **4.77**	2.85 **4.44**	2.74 **4.20**	2.66 **4.03**	2.59 **3.89**	2.54 **3.78**	2.49 **3.69**	2.45 **3.61**	2.42 **3.55**	2.37 **3.45**	2.33 **3.37**	2.28 **3.25**	2.24 **3.18**	2.20 **3.10**	2.16 **3.01**	2.13 **2.96**	2.09 **2.98**	2.07 **2.86**	2.04 **2.80**	2.02 **2.77**	2.01 **2.75**
17	4.45 **8.40**	3.59 **6.11**	3.20 **5.18**	2.96 **4.67**	2.81 **4.34**	2.70 **4.10**	2.62 **3.93**	2.55 **3.79**	2.50 **3.68**	2.45 **3.59**	2.41 **3.52**	2.38 **3.45**	2.33 **3.35**	2.29 **3.27**	2.23 **3.16**	2.19 **3.08**	2.15 **3.00**	2.11 **2.92**	2.08 **2.86**	2.04 **2.79**	2.02 **2.76**	1.99 **2.70**	1.97 **2.67**	1.96 **2.65**
18	4.41 **8.28**	3.55 **6.01**	3.16 **5.09**	2.93 **4.58**	2.77 **4.25**	2.66 **4.01**	2.58 **3.85**	2.51 **3.71**	2.46 **3.60**	2.41 **3.51**	2.37 **3.44**	2.34 **3.37**	2.29 **3.27**	2.25 **3.19**	2.19 **3.07**	2.15 **3.00**	2.11 **2.91**	2.07 **2.83**	2.04 **2.78**	2.00 **2.71**	1.98 **2.68**	1.95 **2.62**	1.93 **2.59**	1.92 **2.57**
19	4.38 **8.18**	3.52 **5.93**	3.13 **5.01**	2.90 **4.50**	2.74 **4.17**	2.63 **3.94**	2.55 **3.77**	2.48 **3.63**	2.43 **3.52**	2.38 **3.43**	2.34 **3.36**	2.31 **3.30**	2.26 **3.19**	2.21 **3.12**	2.15 **3.00**	2.11 **2.92**	2.07 **2.84**	2.02 **2.76**	2.00 **2.70**	1.96 **2.63**	1.94 **2.60**	1.91 **2.54**	1.90 **2.51**	1.88 **2.49**
20	4.35 **8.10**	3.49 **5.85**	3.10 **4.94**	2.87 **4.43**	2.71 **4.10**	2.60 **3.87**	2.52 **3.71**	2.45 **3.56**	2.40 **3.45**	2.35 **3.37**	2.31 **3.30**	2.28 **3.23**	2.23 **3.13**	2.18 **3.05**	2.12 **2.94**	2.08 **2.86**	2.04 **2.77**	1.99 **2.69**	1.96 **2.63**	1.92 **2.56**	1.90 **2.53**	1.87 **2.47**	1.85 **2.44**	1.84 **2.42**
21	4.32 **8.02**	3.47 **5.78**	3.07 **4.87**	2.84 **4.37**	2.68 **4.04**	2.57 **3.81**	2.49 **3.65**	2.42 **3.51**	2.37 **3.40**	2.32 **3.31**	2.28 **3.24**	2.25 **3.17**	2.20 **3.07**	2.15 **2.99**	2.09 **2.88**	2.05 **2.80**	2.00 **2.72**	1.96 **2.63**	1.93 **2.58**	1.89 **2.51**	1.87 **2.47**	1.84 **2.42**	1.82 **2.38**	1.81 **2.36**

continued

	22	23	24	25	26	27	28	29	30	32	34	36	38	40	42	44	46	48	50	55	60	65	70	80
22	1.78 / **2.31**	1.76 / **2.26**	1.73 / **2.21**	1.71 / **2.17**	1.69 / **2.13**	1.67 / **2.10**	1.65 / **2.06**	1.64 / **2.03**	1.62 / **2.01**	1.59 / **1.96**	1.57 / **1.91**	1.55 / **1.87**	1.53 / **1.84**	1.51 / **1.81**	1.49 / **1.78**	1.48 / **1.75**	1.46 / **1.72**	1.45 / **1.70**	1.44 / **1.68**	1.41 / **1.64**	1.39 / **1.60**	1.37 / **1.56**	1.35 / **1.53**	1.32 / **1.49**
23	1.80 / **2.33**	1.77 / **2.28**	1.74 / **2.23**	1.72 / **2.19**	1.70 / **2.15**	1.68 / **2.12**	1.67 / **2.09**	1.65 / **2.06**	1.64 / **2.03**	1.61 / **1.98**	1.59 / **1.94**	1.56 / **1.90**	1.54 / **1.89**	1.53 / **1.84**	1.51 / **1.90**	1.50 / **1.78**	1.48 / **1.76**	1.47 / **1.73**	1.46 / **1.71**	1.43 / **1.66**	1.41 / **1.63**	1.39 / **1.60**	1.37 / **1.56**	1.35 / **1.52**
24	1.81 / **2.37**	1.79 / **2.32**	1.76 / **2.27**	1.74 / **2.23**	1.72 / **2.19**	1.71 / **2.16**	1.69 / **2.13**	1.68 / **2.10**	1.66 / **2.07**	1.64 / **2.02**	1.61 / **1.98**	1.59 / **1.94**	1.57 / **1.90**	1.55 / **1.98**	1.54 / **1.85**	1.52 / **1.82**	1.51 / **1.80**	1.50 / **1.78**	1.48 / **1.76**	1.46 / **1.71**	1.44 / **1.68**	1.42 / **1.64**	1.40 / **1.62**	1.38 / **1.57**
25	1.84 / **2.42**	1.82 / **2.37**	1.80 / **2.33**	1.77 / **2.29**	1.76 / **2.25**	1.74 / **2.21**	1.72 / **2.18**	1.71 / **2.15**	1.69 / **2.13**	1.67 / **2.08**	1.64 / **2.04**	1.62 / **2.00**	1.60 / **1.97**	1.59 / **1.94**	1.57 / **1.91**	1.56 / **1.88**	1.54 / **1.86**	1.53 / **1.84**	1.52 / **1.82**	1.50 / **1.78**	1.48 / **1.74**	1.46 / **1.71**	1.45 / **1.69**	1.42 / **1.65**
26	1.87 / **2.46**	1.84 / **2.41**	1.82 / **2.36**	1.80 / **2.32**	1.78 / **2.28**	1.76 / **2.25**	1.75 / **2.22**	1.73 / **2.19**	1.72 / **2.16**	1.69 / **2.12**	1.67 / **2.08**	1.65 / **2.04**	1.63 / **2.00**	1.61 / **1.97**	1.60 / **1.94**	1.58 / **1.92**	1.57 / **1.90**	1.56 / **1.88**	1.55 / **1.86**	1.52 / **1.82**	1.50 / **1.79**	1.49 / **1.76**	1.47 / **1.74**	1.45 / **1.70**
27	1.91 / **2.53**	1.88 / **2.48**	1.86 / **2.44**	1.84 / **2.40**	1.82 / **2.36**	1.80 / **2.33**	1.78 / **2.30**	1.77 / **2.27**	1.76 / **2.24**	1.74 / **2.20**	1.71 / **2.15**	1.69 / **2.12**	1.67 / **2.08**	1.66 / **2.05**	1.64 / **2.02**	1.63 / **2.00**	1.62 / **1.98**	1.61 / **1.96**	1.60 / **1.94**	1.58 / **1.90**	1.56 / **1.87**	1.54 / **1.84**	1.53 / **1.82**	1.51 / **1.78**
28	1.93 / **2.55**	1.91 / **2.53**	1.89 / **2.49**	1.87 / **2.45**	1.85 / **2.41**	1.84 / **2.38**	1.81 / **2.35**	1.80 / **2.32**	1.79 / **2.29**	1.76 / **2.25**	1.74 / **2.21**	1.72 / **2.17**	1.71 / **2.14**	1.69 / **2.11**	1.68 / **2.08**	1.66 / **2.06**	1.65 / **2.04**	1.64 / **2.02**	1.63 / **2.00**	1.61 / **1.96**	1.59 / **1.93**	1.57 / **1.90**	1.56 / **1.88**	1.54 / **1.84**
29	1.98 / **2.67**	1.96 / **2.62**	1.94 / **2.58**	1.92 / **2.54**	1.90 / **2.50**	1.88 / **2.47**	1.87 / **2.44**	1.85 / **2.41**	1.84 / **2.38**	1.82 / **2.34**	1.80 / **2.30**	1.78 / **2.26**	1.76 / **2.22**	1.74 / **2.20**	1.73 / **2.17**	1.72 / **2.15**	1.71 / **2.13**	1.70 / **2.11**	1.69 / **2.10**	1.67 / **2.06**	1.65 / **2.03**	1.63 / **2.00**	1.62 / **1.98**	1.60 / **1.94**
30	2.03 / **2.75**	2.00 / **2.70**	1.98 / **2.66**	1.96 / **2.62**	1.95 / **2.58**	1.93 / **2.55**	1.91 / **2.52**	1.90 / **2.49**	1.89 / **2.47**	1.86 / **2.42**	1.84 / **2.38**	1.82 / **2.35**	1.80 / **2.32**	1.79 / **2.29**	1.78 / **2.26**	1.76 / **2.24**	1.75 / **2.22**	1.74 / **2.20**	1.74 / **2.18**	1.72 / **2.15**	1.70 / **2.12**	1.68 / **2.09**	1.67 / **2.07**	1.65 / **2.03**
32	2.07 / **2.83**	2.04 / **2.78**	2.02 / **2.74**	2.00 / **2.70**	1.99 / **2.66**	1.97 / **2.63**	1.96 / **2.60**	1.94 / **2.57**	1.93 / **2.55**	1.91 / **2.51**	1.89 / **2.47**	1.87 / **2.43**	1.85 / **2.40**	1.84 / **2.37**	1.82 / **2.35**	1.81 / **2.32**	1.80 / **2.30**	1.79 / **2.29**	1.78 / **2.26**	1.76 / **2.23**	1.75 / **2.20**	1.73 / **2.18**	1.72 / **2.15**	1.70 / **2.11**
34	2.13 / **2.94**	2.10 / **2.89**	2.09 / **2.85**	2.06 / **2.81**	2.05 / **2.77**	2.03 / **2.74**	2.02 / **2.71**	2.00 / **2.68**	1.99 / **2.66**	1.97 / **2.62**	1.95 / **2.58**	1.93 / **2.54**	1.92 / **2.51**	1.90 / **2.49**	1.89 / **2.46**	1.88 / **2.44**	1.87 / **2.42**	1.86 / **2.40**	1.85 / **2.39**	1.83 / **2.35**	1.81 / **2.32**	1.80 / **2.30**	1.79 / **2.28**	1.77 / **2.24**
36	2.18 / **3.02**	2.14 / **2.97**	2.13 / **2.93**	2.11 / **2.89**	2.10 / **2.86**	2.08 / **2.83**	2.06 / **2.80**	2.05 / **2.77**	2.04 / **2.74**	2.02 / **2.70**	2.00 / **2.66**	1.98 / **2.62**	1.96 / **2.59**	1.95 / **2.56**	1.94 / **2.54**	1.92 / **2.52**	1.91 / **2.50**	1.90 / **2.48**	1.90 / **2.46**	1.88 / **2.43**	1.86 / **2.40**	1.85 / **2.37**	1.84 / **2.35**	1.82 / **2.32**
38	2.23 / **3.12**	2.20 / **3.07**	2.18 / **3.03**	2.16 / **2.99**	2.15 / **2.95**	2.13 / **2.93**	2.12 / **2.90**	2.10 / **2.87**	2.09 / **2.84**	2.07 / **2.80**	2.05 / **2.76**	2.03 / **2.72**	2.02 / **2.69**	2.00 / **2.66**	1.99 / **2.64**	1.98 / **2.62**	1.97 / **2.60**	1.96 / **2.58**	1.95 / **2.56**	1.93 / **2.53**	1.92 / **2.50**	1.90 / **2.47**	1.89 / **2.45**	1.88 / **2.41**
40	2.26 / **3.18**	2.24 / **3.14**	2.22 / **3.09**	2.20 / **3.05**	2.18 / **3.02**	2.16 / **2.98**	2.15 / **2.95**	2.14 / **2.92**	2.12 / **2.90**	2.10 / **2.86**	2.08 / **2.82**	2.06 / **2.78**	2.05 / **2.75**	2.04 / **2.73**	2.02 / **2.70**	2.01 / **2.68**	2.00 / **2.66**	1.99 / **2.64**	1.98 / **2.62**	1.97 / **2.59**	1.95 / **2.56**	1.94 / **2.54**	1.93 / **2.51**	1.91 / **2.48**
42	2.30 / **3.26**	2.28 / **3.21**	2.26 / **3.17**	2.24 / **3.13**	2.22 / **3.09**	2.20 / **3.06**	2.19 / **3.03**	2.18 / **3.00**	2.16 / **2.98**	2.14 / **2.94**	2.12 / **2.89**	2.10 / **2.86**	2.09 / **2.82**	2.07 / **2.80**	2.06 / **2.77**	2.05 / **2.75**	2.04 / **2.73**	2.03 / **2.71**	2.02 / **2.70**	2.00 / **2.66**	1.99 / **2.63**	1.98 / **2.61**	1.97 / **2.59**	1.95 / **2.55**
44	2.35 / **3.35**	2.32 / **3.30**	2.30 / **3.25**	2.28 / **3.21**	2.27 / **3.17**	2.25 / **3.14**	2.24 / **3.11**	2.22 / **3.08**	2.21 / **3.06**	2.19 / **3.01**	2.17 / **2.97**	2.15 / **2.94**	2.14 / **2.91**	2.12 / **2.88**	2.11 / **2.86**	2.10 / **2.84**	2.09 / **2.82**	2.08 / **2.80**	2.07 / **2.78**	2.05 / **2.75**	2.04 / **2.72**	2.02 / **2.70**	2.01 / **2.67**	1.99 / **2.64**
46	2.40 / **3.45**	2.38 / **3.41**	2.36 / **3.36**	2.34 / **3.32**	2.32 / **3.29**	2.30 / **3.26**	2.29 / **3.23**	2.28 / **3.20**	2.27 / **3.17**	2.25 / **3.12**	2.23 / **3.08**	2.21 / **3.04**	2.19 / **3.02**	2.18 / **2.99**	2.17 / **2.96**	2.16 / **2.94**	2.14 / **2.92**	2.14 / **2.90**	2.13 / **2.88**	2.11 / **2.85**	2.10 / **2.82**	2.09 / **2.79**	2.07 / **2.77**	2.05 / **2.74**
48	2.47 / **3.59**	2.45 / **3.54**	2.43 / **3.50**	2.41 / **3.46**	2.39 / **3.42**	2.37 / **3.39**	2.36 / **3.36**	2.35 / **3.33**	2.34 / **3.30**	2.32 / **3.25**	2.30 / **3.21**	2.28 / **3.18**	2.26 / **3.15**	2.25 / **3.12**	2.24 / **3.10**	2.23 / **3.07**	2.22 / **3.05**	2.21 / **3.04**	2.20 / **3.02**	2.18 / **2.98**	2.17 / **2.95**	2.15 / **2.93**	2.14 / **2.91**	2.12 / **2.87**
50	2.55 / **3.76**	2.53 / **3.71**	2.51 / **3.67**	2.49 / **3.63**	2.47 / **3.59**	2.46 / **3.56**	2.44 / **3.53**	2.43 / **3.50**	2.42 / **3.47**	2.40 / **3.42**	2.38 / **3.38**	2.36 / **3.35**	2.35 / **3.32**	2.34 / **3.29**	2.32 / **3.26**	2.31 / **3.24**	2.30 / **3.22**	2.30 / **3.20**	2.29 / **3.18**	2.27 / **3.15**	2.25 / **3.12**	2.24 / **3.09**	2.23 / **3.07**	2.21 / **3.04**
55	2.66 / **3.99**	2.64 / **3.94**	2.62 / **3.90**	2.60 / **3.86**	2.59 / **3.82**	2.57 / **3.79**	2.56 / **3.76**	2.54 / **3.73**	2.53 / **3.70**	2.51 / **3.66**	2.49 / **3.61**	2.48 / **3.58**	2.46 / **3.54**	2.45 / **3.51**	2.44 / **3.49**	2.43 / **3.46**	2.42 / **3.44**	2.41 / **3.42**	2.40 / **3.41**	2.38 / **3.37**	2.37 / **3.34**	2.36 / **3.31**	2.35 / **3.29**	2.33 / **3.25**
60	2.82 / **4.31**	2.80 / **4.26**	2.78 / **4.22**	2.76 / **4.18**	2.74 / **4.14**	2.73 / **4.11**	2.71 / **4.07**	2.70 / **4.04**	2.69 / **4.02**	2.67 / **3.97**	2.65 / **3.93**	2.63 / **3.89**	2.62 / **3.86**	2.61 / **3.83**	2.59 / **3.80**	2.58 / **3.78**	2.57 / **3.76**	2.56 / **3.74**	2.56 / **3.72**	2.54 / **3.68**	2.52 / **3.65**	2.51 / **3.62**	2.50 / **3.60**	2.48 / **3.56**
65	3.05 / **4.82**	3.03 / **4.76**	3.01 / **4.72**	2.99 / **4.68**	2.98 / **4.64**	2.96 / **4.60**	2.95 / **4.57**	2.93 / **4.54**	2.92 / **4.51**	2.90 / **4.46**	2.88 / **4.42**	2.86 / **4.38**	2.85 / **4.34**	2.84 / **4.31**	2.83 / **4.29**	2.82 / **4.26**	2.81 / **4.24**	2.80 / **4.22**	2.79 / **4.20**	2.78 / **4.16**	2.76 / **4.13**	2.75 / **4.10**	2.74 / **4.08**	2.72 / **4.04**
70	3.44 / **5.72**	3.42 / **5.66**	3.40 / **5.61**	3.38 / **5.57**	3.37 / **5.53**	3.35 / **5.49**	3.34 / **5.45**	3.33 / **5.42**	3.32 / **5.39**	3.30 / **5.34**	3.28 / **5.29**	3.26 / **5.25**	3.25 / **5.21**	3.23 / **5.18**	3.22 / **5.15**	3.21 / **5.12**	3.20 / **5.10**	3.19 / **5.08**	3.18 / **5.06**	3.17 / **5.01**	3.15 / **4.98**	3.14 / **4.95**	3.13 / **4.92**	3.11 / **4.88**
80	4.30 / **7.94**	4.28 / **7.88**	4.26 / **7.82**	4.24 / **7.77**	4.22 / **7.72**	4.21 / **7.68**	4.20 / **7.64**	4.18 / **7.60**	4.17 / **7.56**	4.15 / **7.50**	4.13 / **7.44**	4.11 / **7.39**	4.10 / **7.35**	4.08 / **7.31**	4.07 / **7.27**	4.06 / **7.24**	4.05 / **7.21**	4.04 / **7.19**	4.03 / **7.17**	4.02 / **7.12**	4.00 / **7.08**	3.99 / **7.04**	3.98 / **7.01**	3.96 / **6.96**

continued

TABLE C
(Continued)

f_1 Degrees of Freedom (for greater mean square)

f_2	1	2	3	4	5	6	7	8	9	10	11	12	14	16	20	24	30	40	50	75	100	200	500	∞	f_2
100	3.94 / **6.90**	3.09 / **4.82**	2.70 / **3.98**	2.46 / **3.51**	2.30 / **3.20**	2.19 / **2.99**	2.10 / **2.82**	2.03 / **2.69**	1.97 / **2.59**	1.92 / **2.51**	1.88 / **2.43**	1.85 / **2.36**	1.79 / **2.26**	1.75 / **2.19**	1.68 / **2.06**	1.63 / **1.98**	1.57 / **1.89**	1.51 / **1.79**	1.48 / **1.73**	1.42 / **1.64**	1.39 / **1.59**	1.34 / **1.51**	1.30 / **1.46**	1.28 / **1.43**	100
125	3.92 / **6.84**	3.07 / **4.78**	2.68 / **3.94**	2.44 / **3.47**	2.29 / **3.17**	2.17 / **2.95**	2.08 / **2.79**	2.01 / **2.65**	1.95 / **2.56**	1.90 / **2.47**	1.86 / **2.40**	1.83 / **2.33**	1.77 / **2.23**	1.72 / **2.15**	1.65 / **2.03**	1.60 / **1.94**	1.55 / **1.85**	1.49 / **1.75**	1.45 / **1.68**	1.39 / **1.59**	1.36 / **1.54**	1.31 / **1.46**	1.27 / **1.40**	1.25 / **1.37**	125
150	3.91 / **6.81**	3.06 / **4.75**	2.67 / **3.91**	2.43 / **3.44**	2.27 / **3.14**	2.16 / **2.92**	2.07 / **2.76**	2.00 / **2.62**	1.94 / **2.53**	1.89 / **2.44**	1.85 / **2.37**	1.82 / **2.30**	1.76 / **2.20**	1.71 / **2.12**	1.64 / **2.00**	1.59 / **1.91**	1.54 / **1.83**	1.47 / **1.72**	1.44 / **1.66**	1.37 / **1.56**	1.34 / **1.51**	1.29 / **1.43**	1.25 / **1.37**	1.22 / **1.33**	150
200	3.89 / **6.76**	3.04 / **4.71**	2.65 / **3.88**	2.41 / **3.41**	2.26 / **3.11**	2.14 / **2.90**	2.05 / **2.73**	1.98 / **2.60**	1.92 / **2.50**	1.87 / **2.41**	1.83 / **2.34**	1.80 / **2.28**	1.74 / **2.17**	1.69 / **2.09**	1.62 / **1.97**	1.57 / **1.88**	1.52 / **1.79**	1.45 / **1.69**	1.42 / **1.62**	1.35 / **1.53**	1.32 / **1.48**	1.26 / **1.39**	1.22 / **1.33**	1.19 / **1.28**	200
400	3.86 / **6.70**	3.02 / **4.66**	2.62 / **3.83**	2.39 / **3.36**	2.23 / **3.06**	2.12 / **2.85**	2.03 / **2.69**	1.96 / **2.55**	1.90 / **2.46**	1.85 / **2.37**	1.81 / **2.29**	1.79 / **2.23**	1.72 / **2.12**	1.67 / **2.04**	1.60 / **1.92**	1.54 / **1.84**	1.49 / **1.74**	1.42 / **1.64**	1.38 / **1.57**	1.32 / **1.47**	1.28 / **1.42**	1.22 / **1.32**	1.16 / **1.24**	1.13 / **1.19**	400
1000	3.85 / **6.66**	3.00 / **4.62**	2.61 / **3.80**	2.38 / **3.34**	2.22 / **3.04**	2.10 / **2.82**	2.02 / **2.66**	1.95 / **2.53**	1.89 / **2.43**	1.84 / **2.34**	1.80 / **2.26**	1.76 / **2.20**	1.70 / **2.09**	1.65 / **2.01**	1.58 / **1.89**	1.53 / **1.81**	1.47 / **1.71**	1.41 / **1.61**	1.36 / **1.54**	1.30 / **1.44**	1.26 / **1.38**	1.19 / **1.28**	1.13 / **1.19**	1.09 / **1.11**	1000
∞	3.84 / **6.63**	2.99 / **4.60**	2.60 / **3.78**	2.37 / **3.32**	2.21 / **3.02**	2.09 / **2.80**	2.01 / **2.64**	1.94 / **2.51**	1.88 / **2.41**	1.83 / **2.32**	1.79 / **2.24**	1.75 / **2.18**	1.69 / **2.07**	1.64 / **1.99**	1.57 / **1.87**	1.52 / **1.79**	1.46 / **1.69**	1.40 / **1.59**	1.35 / **1.52**	1.28 / **1.41**	1.24 / **1.36**	1.17 / **1.25**	1.11 / **1.15**	1.00 / **1.00**	∞

The function, $F = i$ with exponent $2z$, is computed in part from Fisher's table VI (7). Additional entries are by interpolation, mostly graphical.

TABLE C – PART II
25%, 10%, 2.5%, and 0.5% Points for the Distribution of F*

f_1 Degrees of Freedom (for greater mean square)

f_2	P	1	2	3	4	5	6	7	8	9	10	12	15	20	24	30	40	60	120	∞
1	.250	5.83	7.50	8.20	8.58	8.82	8.98	9.10	9.19	9.26	9.32	9.41	9.49	9.59	9.63	9.67	9.71	9.76	9.80	9.85
	.100	39.86	49.50	53.59	55.83	57.2	58.20	58.91	59.44	59.86	60.2	60.70	61.22	61.74	62.00	62.26	62.53	62.79	63.06	63.33
	.025	648	800	864	900	924	937	948	957	963	969	977	985	993	997	1,001	1,006	1,010	1,014	1,018
	.005	16,211	20,000	21,615	22,500	23,056	23,437	23,715	23,925	24,091	24,224	24,426	24,630	24,836	24,940	25,044	25,148	25,253	25,359	25,465
2	.250	2.57	3.00	3.15	3.23	3.28	3.31	3.34	3.35	3.37	3.38	3.39	3.41	3.43	3.43	3.44	3.45	3.46	3.47	3.48
	.100	8.53	9.00	9.16	9.24	9.29	9.33	9.35	9.37	9.38	9.39	9.41	9.42	9.44	9.45	9.46	9.47	9.47	9.48	9.49
	.025	38.51	39.00	39.16	39.25	39.30	39.33	39.36	39.37	39.39	39.40	39.42	39.43	39.45	39.46	39.46	39.47	39.48	39.49	39.50
	.005	198	199	199	199	199	199	199	199	199	199	199	199	199	199	199	199	199	199	200
3	.250	2.02	2.28	2.36	2.39	2.41	2.42	2.43	2.44	2.44	2.44	2.45	2.46	2.46	2.46	2.46	2.47	2.47	2.47	2.47
	.100	5.54	5.46	5.39	5.34	5.31	5.28	5.27	5.25	5.24	5.23	5.22	5.20	5.18	5.18	5.17	5.16	5.15	5.14	5.13
	.025	17.44	16.04	15.44	15.10	14.88	14.74	14.62	14.54	14.47	14.42	14.34	14.25	14.17	14.12	14.08	14.04	13.99	13.95	13.90
	.005	55.55	49.80	47.47	46.20	45.39	44.84	44.43	44.13	43.88	43.69	43.39	43.08	42.78	42.62	42.47	42.31	42.15	41.99	41.83
4	.250	1.81	2.00	2.05	2.06	2.07	2.08	2.08	2.08	2.08	2.08	2.08	2.08	2.08	2.08	2.08	2.08	2.08	2.08	2.08
	.100	4.54	4.32	4.19	4.11	4.05	4.01	3.98	3.95	3.94	3.92	3.90	3.87	3.84	3.83	3.82	3.80	3.79	3.78	3.76
	.025	12.22	10.65	9.98	9.60	9.36	9.20	9.07	8.98	8.90	8.84	8.75	8.66	8.56	8.51	8.46	8.41	8.36	8.31	8.26
	.005	31.33	26.28	24.26	23.16	22.46	21.98	21.62	21.35	21.14	20.97	20.70	20.44	20.17	20.03	19.89	19.75	19.61	19.47	19.32
5	.250	1.69	1.85	1.88	1.89	1.89	1.89	1.89	1.89	1.89	1.89	1.89	1.89	1.88	1.88	1.88	1.88	1.87	1.87	1.87
	.100	4.06	3.78	3.62	3.52	3.45	3.40	3.37	3.34	3.32	3.30	3.27	3.24	3.21	3.19	3.17	3.16	3.14	3.12	3.10
	.025	10.01	8.43	7.76	7.39	7.15	6.98	6.85	6.76	6.68	6.62	6.52	6.43	6.33	6.28	6.23	6.18	6.12	6.07	6.02
	.005	22.78	18.31	16.53	15.56	14.94	14.51	14.20	13.96	13.77	13.62	13.38	13.15	12.90	12.78	12.66	12.53	12.40	12.27	12.14
6	.250	1.62	1.76	1.78	1.79	1.79	1.78	1.78	1.78	1.77	1.77	1.77	1.76	1.76	1.75	1.75	1.75	1.74	1.74	1.74
	.100	3.78	3.46	3.29	3.18	3.11	3.05	3.01	2.98	2.96	2.94	2.90	2.87	2.84	2.82	2.80	2.78	2.76	2.74	2.72
	.025	8.81	7.26	6.60	6.23	5.99	5.82	5.70	5.60	5.52	5.46	5.37	5.27	5.17	5.12	5.07	5.01	4.96	4.90	4.85
	.005	18.64	14.54	12.92	12.03	11.46	11.07	10.79	10.57	10.39	10.25	10.03	9.81	9.59	9.47	9.36	9.24	9.12	9.00	8.88
7	.250	1.57	1.70	1.72	1.72	1.71	1.71	1.70	1.70	1.69	1.69	1.68	1.68	1.67	1.67	1.66	1.66	1.65	1.65	1.65
	.100	3.59	3.26	3.07	2.96	2.88	2.83	2.78	2.75	2.72	2.70	2.67	2.63	2.59	2.58	2.56	2.54	2.51	2.49	2.47
	.025	8.07	6.54	5.89	5.52	5.29	5.12	4.99	4.90	4.82	4.76	4.67	4.57	4.47	4.42	4.36	4.31	4.25	4.20	4.14
	.005	16.24	12.40	10.88	10.05	9.52	9.16	8.89	8.68	8.51	8.38	8.18	7.97	7.75	7.64	7.53	7.42	7.31	7.19	7.08
8	.250	1.54	1.66	1.67	1.66	1.66	1.65	1.64	1.64	1.64	1.63	1.62	1.62	1.62	1.60	1.60	1.59	1.59	1.58	1.58
	.100	3.46	3.11	2.92	2.81	2.73	2.67	2.62	2.59	2.56	2.54	2.50	2.46	2.42	2.40	2.38	2.36	2.34	2.32	2.29
	.025	7.57	6.06	5.42	5.05	4.82	4.65	4.53	4.43	4.36	4.30	4.20	4.10	4.00	3.95	3.89	3.84	3.78	3.73	3.67
	.005	14.69	11.04	9.60	8.81	8.30	7.95	7.69	7.50	7.34	7.21	7.01	6.81	6.61	6.50	6.40	6.29	6.18	6.06	5.95
9	.250	1.51	1.62	1.63	1.63	1.62	1.61	1.60	1.60	1.59	1.59	1.58	1.57	1.56	1.56	1.55	1.54	1.54	1.53	1.53
	.100	3.36	3.01	2.81	2.69	2.61	2.55	2.51	2.47	2.44	2.42	2.38	2.34	2.30	2.28	2.25	2.23	2.21	2.18	2.16
	.025	7.21	5.71	5.08	4.72	4.48	4.32	4.20	4.10	4.03	3.96	3.87	3.77	3.67	3.61	3.56	3.51	3.45	3.39	3.33
	.005	13.61	10.11	8.72	7.96	7.47	7.13	6.88	6.69	6.54	6.42	6.23	6.03	5.83	5.73	5.62	5.52	5.41	5.30	5.19
10	.250	1.49	1.60	1.60	1.59	1.59	1.58	1.57	1.56	1.56	1.55	1.54	1.53	1.52	1.52	1.51	1.51	1.50	1.49	1.48
	.100	3.28	2.92	2.73	2.61	2.52	2.46	2.41	2.38	2.35	2.32	2.28	2.24	2.20	2.18	2.16	2.13	2.11	2.08	2.06
	.025	6.94	5.46	4.83	4.47	4.24	4.07	3.95	3.85	3.78	3.72	3.62	3.52	3.42	3.37	3.31	3.26	3.20	3.14	3.08
	.005	12.83	9.43	8.08	7.34	6.87	6.54	6.30	6.12	5.97	5.85	5.66	5.47	5.27	5.17	5.07	4.97	4.86	4.75	4.64
11	.250	1.47	1.58	1.58	1.57	1.56	1.55	1.54	1.53	1.53	1.52	1.51	1.50	1.49	1.49	1.48	1.47	1.47	1.46	1.45
	.100	3.23	2.86	2.66	2.54	2.45	2.39	2.34	2.30	2.27	2.25	2.21	2.17	2.12	2.10	2.08	2.05	2.03	2.00	1.97
	.025	6.72	5.26	4.63	4.28	4.04	3.88	3.76	3.66	3.59	3.53	3.43	3.33	3.23	3.17	3.12	3.06	3.00	2.94	2.83
	.005	12.23	8.91	7.60	6.88	6.42	6.10	5.86	5.68	5.54	5.42	5.24	5.05	4.86	4.76	4.65	4.55	4.44	4.34	4.23
12	.250	1.46	1.56	1.56	1.55	1.54	1.53	1.52	1.51	1.51	1.50	1.49	1.48	1.47	1.46	1.45	1.45	1.44	1.43	1.42
	.100	3.18	2.81	2.61	2.48	2.39	2.33	2.28	2.24	2.21	2.19	2.15	2.10	2.06	2.04	2.01	1.99	1.96	1.93	1.90
	.025	6.55	5.10	4.47	4.12	3.89	3.73	3.61	3.51	3.44	3.37	3.28	3.18	3.07	3.02	2.96	2.91	2.85	2.79	2.72
	.005	11.75	8.51	7.23	6.52	6.07	5.76	5.52	5.35	5.20	5.09	4.91	4.72	4.53	4.43	4.33	4.23	4.12	4.01	3.90

continued

TABLE C
(Continued)

f_1 Degrees of Freedom (for greater mean square)

f_2	P	1	2	3	4	5	6	7	8	9	10	12	15	20	24	30	40	60	120	∞
13	.250	1.45	1.55	1.55	1.53	1.52	1.51	1.50	1.49	1.49	1.48	1.47	1.46	1.45	1.44	1.43	1.42	1.42	1.41	1.40
	.100	3.14	2.76	2.56	2.43	2.35	2.28	2.23	2.20	2.16	2.14	2.10	2.05	2.01	1.98	1.96	1.93	1.90	1.88	1.85
	.025	6.41	4.97	4.35	4.00	3.77	3.60	3.48	3.39	3.31	3.25	3.15	3.05	2.95	2.89	2.84	2.78	2.72	2.66	2.60
	.005	11.37	8.19	6.93	6.23	5.79	5.48	5.25	5.08	4.94	4.82	4.64	4.46	4.27	4.17	4.07	3.97	3.87	3.76	3.65
14	.250	1.44	1.53	1.53	1.52	1.51	1.50	1.49	1.48	1.47	1.46	1.45	1.44	1.43	1.42	1.41	1.41	1.40	1.39	1.38
	.100	3.10	2.73	2.52	2.39	2.31	2.24	2.19	2.15	2.12	2.10	2.05	2.01	1.96	1.94	1.91	1.89	1.86	1.83	1.80
	.025	6.30	4.86	4.24	3.89	3.66	3.50	3.38	3.29	3.21	3.15	3.05	2.95	2.84	2.79	2.73	2.67	2.61	2.55	2.49
	.005	11.06	7.92	6.68	6.00	5.56	5.26	5.03	4.86	4.72	4.60	4.43	4.25	4.06	3.96	3.86	3.76	3.66	3.55	3.44
15	.250	1.43	1.52	1.52	1.51	1.49	1.48	1.47	1.46	1.46	1.45	1.44	1.43	1.41	1.41	1.40	1.39	1.38	1.37	1.36
	.100	3.07	2.70	2.49	2.36	2.27	2.21	2.16	2.12	2.09	2.06	2.02	1.97	1.92	1.90	1.87	1.85	1.82	1.79	1.76
	.025	6.20	4.76	4.15	3.80	3.58	3.41	3.29	3.20	3.12	3.06	2.96	2.86	2.76	2.70	2.64	2.58	2.52	2.46	2.40
	.005	10.80	7.70	6.48	5.80	5.37	5.07	4.85	4.67	4.54	4.42	4.25	4.07	3.88	3.79	3.69	3.58	3.48	3.37	3.26
16	.250	1.42	1.51	1.51	1.50	1.48	1.47	1.46	1.45	1.44	1.44	1.43	1.41	1.40	1.39	1.38	1.37	1.36	1.35	1.34
	.100	3.05	2.67	2.46	2.33	2.24	2.18	2.13	2.09	2.06	2.03	1.99	1.94	1.89	1.87	1.84	1.81	1.78	1.75	1.72
	.025	6.12	4.69	4.08	3.73	3.50	3.34	3.22	3.12	3.05	2.99	2.89	2.79	2.68	2.63	2.57	2.51	2.45	2.38	2.32
	.005	10.58	7.51	6.30	5.64	5.21	4.91	4.69	4.52	4.38	4.27	4.10	3.92	3.73	3.64	3.54	3.44	3.33	3.22	3.11
17	.250	1.42	1.51	1.50	1.49	1.47	1.46	1.45	1.44	1.43	1.43	1.41	1.40	1.39	1.38	1.37	1.36	1.35	1.34	1.33
	.100	3.03	2.64	2.44	2.31	2.22	2.15	2.10	2.06	2.03	2.00	1.96	1.91	1.86	1.84	1.81	1.78	1.75	1.72	1.69
	.025	6.04	4.62	4.01	3.66	3.44	3.28	3.16	3.06	2.98	2.92	2.82	2.72	2.62	2.56	2.50	2.44	2.38	2.32	2.25
	.005	10.38	7.35	6.16	5.50	5.07	4.78	4.56	4.39	4.25	4.14	3.97	3.79	3.61	3.51	3.41	3.31	3.21	3.10	2.98
18	.250	1.41	1.50	1.49	1.48	1.46	1.45	1.44	1.43	1.42	1.42	1.40	1.39	1.38	1.37	1.36	1.35	1.34	1.33	1.32
	.100	3.01	2.62	2.42	2.29	2.20	2.13	2.08	2.04	2.00	1.98	1.93	1.89	1.84	1.81	1.78	1.75	1.72	1.69	1.66
	.025	5.98	4.56	3.95	3.61	3.38	3.22	3.10	3.01	2.93	2.87	2.77	2.67	2.56	2.50	2.44	2.38	2.32	2.26	2.19
	.005	10.22	7.21	6.03	5.37	4.96	4.66	4.44	4.28	4.14	4.03	3.86	3.68	3.50	3.40	3.30	3.20	3.10	2.99	2.87
19	.250	1.41	1.49	1.49	1.47	1.46	1.44	1.43	1.42	1.41	1.41	1.40	1.38	1.37	1.36	1.35	1.34	1.33	1.32	1.30
	.100	2.99	2.61	2.40	2.27	2.18	2.11	2.06	2.02	1.98	1.96	1.91	1.86	1.81	1.79	1.76	1.73	1.70	1.67	1.63
	.025	5.92	4.51	3.90	3.56	3.33	3.17	3.05	2.96	2.88	2.82	2.72	2.62	2.51	2.45	2.39	2.33	2.27	2.20	2.13
	.005	10.07	7.09	5.92	5.27	4.85	4.56	4.34	4.18	4.04	3.93	3.76	3.59	3.40	3.31	3.21	3.11	3.00	2.89	2.78
20	.250	1.40	1.49	1.48	1.47	1.45	1.44	1.43	1.42	1.41	1.40	1.39	1.37	1.36	1.35	1.34	1.33	1.32	1.31	1.29
	.100	2.97	2.59	2.38	2.25	2.16	2.09	2.04	2.00	1.96	1.94	1.89	1.84	1.79	1.77	1.74	1.71	1.68	1.64	1.61
	.025	5.87	4.46	3.86	3.51	3.29	3.13	3.01	2.91	2.84	2.77	2.68	2.57	2.46	2.41	2.35	2.29	2.22	2.16	2.09
	.005	9.94	6.99	5.82	5.17	4.76	4.47	4.26	4.09	3.96	3.85	3.68	3.50	3.32	3.22	3.12	3.02	2.92	2.81	2.69
21	.250	1.40	1.48	1.48	1.46	1.44	1.43	1.42	1.41	1.40	1.39	1.38	1.37	1.35	1.34	1.33	1.32	1.31	1.30	1.28
	.100	2.96	2.57	2.36	2.23	2.14	2.08	2.02	1.98	1.95	1.92	1.88	1.83	1.78	1.75	1.72	1.69	1.66	1.62	1.59
	.025	5.83	4.42	3.82	3.48	3.25	3.09	2.97	2.87	2.80	2.73	2.64	2.53	2.42	2.37	2.31	2.25	2.18	2.11	2.04
	.005	9.83	6.89	5.73	5.09	4.68	4.39	4.18	4.01	3.88	3.77	3.60	3.43	3.24	3.15	3.05	2.95	2.84	2.73	2.61
22	.250	1.40	1.48	1.47	1.45	1.44	1.42	1.41	1.40	1.39	1.39	1.37	1.36	1.34	1.33	1.32	1.31	1.30	1.29	1.28
	.100	2.95	2.56	2.35	2.22	2.13	2.06	2.01	1.97	1.93	1.90	1.86	1.81	1.76	1.73	1.70	1.67	1.64	1.60	1.57
	.025	5.79	4.38	3.78	3.44	3.22	3.05	2.93	2.84	2.76	2.70	2.60	2.50	2.39	2.33	2.27	2.21	2.14	2.08	2.00
	.005	9.73	6.81	5.65	5.02	4.61	4.32	4.11	3.94	3.81	3.70	3.54	3.36	3.19	3.08	2.98	2.88	2.77	2.66	2.55
23	.250	1.39	1.47	1.47	1.45	1.43	1.42	1.41	1.40	1.39	1.38	1.37	1.35	1.34	1.33	1.32	1.31	1.30	1.28	1.27
	.100	2.94	2.55	2.34	2.21	2.11	2.05	1.99	1.95	1.92	1.89	1.84	1.80	1.74	1.72	1.69	1.66	1.62	1.59	1.55
	.025	5.75	4.35	3.75	3.41	3.18	3.02	2.90	2.81	2.73	2.67	2.57	2.47	2.36	2.30	2.24	2.18	2.11	2.04	1.97
	.005	9.63	6.73	5.58	4.95	4.54	4.26	4.05	3.88	3.75	3.64	3.47	3.30	3.12	3.02	2.92	2.82	2.71	2.60	2.48
24	.250	1.39	1.47	1.46	1.44	1.43	1.41	1.40	1.39	1.38	1.38	1.36	1.35	1.33	1.32	1.31	1.30	1.29	1.28	1.26
	.100	2.93	2.54	2.33	2.19	2.10	2.04	1.98	1.94	1.91	1.88	1.83	1.78	1.73	1.70	1.67	1.64	1.61	1.57	1.53
	.015	5.72	4.32	3.72	3.38	3.15	2.99	2.87	2.78	2.70	2.64	2.54	2.44	2.33	2.27	2.21	2.15	2.08	2.01	1.94
	.005	9.55	6.66	5.52	4.89	4.49	4.20	3.99	3.83	3.69	3.59	3.42	3.25	3.06	2.97	2.87	2.77	2.66	2.55	2.43

continued

df	α	1	2	3	4	5	6	7	8	9	10	12	15	20	24	30	40	60	120	∞
25	.250	1.39	1.47	1.46	1.44	1.42	1.41	1.40	1.39	1.38	1.37	1.36	1.34	1.33	1.32	1.31	1.29	1.28	1.27	1.25
	.100	2.92	2.53	2.32	2.18	2.09	2.02	1.97	1.93	1.89	1.87	1.82	1.77	1.72	1.69	1.66	1.63	1.59	1.56	1.52
	.025	5.69	4.29	3.69	3.35	3.13	2.97	2.85	2.75	2.68	2.61	2.51	2.41	2.30	2.24	2.18	2.12	2.05	1.98	1.91
	.005	9.48	6.60	5.46	4.84	4.43	4.15	3.94	3.78	3.64	3.54	3.37	3.20	3.02	2.92	2.82	2.72	2.61	2.50	2.38
26	.250	1.38	1.46	1.45	1.44	1.42	1.41	1.39	1.38	1.37	1.37	1.35	1.34	1.32	1.31	1.30	1.28	1.27	1.26	1.25
	.100	2.91	2.52	2.31	2.17	2.08	2.01	1.96	1.92	1.88	1.86	1.81	1.76	1.71	1.68	1.65	1.61	1.58	1.54	1.50
	.025	5.66	4.27	3.67	3.33	3.10	2.94	2.82	2.73	2.65	2.59	2.49	2.39	2.28	2.22	2.16	2.09	2.03	1.95	1.88
	.005	9.41	6.54	5.41	4.79	4.38	4.10	3.89	3.73	3.60	3.49	3.33	3.15	2.97	2.87	2.77	2.67	2.56	2.45	2.33
27	.250	1.38	1.46	1.45	1.43	1.42	1.40	1.39	1.38	1.37	1.36	1.35	1.33	1.32	1.31	1.30	1.28	1.27	1.26	1.24
	.100	2.90	2.51	2.30	2.17	2.07	2.00	1.95	1.91	1.87	1.85	1.80	1.75	1.70	1.67	1.64	1.60	1.57	1.53	1.49
	.025	5.63	4.24	3.65	3.31	3.08	2.92	2.80	2.71	2.63	2.57	2.47	2.36	2.25	2.19	2.13	2.07	2.00	1.93	1.85
	.005	9.34	6.49	5.36	4.74	4.34	4.06	3.85	3.69	3.56	3.45	3.28	3.11	2.93	2.83	2.73	2.63	2.52	2.41	2.29
28	.250	1.38	1.46	1.45	1.43	1.41	1.40	1.39	1.38	1.37	1.36	1.34	1.33	1.31	1.30	1.29	1.27	1.26	1.25	1.24
	.100	2.89	2.50	2.29	2.16	2.06	2.00	1.94	1.90	1.87	1.84	1.79	1.74	1.69	1.66	1.63	1.59	1.56	1.52	1.48
	.025	5.61	4.22	3.63	3.29	3.06	2.90	2.78	2.69	2.61	2.55	2.45	2.34	2.23	2.17	2.11	2.05	1.98	1.91	1.83
	.005	9.28	6.44	5.32	4.70	4.30	4.02	3.81	3.65	3.52	3.41	3.25	3.07	2.89	2.79	2.69	2.59	2.48	2.37	2.25
29	.250	1.38	1.45	1.45	1.43	1.41	1.40	1.38	1.37	1.36	1.35	1.34	1.32	1.31	1.30	1.29	1.27	1.26	1.25	1.23
	.100	2.89	2.50	2.28	2.15	2.06	1.99	1.93	1.89	1.86	1.83	1.78	1.73	1.68	1.65	1.62	1.58	1.55	1.51	1.47
	.025	5.59	4.20	3.61	3.27	3.04	2.88	2.76	2.67	2.59	2.53	2.43	2.32	2.21	2.15	2.09	2.03	1.96	1.89	1.81
	.005	9.23	6.40	5.28	4.66	4.26	3.98	3.77	3.61	3.48	3.38	3.21	3.04	2.86	2.76	2.66	2.56	2.45	2.33	2.21
30	.250	1.38	1.45	1.44	1.42	1.41	1.39	1.38	1.37	1.36	1.35	1.34	1.32	1.30	1.29	1.28	1.27	1.26	1.24	1.23
	.100	2.88	2.49	2.28	2.14	2.05	1.98	1.93	1.88	1.85	1.82	1.77	1.72	1.67	1.64	1.61	1.57	1.54	1.50	1.46
	.025	5.57	4.18	3.59	3.25	3.03	2.87	2.75	2.65	2.57	2.51	2.41	2.31	2.20	2.14	2.07	2.01	1.94	1.87	1.79
	.005	9.18	6.35	5.24	4.62	4.23	3.95	3.74	3.58	3.45	3.34	3.18	3.01	2.82	2.73	2.63	2.52	2.42	2.30	2.18
40	.250	1.36	1.44	1.42	1.40	1.39	1.37	1.36	1.35	1.34	1.33	1.31	1.30	1.28	1.26	1.25	1.24	1.22	1.21	1.19
	.100	2.84	2.44	2.23	2.09	2.00	1.93	1.87	1.83	1.79	1.76	1.71	1.66	1.61	1.57	1.54	1.51	1.47	1.42	1.38
	.025	5.42	4.05	3.46	3.13	2.90	2.74	2.62	2.53	2.45	2.39	2.29	2.18	2.07	2.01	1.94	1.88	1.80	1.72	1.64
	.005	8.83	6.07	4.98	4.37	3.99	3.71	3.51	3.35	3.22	3.12	2.95	2.78	2.60	2.50	2.40	2.30	2.18	2.06	1.93
60	.250	1.35	1.42	1.41	1.38	1.37	1.35	1.33	1.32	1.31	1.30	1.29	1.27	1.25	1.24	1.22	1.22	1.19	1.17	1.15
	.100	2.79	2.39	2.18	2.04	1.95	1.87	1.82	1.77	1.74	1.71	1.66	1.60	1.54	1.51	1.48	1.44	1.40	1.35	1.29
	.025	5.29	3.93	3.34	3.01	2.79	2.63	2.51	2.41	2.33	2.27	2.17	2.06	1.94	1.88	1.82	1.74	1.67	1.58	1.48
	.005	8.49	5.80	4.73	4.14	3.76	3.49	3.29	3.13	3.01	2.90	2.74	2.57	2.39	2.29	2.19	2.08	1.96	1.83	1.69
120	.250	1.34	1.40	1.39	1.37	1.35	1.33	1.31	1.30	1.29	1.28	1.26	1.24	1.22	1.21	1.19	1.18	1.16	1.13	1.10
	.100	2.75	2.35	2.13	1.99	1.90	1.82	1.77	1.72	1.68	1.65	1.60	1.54	1.48	1.45	1.41	1.37	1.32	1.26	1.19
	.025	5.15	3.80	3.23	2.89	2.67	2.52	2.39	2.30	2.22	2.16	2.05	1.94	1.82	1.76	1.69	1.61	1.53	1.43	1.31
	.005	8.18	5.54	4.50	3.92	3.55	3.28	3.09	2.93	2.81	2.71	2.54	2.37	2.19	2.09	1.98	1.87	1.75	1.61	1.43
∞	.250	1.32	1.39	1.37	1.35	1.33	1.31	1.29	1.28	1.27	1.25	1.24	1.22	1.19	1.18	1.16	1.14	1.12	1.08	1.00
	.100	2.71	2.30	2.08	1.94	1.85	1.77	1.72	1.67	1.63	1.60	1.55	1.49	1.42	1.38	1.34	1.30	1.24	1.17	1.00
	.025	5.02	3.69	3.12	2.79	2.57	2.41	2.29	2.19	2.11	2.05	1.94	1.83	1.71	1.64	1.57	1.48	1.39	1.27	1.00
	.005	7.88	5.30	4.28	3.72	3.35	3.09	2.90	2.74	2.62	2.52	2.36	2.19	2.00	1.90	1.79	1.67	1.53	1.36	1.00

*Reprinted from "Tables of percentage points of the inverted beta (F) distribution," by Maxine Merrington and Catherine M. Thompson, Biometrika, 33, 73 (1943) by permission of the authors and the editor.

Source: Snedecor, G. W. and W. G. Cochran. 1967. Statistical Methods, 6th ed. Ames: The Iowa State University Press.

TABLE D

Cumulative Normal Frequency Distribution (area under the standard normal curve from 0 to Z)

Z	0.00	0.01	0.02	0.03	0.04	0.05	0.06	0.07	0.08	0.09
0.0	0.0000	0.0040	0.0080	0.0120	0.0160	0.0199	0.0239	0.0279	0.0319	0.0359
0.1	.0398	.0438	.0478	.0517	.0557	.0596	.0636	.0675	.0714	.0753
0.2	.0793	.0832	.0871	.0910	.0948	.0987	.1026	.1064	.1103	.1141
0.3	.1179	.1217	.1255	.1293	.1331	.1368	.1406	.1443	.1480	.1517
0.4	.1554	.1591	.1628	.1664	.1700	.1736	.1772	.1808	.1844	.1879
0.5	.1915	.1950	.1985	.2019	.2054	.2088	.2123	.2157	.2190	.2224
0.6	.2257	.2291	.2324	.2357	.2389	.2422	.2454	.2486	.2517	.2549
0.7	.2580	.2611	.2642	.2673	.2704	.2734	.2764	.2794	.2823	.2852
0.8	.2881	.2910	.2939	.2967	.2995	.3023	.3051	.3078	.3106	.3133
0.9	.3159	.3186	.3212	.3238	.3264	.3289	.3315	.3340	.3365	.3389
1.0	.3413	.3438	.3461	.3485	.3508	.3531	.3554	.3577	.3599	.3621
1.1	.3643	.3665	.3686	.3708	.3729	.3749	.3770	.3790	.3810	.3830
1.2	.3849	.3869	.3888	.3907	.3925	.3944	.3962	.3980	.3997	.4015
1.3	.4032	.4049	.4066	.4082	.4099	.4115	.4131	.4147	.4162	.4177
1.4	.4192	.4207	.4222	.4236	.4251	.4265	.4279	.4292	.4306	.4319
1.5	.4332	.4345	.4357	.4370	.4382	.4394	.4406	.4418	.4429	.4441
1.6	.4452	.4463	.4474	.4484	.4495	.4505	.4515	.4525	.4535	.4545
1.7	.4554	.4564	.4573	.4582	.4591	.4599	.4608	.4616	.4625	.4633
1.8	.4641	.4649	.4656	.4664	.4671	.4678	.4686	.4693	.4699	.4706
1.9	.4713	.4719	.4726	.4732	.4738	.4744	.4750	.4756	.4761	.4767
2.0	.4772	.4778	.4783	.4788	.4793	.4798	.4803	.4808	.4812	.4817
2.1	.4821	.4826	.4830	.4834	.4838	.4842	.4846	.4850	.4854	.4857
2.2	.4861	.4864	.4868	.4871	.4875	.4878	.4881	.4884	.4887	.4890
2.3	.4893	.4896	.4898	.4901	.4904	.4906	.4909	.4911	.4913	.4916
2.4	.4918	.4920	.4922	.4925	.4927	.4929	.4931	.4932	.4934	.4936
2.5	.4938	.4940	.4941	.4943	.4945	.4946	.4948	.4949	.4951	.4952
2.6	.4953	.4955	.4956	.4957	.4959	.4960	.4961	.4962	.4963	.4964
2.7	.4965	.4966	.4967	.4968	.4969	.4970	.4971	.4972	.4973	.4974
2.8	.4974	.4975	.4976	.4977	.4977	.4978	.4979	.4979	.4980	.4981
2.9	.4981	.4982	.4982	.4983	.4984	.4984	.4985	.4985	.4986	.4986
3.0	.4987	.4987	.4987	.4988	.4988	.4989	.4989	.4989	.4990	.4990
3.1	.4990	.4991	.4991	.4991	.4992	.4992	.4992	.4992	.4993	.4993
3.2	.4993	.4993	.4994	.4994	.4994	.4994	.4994	.4995	.4995	.4995
3.3	.4995	.4995	.4995	.4996	.4996	.4996	.4996	.4996	.4996	.4997
3.4	.4997	.4997	.4997	.4997	.4997	.4997	.4997	.4997	.4997	.4998
3.6	.4998	.4998	.4999	.4999	.4999	.4999	.4999	.4999	.4999	.4999
3.9	.5000									

Source: Snedecor, G. W. and W. G. Cochran. 1967. *Statistical Methods, 6th ed.* Ames: The Iowa State University Press.

CASE CONTROL STUDIES

Steven T. Fleming

Introduction

One of the classic study designs used in epidemiological research is the retrospective or **case control study**. With this mode of investigation, one identifies a group of subjects with a particular outcome, such as a disease or condition (the **cases**), and compares them to a group without the disease or condition (the **controls**). The comparison is made by looking back in time—that is, retrospectively (Gr. *retro spicere*: to look back)—at the risk(s) to which each group was exposed. Case control studies are sometimes referred to as retrospective observational studies.

Most epidemiological studies compare one group to another to determine the effect of risk factors (i.e., exposures) or treatments (i.e., interventions) on the incidence or course of disease. The studies can be classified on the basis of (1) the date when the disease is identified; (2) the date of exposure or treatment recognition; (3) the time frame used in conducting the analysis. Figure 4.1 illustrates this paradigm for the case control study. The identification of cases (with a particular outcome) and controls (without the outcome) is done in the present. Researchers look to the past for exposure to a risk factor and classify each case and control into exposed or unexposed groups. The analysis is typically accomplished in the present.

Selection of Cases

In most case control studies, cases are patients who have developed a particular disease, condition, or disability. In order to be identified as such, most of these

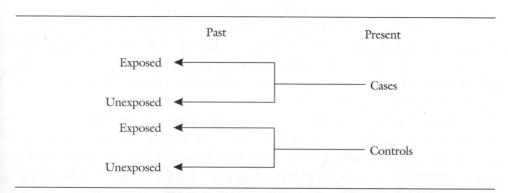

FIGURE 4.1
Schematic for Case-Control Studies

patients have had access to the healthcare system at some point in time. For example, they have become hospitalized or they have been seen by their primary care physician. Notice the definition of cases in this list of five studies:

1. "Cases ($n = 4,083$) were women with a first primary breast cancer diagnosed between 1966 and 1989" (Slattery and Kerber 1993).
2. "A total of 1,500 subjects 35–74 years old with primary cancer of the bronchus or lung . . . . diagnosed from January 1, 1980, through December 31, 1984 were selected from the Swedish Cancer Registry" (Pershagen et al. 1994).
3. "Case patients for the study consisted of all adult in-patient trauma deaths ($n = 3,074$) that occurred in California" (Morris, MacKenzie, and Edelstein 1990).
4. "The cases or claimants ($n = 51$) were identified as those study patients who filed malpractice claims referring to allegedly negligent care that was provided during the sampled hospitalization" (Burstin et al. 1993).
5. "The case patient had to have ESRD [end stage renal dialysis] and had to have started long-term dialysis between January and July 1991." (Perneger, Whelton, and Klag 1994).

It is important to be specific in terms of patient characteristics (age, diagnosis, even severity of illness) and the period of time during which patients present themselves for medical care. Cases may even be defined over an extended period of time (e.g., Study no. 1).

Selection of Controls

Control groups are necessary in most epidemiological studies to account for the underlying propensity of people to develop disease, even without a particular exposure, or recover from illness, even without a particular treatment. In a case control study, researchers determine the exposure status of the subjects in the case group (those who have developed disease) and compare that with the exposure status of the control group (those who have not developed disease). The purpose is to measure the extent to which cases are more likely than controls are to be exposed to risk factor(s). The control group should be representative of the general population and should have the same probability of selection into the sample and exposure to the risk factor(s) as the cases are (Timmreck 1998). Control groups are typically matched to cases using a matching strategy. For example, cases may be **pair matched** to controls along a number of relevant dimensions. This means that the researcher must match one control (with specific characteristics, such as age and sex) with each case. Alternatively, the controls may be **group** or **frequency matched**. This strategy involves no one-to-one matching, but it requires that controls as a group be similar to the case group in terms of certain characteristics (e.g., the percentage of cases age 65 and older should be the same as that of the control group). Notice how controls were chosen in this next list of studies:

1. "[C]ontrols were ascertained for each study site . . . using random digit dialing with frequency-matching to ensure an age distribution comparable to that of cases" (Daling et al. 1996).
2. "We selected as controls patients aged 40–69 years who had been admitted for nonmalignant conditions judged to be unrelated to the use of antihypertensive drugs" (Rosenberg et al. 1998).
3. "Controls were white women hospitalized in either a general surgical or an orthopedic service who had not had a previous hip fracture or hip replacement and who lived within the geographic areas included in the study" (Grisso et al. 1991).
4. "Four control patients were sought for each patient with primary pulmonary hypertension. The controls were randomly selected from lists of consecutive patients seen by the same general practitioner" (Abenhaim et al. 1996).
5. "For each woman with stroke, three controls, matched for year of birth and location of the facility where care was received were randomly selected from among the female members of the program" (Pettiti et al. 1996).

Typically, the desire to match cases to controls along a number of potentially relevant characteristics must be balanced against the practicality of being able to locate controls who meet the necessary criteria for inclusion in the study. Thus, most studies seek controls of the same age and gender, without the disease, and from the same general geographical area or with some history of treatment in the same facility. It should also be pointed out that the influence of a particular variable (e.g., income) can be measured later on, in the statistical analysis, and need not be included in the matching strategy (Lilienfeld and Stolley 1994).

Selection of a control group(s) is a critical component of the research. If the control group is not representative of the general population for some reason and/or is more likely to have characteristics associated with the disease under study, or if it is biased in any other way, the study is flawed. This means that the results and interpretations may be misleading. For example, Grisso and colleagues (1991) studied risk factors for falls as a cause of hip fracture in women and recognized that the control group "may have a greater prevalence of risk factors for falls, such as neurologic illnesses, lower limb disability, use of psychoactive medications, and alcohol use, than the general population [and] thus the comparison of case patients with hospitalized controls is likely to underestimate the effect of these factors on the risk of hip fracture."

Cross-Sectional Studies

Cross-sectional studies, or prevalence surveys, associate the presence or absence of disease in a population with potential risk factors such as age or gender (Lilienfeld and Stolley 1994). Such studies could be conducted based on data gathered from national surveys, such as the United States National Health Interview Survey (NHIS), and other surveys conducted by the National Center for Health Statistics. The findings of these surveys are routinely reported in the popular "rainbow series" booklets. The main difference between cross-sectional studies and case control studies is that case control studies look back in time to determine exposure history. Presumably, exposure precedes the onset of disease as assumed in the study design. With the cross-sectional study, typically based on survey information, one is attempting to estimate the prevalence of disease and to associate disease patterns with demographic, health behavior, and other information. For example, The NHIS collects data on various acute and chronic conditions, such as ulcers, and on demographic data, including marital status. While it may be possible to associate ulcers with stressful events such as divorce and losing a spouse, it is impossible with cross-sectional studies to establish causality. Stomach problems may have preceded or followed the stressful event. The case control study is more robust than the cross-sectional study to the extent that causality can be demonstrated by the methodology.

Exposure

Any characteristic or event that either increases or decreases the probability of disease, disability, death, or other adverse outcome can be referred to as an **exposure** (Norell 1995).

Although an exposure can also be called a **risk factor**, please note that exposures can either increase or decrease the risk of disease. Thus, some exposures are protective, whereas others are malicious. Exposures may be characterized in terms of magnitude and duration for the purpose of determining whether a **dose-response** relationship exists. A higher dose may be of higher magnitude, longer duration, or both. With a dose-response relationship, a higher dose of exposure results in a larger response (or effect), in terms of its impact on the outcome in question. Consider the following examples of exposures:

1. "We observed a positive association between adult height and breast cancer risk" (Swanson et al. 1996).
2. "[The] risk associated with obesity is, in most studies, limited to older postmenopausal women. In younger women . . . . obesity appears to be inversely related to the risk of disease" (Swanson et al. 1996).
3. "Pregnancy has a dual effect on the risk of breast cancer: it transiently increases the risk after childbirth but reduces the risk in later years" (Lambe et al. 1994).
4. "Women with a family history of breast cancer, even if the nearest relative with breast cancer is a third-degree relative, are at increased risk of the disease" (Slattery and Kerber 1994).

Each of the above studies concerns an exposure that is associated with the risk of developing breast cancer. These studies illustrate the inherent complexity in defining exposure. Height is simply a characteristic that appears to be associated with the risk of breast cancer. The authors hypothesize that height may represent some other underlying risk factor such as surface area or metabolic rate. Obesity is a risk factor that appears to be protective in younger women, but malicious in older women, with an underlying hormonal basis that is only speculative. With regard to pregnancy, the element of time affects the risk of disease rather than the exposure to it. The risk of breast cancer associated with pregnancy is initially higher, immediately following the pregnancy, but lower thereafter. Finally, family history is an exposure related to one's pedigree, which may have underlying genetic and environmental components.

The diversity, definitions, and distinctions of exposure can be explored in the following studies. According to Perneger (1994), "Both heavy average intake . . . and medium-to-high cumulative intake . . . of acetaminophen [Tylenol] appeared to double the odds of ESRD [end stage renal disease]." The results of this study would indicate a dose-response relationship with the exposure (acetaminophen) and disease (ESRD) in terms of both magnitude ("average intake") and duration ("cumulative intake").

Grisso and colleagues (1994), who studied the risk of hip fracture in women, showed that "among black women thinness, previous stroke, use of aids in walking, and alcohol consumption are associated with an increased risk of hip fracture." Here the four exposures are a body characteristic, a medical history event, a therapeutic device, and a behavior.

Eskenazi, Fenster, and Sidney (1991) examined the risks of preeclampsia, which is a hypertensive disorder of pregnancy, and found that "being nulliparous [childless] and having a previous history of preeclampsia greatly increased a women's risk for preeclampsia . . . working during pregnancy more than doubled the risk for preeclampsia . . . . cigarette smoking tended to protect against preeclampsia . . . alcohol consumption was protective . . . having a history of spontaneous abortion may be protective and being black may be a risk." With this study the protective exposures are a condition (pregnancy), two behaviors (smoking and alcohol use), and a history of medical events (miscarriages).

The relationship between baldness in men and myocardial infarction (heart attack) was the topic of a study by Lesko, Rosenberg, and Shapiro (1993) who reported a dose-response relationship, since "the results support the hypothesis that MPB [male pattern baldness] is associated with an increased risk of MI [myocardial infarction] in men under the age of 55 years . . . the RR [relative risk] estimate for men with extreme vertex baldness compared with men with no baldness was approximately 3.0; for lesser degrees of hair loss, the risk was lower." Clearly, it is not baldness in itself that predisposes one to these cardiovascular events but rather some underlying physiological mechanism (e.g., level of testosterone) for which baldness is the observable measure.

These examples were offered to alert the reader to the breadth of possible exposures and to the difficulty of distinguishing exposures as derivative risks, in the sense that they represent a more cellular, biochemical, or physiological basis of disease than that found in the exposures themselves. It should also be clear that both exposure and risk operate within the context of time. A dose-response relationship may reflect either (or both) the magnitude or the duration of exposure. Further, the increase or decrease in the probability of disease brought about by an exposure may vary across time, as was the case with the effect of pregnancy on breast cancer.

Relative Risk in a Case Control Study

The purpose of most case control studies is to assess the degree of risk, in terms of disease, disability, or other adverse outcome, that is associated with a particular exposure to a risk factor. The data are typically presented in a two-by-two table (Table 4.1) with the presence or absence of a characteristic or risk factor (the exposure) as rows, and the presence (cases) or absence (controls) of disease as columns.

With most epidemiological studies, the interest is in measuring the number of times more likely that one is to develop disease after exposure to a particular risk factor. This concept is referred to as **relative risk**. With a case control study design, one can estimate the relative risk by the **odds ratio (OR),** which is defined as the cross-product of the entries in Table 4.1—ad/bc. The odds ratio is only an estimate of the relative risk. The degree to which the estimate of relative risk is valid depends on (1) whether cases and controls are truly representative of the population from which they are drawn and (2) whether the frequency of disease in the population is small (see Lilienfeld and Stolley 1994, on pages 316–317, for a derivation of the odds ratio as a good estimate of relative risk under these circumstances). Relative risk cannot be calculated directly from the data typically presented in case control studies because we are not supplied with information on the incidence of disease in the population, nor can we calculate the incidence of disease among persons who were exposed or unexposed to a particular risk factor. That is, with a case control study, we have no cohorts who develop disease and no cohorts from whom incidence rates can be calculated.

An odds ratio greater than 1.0 indicates the number of times more likely that one is to develop disease given exposure to a risk factor; a value of 1.0 means that the disease is unaffected by the risk factor; a value of less than one implies that the risk factor is actually protective—that one is less likely to develop disease if exposed. For example, when Slattery and Kerber (1993) evaluated family history and breast cancer risk, they considered, among other things, the risk of having

TABLE 4.1
Case-Control Study
Design

	Cases	Controls
Exposure		
Yes	a	b
No	c	d

a mother who had suffered breast cancer. Table 4.2 reports these results. In this example the exposure is to have a mother who had suffered breast cancer. Cases are those with breast cancer; controls are those without the disease. According to the odds ratio, a woman is 2.4 times as likely to get breast cancer if her mother had the disease.

Table 4.3 illustrates the risk of breast cancer reported by Daling and colleagues (1996) among nulliparous women associated with induced abortion. The exposure here is induced abortion. The odds ratio would indicate that women who remain childless but undergo an induced abortion are 1.3 times as likely (or 30 percent more likely) to develop breast cancer than those who do not. Table 4.4, on the other hand, illustrates the protective effect of lactation on breast cancer risk as well as a dose-response relationship, from a study by Newcomb and colleagues (1994). In this study the hypothesis was that lactation duration may be associated with reduced risk of premenopausal breast cancer.

As the odds ratio decreases (from 1.0 toward 0), the protective effect increases. In other words, women who lactate for a year or two are .71 times as likely (or 29 percent less likely) to suffer premenopausal breast cancer compared with women who do not lactate at all. The protective effect of lactation decreases (OR increases) as the dose of the exposure decreases.

	Cases	Controls
Exposure		
Yes	123	51
No	3,960	4,032

$OR = 123 \times 4032/51 \times 3960 = 2.4$

TABLE 4.2
Family History and Breast Cancer Risk

	Cases	Controls
Exposure		
Yes	95	63
No	208	181

$OR = 95 \times 181/63 \times 208 = 1.3$

TABLE 4.3
Induced Abortion and Breast Cancer Risk

TABLE 4.4
Dose-Response
Relationship
Between Duration
of Lactation and
Premenopausal
Breast Cancer

	Cases	Controls		Cases	Controls		Cases	Controls
	Exposure ≤ 3 months			Exposure 4–12 months			Exposure 13–24 months	
Yes	203	375		195	390		106	251
No	602	1009		602	1009		602	1009
	OR = 0.91			OR = 0.84			OR = 0.71	

Confounding

Factors or variables other than the exposures in question may influence the probability of developing the disease under study. These **confounding variables** complicate and confuse the analysis. According to Timmreck (1998):

> Confounding variables can affect controls and may lead to biased or misguided association between disease and cause, the agents or risk factors. Any characteristic, trait, or other factor that can distort or slant the results of the study can be a confounding variable if not taken into account or considered.

Thompson (1994) makes four points with regard to confounding: (1) the size of the bias in the odds ratio depends on the level of confounder association with the exposure and the disease; (2) confounders may be causally related to the disease or are associated with the exposure as proxies for unmeasured causes; (3) if an exposure has a causal effect on another variable, that variable is an intervening variable rather than a confounder; and (4) the aggregate effect of multiple confounders may be substantial even though the effect of each is small. For example, consider the relationship between smoking (an exposure) and coronary heart disease (CHD). Confounders may include variables such as stress. Stress may be causally related to CHD, or it may be a proxy for some unmeasured variable such as personality. Moreover, stress may be related to the exposure, to the extent that smokers are more likely to smoke under stress. In any event, failure to measure stress could distort or bias the results. If the exposed group (smokers) is more likely to be under stress than the unexposed group (nonsmokers), then an exaggerated incidence of CHD could be the result of both smoking and stress.

At least two ways have been developed to deal with confounding: **multivariate analysis** and **stratification**. The former is appropriate when many known risk factors can be measured and included in the analysis. The latter can be useful with a small number of risk factors. Newcomb et al. (1994) studied the hypothesis that lactation may be a protective factor for breast cancer. These authors chose to use a multivariate logistic regression that includes a number of well-established risk factors for breast cancer, such as subjects' age at birth of first child and family history of breast cancer. Cases and controls may differ in exposure to these other risk factors (e.g., in the Newcomb study, 18 percent of cases had a family history of breast cancer compared with 11 percent of controls). If these confounding variables are related to the exposure in question, the results may be biased or misleading. Suppose that older mothers are more likely to breast-feed their babies. The protective effect of lactation may be mitigated by delivery of the first child at a later age (a risk factor). The logistic regression calculates an adjusted odds ratio that compensates or controls for the influence of these other risk factors.

The other approach is to stratify the results by the confounding variable in question. Pershagen and colleagues (1994), for instance, were interested is residential radon exposure as a risk factor for lung cancer in Sweden. Strong evidence would suggest that smoking is a behemoth of a risk factor for lung cancer, the protests of the tobacco industry to the contrary notwithstanding. If cases (those with lung cancer) were more likely to be smokers than controls, and smoking was associated with radon exposure, it would be difficult to disentangle the effects of smoking versus radon exposure in the analysis. One solution would be to stratify the analysis as in Table 4.5. Although the authors used a multivariate logistic regression, the results are stratified by exposure to smoking.

Although there may be some increased risk of lung cancer with radon exposure, the risk of lung cancer for smokers who are exposed to radon grows exponentially. Since the results are stratified by smoking exposure, we are able to see the interaction (and potential confounding) of these two exposures.

Attributable Fraction

Earlier, the odds ratio (OR) was defined as an estimate of the relative risk of disease given exposure to a particular risk factor. To the extent that confounding may occur—especially if there are multiple risk factors, some of which may potentiate or mitigate each another—the odds ratio must be adjusted to compensate for this

Smoking Exposure	Level of Radon in the Home				
	1	2	3	4	5
Never smoked	1	1.1	1.0	1.5	1.2
Exsmoker	2.6	2.4	3.2	4.5	1.1
Current Smoker					
<10 cigarettes/day	6.2	6.0	6.1	7.3	25.1
≥10 cigarettes/day	12.6	11.6	11.8	15.0	32.5

TABLE 4.5
Radon and Risk of Lung Cancer Stratified by Smoking Exposure (adapted from ref)

interaction. Also, one may be interested in determining the extent to which a particular risk factor is responsible for disease in the population. The proportion of disease that is attributed to a particular risk factor is defined as the attributable fraction and is estimated for case control studies here:

$$\text{Attributable fraction } (AF) = \frac{p\,(OR-1)}{p\,(OR-1)+1} \times 100\%$$

where p is the proportion of the population with the risk factor and OR is the odds ratio. For example, in a study of the risk factors for lung cancer among young adults in Germany, Kreuzer and colleagues (1998) report odds ratios of 15.9 and 29.9 for males and females, respectively, who are 45 years old or less and current smokers. Assume that the prevalence of smoking in Germany is 36.8 percent for men and 21.5 percent for women (World Health Organization 1996). The attributable fraction for men and women would be:

$$AF \text{ (males)} = \frac{.368\,(14.9)}{.368\,(14.9)+1} \times 100 = 84.5\%$$

$$AF \text{ (females)} = \frac{.215\,(28.9)}{.215\,(28.9)+1} \times 100 = 86.1\%$$

According to these results, current male smokers are 15.9 times as likely to get lung cancer, with smoking behavior being responsible for 84.5 percent of the disease. Current female smokers are 29.9 times as likely to get lung cancer, with smoking behavior being responsible for 86.1 percent of the disease.

The AF may be very high as in the case with smoking and lung cancer. Another study (Chaouki et al. 1998) reported an odds ratio of 61.6 for human papillovirus and cervical cancer in Morocco with an attributable fraction of 92%. These results would indicate that 92 percent of cervical cancer is attributed to the human papillovirus. On the other hand, the risk factor may be only one of multiple causes of the disease. The AF may be low because of a low odds ratio or a low prevalence of the risk factor in the population, or both. In the Daling study discussed earlier, the risk of breast cancer among childless women who had an induced abortion was 1.3. If we assume that about 30 percent of women in this age group report an induced abortion, the attributable fraction would be $[0.3(0.4)/(0.3(0.4)+1] \times 100 = 10.7\%$.

Attributable risk, on the other hand, is another measure of the degree to which intervention to eliminate a particular risk factor would decrease the incidence of disease. Since it is calculated as a rate difference (incidence in the exposed group minus incidence in the unexposed group), it is more appropriate to discuss in the cohort study (Chapter 5) where incidence rates can be calculated directly.

Sources of Bias

A study design may be subject to one or more sources of bias, which means that the results either underestimate or exaggerate the true effect. **Selection bias** relates to the process by which both cases and controls are selected for the study. Cases and controls should have the same probability of being included in the analysis. This source of bias is especially pronounced in hospital studies where cases (e.g., patients with a hip fracture or hip replacement) are typically compared to a control group of hospitalized patients without that condition. But it can also occur in other settings (e.g., physician offices) where the control group is derived from patients who are seen in that same setting. It can be demonstrated (Lilienfeld and Stolley 1994) that this source of bias, also referred to as **Berksonian bias** may either underestimate or overestimate the relationship between a risk factor and disease (Kraus 1954) if either (1) the rates of admission to the hospital (or visits to a physician) are different for cases and controls or (2) people are hospitalized (or see a physician) simply because they have a particular risk factor. The former is probably true most of the time; the latter is difficult to prove. Thus, selection bias is a very real possibility.

Another important source of bias is referred to as **misclassification bias**. According to Figure 4.1, cases in the present must be compared to a group of controls, with regard to exposure status in the past. Thus, subjects must be classified as either cases or controls, all of whom either were exposed or not exposed to the particular risk factor. To the extent that a subject has been misclassified as a case (when he or she should have been a control) or a control (when he or she should have been a case), this is a potential source of bias that may either underestimate or exaggerate the true effect of the study. Likewise, if either a case (or a control) has been erroneously classified as having been exposed to a risk factor (when he or she was not) or unexposed (when he or she was), this is a source of bias that either underestimates the true effect or exaggerates it. Thus, subjects may be misclassified on the basis of either disease or exposure, or both. See Norell (1995) for an excellent expostulation of these concepts.

Recall bias is a common type of misclassification bias of exposure. This bias is associated with the method by which subjects are asked to report on past exposures, and the period of time between the actual exposure and the information-gathering process. Subjects are often asked to "remember" their history of exposure to risk factors. If subjects misrepresent their exposure history, either intentionally (because of fears, embarrassment, or social expectations) or unintentionally (because of forgetfulness), recall bias rears its ugly head.

Misclassification bias may be **differential** or **nondifferential** depending on the amount and direction of the bias (Norell 1995). Differential bias moves in opposite directions; nondifferential bias moves in the same direction. In other words, if both cases and controls tend to underreport exposure history (e.g., number of sexual contacts), the bias is nondifferential. If one of the groups underreports exposures whereas the other group overreports exposures, the bias is differential. The four types of misclassification bias can be illustrated and described as follows:

1. nondifferential misclassification bias of disease;
2. differential misclassification bias of disease;

3. nondifferential misclassification bias of exposure; and
4. differential misclassification bias of exposure.

With **nondifferential misclassification bias of disease** (or condition), there is a gap between the theoretical and empirical definition of disease that may relate to issues of either definition or measurement. The criteria used to diagnose the disease may be either too narrow or too wide, or the definition of disease may be too narrow or too wide. Consider AIDS, for example, where the definition has widened over the years to include some of the common symptoms of immunodeficiency as manifested in women (e.g., invasive cervical cancer). Suppose that you are engaging in a case control study to determine if promiscuity is a risk factor for AIDS in women. If the definition of AIDS is too narrow (i.e., does not include invasive cervical cancer), then both exposure groups (sexually overactive and never active) are more likely to be classified as controls. The bias is nondifferential because both exposure groups would tend to be classified as controls rather than cases. This type of bias typically results in underestimating the effect by shifting the relative risk (or odds ratio) toward 1.0.

With **differential misclassification bias of disease** (condition), the tendency to classify subjects as either cases or controls depends on the exposure status and typically moves in opposite directions. For example, people who are exposed may more likely be recognized as having the disease, simply because the medical staff who differentiate between cases and controls had prior knowledge of the exposure. Without blinding, the staff would tend to classify the exposed subject with symptoms as a case, and the unexposed subject as a control. The staff may even engage in more thorough diagnostic inquiry for exposed subjects, presupposing that they are cases. Abenhaim and colleagues (1996) studied the risk of primary pulmonary hypertension associated with appetite-suppressant drugs (e.g., Fen-Phen). Had they not blinded the panel of reviewers to the patients' exposure to anorexic drugs, the reviewers might have had a tendency to misclassify patients as either cases or controls, based on presuppositions. With this type of bias the effect is exaggerated by shifting the relative risk toward infinity (larger risk) or zero (larger protection).

Nondifferential misclassification bias of exposure occurs when cases and controls tend to misrepresent (i.e., forget, omit, not want to reveal) their exposure status due to recall bias. Cases and controls may both overestimate or underestimate their exposure as a result of forgetfulness, embarrassment, or social expectations. This type of bias results in underestimating the effect by shifting the relative risk (or odds ratio) toward 1.0. For example, in a hypothetical study that attempts to link vitamin intake during early childhood with colon cancer, both cases and controls may underestimate the exposure (vitamins) due to recall bias.

Differential misclassification bias of exposure occurs if the tendency of cases to misrepresent (i.e., forget, omit, not want to reveal) their exposure status differs from that of controls. Either cases or controls overestimate or underestimate the exposure, or the bias is in different directions. For example, earlier we reported that women were 1.3 times as likely to develop breast cancer if they had an induced abortion (Daling et al. 1996). Suppose that both cases and controls tended to misrepresent this type of exposure for different reasons. Rookus and Leeuwen (1996) examined this question using data from four regions in the Netherlands, two in which Roman Catholics comprised about 63 percent of the population, and two in which the Roman Catholic population comprised only 28 percent of the residents. Presumably, Roman Catholics would be less willing to report an induced abortion because church teaching outlaws the act. Table 4.6 reports these results.

Notice that the odds ratio in the Roman Catholic areas is probably exaggerated because the authors "found evidence that the. . . . increased risk for breast cancer after induced abortion was largely attributable to underreporting of abortion by healthy control subjects." Thus they conclude that cases may be more likely to report an exposure despite social norms and critique, perhaps because of the quest to understanding the peril of disease, whereas controls, on the other hand, may misrepresent exposures that are not consistent with social norms of behavior. With this type of bias the effect will be exaggerated by shifting the relative risk toward infinity (larger risk) or zero (larger protection).

The issue with each of the four biases is whether cases/controls or exposures are misclassified in the same (or the opposite) way. This can be illustrated by Table 4.7, which is the standard two-by-two table used to calculate the odds ratio of a case control study. Each quadrant represents one of two possible diagrams for each of the four types of misclassification bias.

Note that in the case of nondifferential misclassification bias, of disease (I) and of exposure (III), the bias is in the same direction and the effect on the odds ratio (ad/bc) may be minimal (or may shift toward 1.0). In the former, some cases probably should be classified as controls, and in the latter, some of the unexposed were probably truly exposed. With differential misclassification bias, of disease (II) or of exposure (IV), the bias is in opposite directions. The effect is to increase the odd ratios toward infinity (higher risk) or toward zero (higher protection). The product "bc" is probably higher than it should be, with the result

	Low Roman Catholic		High Roman Catholic	
	Cases	Controls	Cases	Controls
Exposure				
Yes	23	22	12	1
No	292	326	213	229
	OR = 1.2		OR = 12.9	

TABLE 4.6
Induced Abortion and Breast Cancer in Two Areas in the Netherlands

TABLE 4.7
Effect of
Misclassification
Bias on the Odds
Ratio

(I) Nondifferential/Disease				(II) Differential/Disease			
	Cases		Controls		Cases		Controls
Exposed	a	⇐	b	Exposed	a	⇒	b
Unexposed	c	⇐	d	Unexposed	c	⇐	d

(III) Nondifferential/Exposure			(IV) Differential/Exposure		
	Cases	Controls		Cases	Controls
Exposed	a	b	Exposed	a	b
	⇓	⇓		⇓	⇑
Unexposed	c	d	Unexposed	c	d

that the odds ratio shifts toward zero. With the arrows reversed in (II) and (IV), the product "bc" would be lower than it should be resulting in a shift of the odds ratio toward infinity.

Case Control Advantages and Disadvantages

The case control study is an inexpensive, relatively efficient approach to measuring the effect of exposures, and it is particularly suited for rare diseases with long latency periods or exposures over a long period of time. For example, in a study of the effects of environmental tobacco smoke (passive smoking) on lung cancer in nonsmoking women (Fondham et al. 1994), the authors describe the process:

> In-person interviews followed by an extensive structured questionnaire designed to obtain information on household, occupational, and other exposures to ETS [environmental tobacco smoke] during each study subject's lifetime, as well as other exposures associated with lung cancer. Exposure to ETS was examined by source during childhood . . . and during adult life.

Lung cancer is a relatively rare disease (incidence of 56 per 100,000 population in 1994) with a long latency period. Exposure to environmental tobacco smoking was measured over the entire lifetime of the subjects. A cohort study would have to be much larger (because of the low incidence of disease) and more expensive, and it would take years to accomplish given the long-term latency of the disease.

Case control studies are not without disadvantages, however. The configuration of the control group, a critical element in this design, may become the Achille's heel of study validity if it is not structured correctly. Moreover, a sufficient number of controls willing to participate in the study may be difficult to find. Furthermore, whether or not the exposure preceded the disease may be difficult to ascertain in many studies, that is, the extent to which causality can be inferred from the results. The classic example of the latter is whether inactivity leads to heart disease or whether heart disease results in an inactive lifestyle. In another example the authors state:

> Establishing the causality of the association between acetaminophen [Tylenol] use and ESRD [end stage renal disease] is critical. The association was dose-dependent, specific . . . consistent with several previous reports, and biologically plausible. . . . Thus several criteria for causality were fulfilled. Nevertheless, the temporal precedence of the presumed cause still needs to be demonstrated. (Perneger et al. 1994)

The case control study may be subject to a number of biases discussed earlier: selection, recall, and misclassification biases, for example. Many researchers recognize these as potential flaws and try to ascertain whether these biases are real and the degree to which these biases could have affected the results:

> We also examined potential sources of misclassification of the exposure to anorexic agents. Patients with primary pulmonary hypertension might be more likely to remember using anorexic agents than controls (recall bias) (Abenhaim et al. 1996).
>
> It could be that those women with breast cancer whom we were unable to interview because of serious illness or death may have been more likely to have had an induced abortion than the women we did interview (Daling et al. 1996).
>
> It is possible that a woman diagnosed with a life-threatening disease such as breast cancer might report a history of induced abortion more completely than a healthy control woman contacted at random (Daling et al. 1996).
>
> Other data suggest that lung cancer cases who are ever smokers may be less inclined to misreport smoking status than others in the general population (Fontham et al. 1994).

The case control study does not directly report the incidence of disease among those exposed and not exposed to a presumed risk factor, as does the cohort study. Thus, the odds ratio is only an estimate of relative risk, the validity of which depends on the incidence of disease in the population.

The validity of inferences drawn from case control studies depends on the purity of the study design. Flawed studies can be somewhat biased at best and seriously misleading at worst. Armenian and Shapiro (1998) have suggested asking eight questions to assess the integrity of any particular case control study with respect to the following issues: (1) clarity of problem definition; (2) consistency between the definition of cases and the problem; (3) selection of cases and controls from the same base population; (4) validity of the measurement of exposure; (5) case/control selection independent of exposure assessment; (6) alternative explanations, such as confounding; (7) factor interactions; and (8) value of the study for health services decision making.

Summary

Although the case control study is not the gold standard approach to determining causality in epidemiological research (that distinction belongs to the randomized clinical trial), it is an efficient, inexpensive approach to determining the extent of relationships between risk factors and outcomes. With this study design, a group of subjects with a particular outcome is compared to a group of subjects selected because of the absence of the outcome on the basis of exposure (in the past) to specific risk factors. The odds ratio, which is an estimate of relative risk, measures the number of times that one is more or less likely to suffer a particular outcome if exposed to the risk factor. Although these studies are inexpensive and particularly appropriate for rare outcomes with long latency periods and lengthy exposures, they may be flawed by various types of bias such as misclassification bias, which occurs when subjects are incorrectly classified in terms of either outcome or exposure. Despite these shortcomings, the case control study remains a fundamental element of epidemiological research.

Case Study 4.1

Considerable controversy has emerged as a result of the alleged link between induced abortions and breast cancer. Much of the controversy is centered around the question of recall bias. The authors of a Swedish study (Lindefors-Harris et al. 1991) hypothesize that "a woman who had recently been given a diagnosis of a malignant disease, contemplating causes of her illness, would remember and report an induced abortion more consistently than would a healthy control." In an effort to deal with this problem these researchers compared two separate epidemiological studies of breast cancer with an overlap sample of 317 cases and 512 controls. One study used interviews to obtain the data on the history of abortion. The second study determined exposure based on a nationwide registry of legally induced abortions. With the first study, the interview revealed that 26 cases and 44 controls had been exposed to an induced abortion. The registry, on the other hand, confirmed that 24 cases and 59 controls had had an abortion. What is the odds ratio for each of the two separate studies? Is there evidence of misclassification bias? What is the effect of this bias on the estimate of relative risk? What other forms of bias might be present in this study?

Case Study 4.2

The popular diet pills (Fen-Phen) were removed from the market after millions of prescriptions were written, based on several studies that indicated serious complications. One study examined whether appetite suppressants (mostly related to fenfluramine, i.e., Fen) are a risk factor in the development of primary pulmonary hypertension (PPH), a rare but often fatal disease (Abenhaim et al. 1996). The study used a case control design conducted in four European countries. The 95 cases were patients diagnosed with primary pulmonary hypertension between September 1992 and September 1994. Four control patients were randomly selected for each case with PPH, based on lists of patients seen by the same physician as the case (total controls = 355). Interviewers of each subject were blinded to the study objectives and asked questions relating to health status and various other exposures. Table 4.8 presents odds ratios that have been adjusted for body mass index (BMI), systemic hypertension, and use of cocaine or intravenous drugs, among other things, for exposure to appetite suppressants for under and over three months. The table also presents the frequency of a high BMI, systemic hypertension, and use of cocaine or intravenous drugs among cases and controls.

How do the unadjusted (crude) odds ratios related to the use of appetite suppressants for under and over three months compare to odds ratios that have been adjusted for several confounders? How can the differences be explained? Explain some of the problems with this study design, particularly the issues of selection and misclassification bias. Given the size of the study, if five control patients were incorrectly classified as unexposed to these appetite suppressants, how would this affect the odds ratios? Some have suggested that because there "was considerable publicity about the possible association between appetite-suppressant drugs with primary pulmonary hypertension, this publicity is likely to have increased the referral of patients treated with such drugs to study hospitals" (Manson and Faich 1996; Brenot et al. 1993; Atanassoff et al. 1992). What kind of bias would be introduced into the study if this were true?

Exposure	Cases (PPH)	Controls	Adjusted OR
≤3 months	7	12	1.8
none	65	329	
>3 months	18	5	23.1
none	65	329	
questionable	5	9	2.6
none	65	329	
Confounders			
BMI ≥ 30	34	65	1.9
systemic hypertension	11	21	2.1
use of concaine/IV drugs	4	4	2.8

TABLE 4.8
Adjusted Odds Ratio for the Risk of Primary Pulmonary Hypertension with the Use of Appetite Suppressants

References

Abenhaim, L., Y. Moride, F. Brenot, S. Rich, J. Benichou, X. Kurz, T. Higenbottam, C. Oakley, E. Wouters, M. Aubier, G. Simonneau, and B. Begaud. 1996. "Appetite-Suppressant Drugs and the Risk of Primary Pulmonary Hypertension. International Primary Pulmonary Hypertension Study Group." *The New England Journal of Medicine* 335 (9): 609–16.

Armenian, H. K., and S. Shapiro. 1997. *Epidemiology and Health Services.* New York: Oxford University Press.

Atanassoff, P. G., B. M. Weiss, E. R. Schmid, and M. Tornic. 1992. "Pulmonary Hypertension and Dexfenfluramine." [letter] *Lancet* 339 (8790): 436.

Brenot, F., P. Herve, P. Petitpretz, F. Parent, P. Duroux, and G. Simonneau. 1993. "Primary Pulmonary Hypertension and Fenfluramine Use." *British Heart Journal* 70 (6): 537–41.

Burstin, H. R., W. G. Johnson, S. R. Lipsitz, and T. A. Brennan. 1993. "Do the Poor Sue More?: A Case-Control Study of Malpractice Claims and Socioeconomic Status." *Journal of the American Medical Association* 270 (14): 1697–701

Chaouki, N., F. X. Bosch, N. Munoz, C. J. Meijer, B. El-Gueddari, A. El-Ghazi, J. Deacon, X. Castellsague, and J. M. Wallboomers. 1998. "The Viral Origin of Cervical Cancer in Rabat, Morocco." *International Journal of Cancer* 75 (4): 546–54.

Daling, J. R., L. A. Brinton, L. F. Voigt, N. S. Weiss, R. J. Coates, K. E. Malone, J. B. Schoenberg, and M. Gammon. 1996. "Risk of Breast Cancer Among White Women Following Induced Abortion." *American Journal of Epidemiology* 144 (4): 373–80.

Eskenazi, B., L. Fenster, and S. Sidney. 1991. "A Multivariate Analysis of Risk Factors for Preeclampsia." *Journal of the American Medical Association* 266 (2): 237–41.

Fontham, E. T., P. Correa, P. Reynolds, A. Wu-Williams, P. A. Buffler, R. S. Greenberg, V. W. Chen, T. Alterman, P. Boyd, D. F. Austin, and J. Liff. 1994. "Environmental Tobacco Smoke and Lung Cancer in Nonsmoking Women: A Multicenter Study." *Journal of the American Medical Association* 271 (22): 1752–59.

Grisso, J. A., J. L. Kelsey, B. L. Strom, G. Y. Chiu, G. Maislin, L. A. O'Brien, S. Hoffman, and F. Kaplan. 1991. "Risk Factors for Falls as a Cause of Hip Fracture in Women." The Northeast Hip Fracture Study Group. *The New England Journal of Medicine* 324 (19): 1326–31.

Grisso, J. A., J. L. Kelsey, B. L. Strom, L. A. O'Brien, G. Maislin, K. LaPann, L. Samelson, and S. Hoffman. 1994. "Risk Factors for Hip Fracture in Black Women." The Northeast Hip Fracture Study Group. *The New England Journal of Medicine* 330 (22): 1555–59.

Kraus, A. S., 1954. "The Use of Hospital Data in Studying the Association Between a Characteristic and a Disease." *Public Health Report* 69 (December): 1211–14.

Kreuzer, M., L. Kreienbrock, M. Gerken, J. Heinrich, I. Bruske-Hohlfeld, K. Muller, and E. Wichmann. 1998. "Risk Factors for Lung Cancer in Young Adults." *American Journal of Epidemiology* 147 (11): 1028–37.

Lambe, M., C. Hsieh, D. Trichopoulos, A. Ekbom, M. Pavia, and H. O. Adami. 1994. "Transient Increase in the Risk of Breast Cancer after Giving Birth." *The New England Journal of Medicine* 331 (1): 5–9.

Lesko, S. M., L. Rosenberg, and S. Shapiro. 1993. "A Case Control Study of Baldness in Relation to Myocardial Infarction in Men," published erratum appears in *Journal of the American Medical Association* 269 (19): 2508, *Journal of the American Medical Association* 269 (8): 998–1003.

Lilienfeld, D. E., and P. D. Stolley. 1994. *Foundations of Epidemiology, 3rd ed.* New York: Oxford University Press.

Lindefors-Harris, B., G. Eklund, H. Adami, and O. Meirik. 1991. "Response Bias in a Case-Control Study: Analysis Utilizing Comparative Data Concerning Legal Abortions from Two Independent Swedish Studies." *American Journal of Epidemiology* 134 (9): 1003–1008.

Manson, J. E., and G. A. Faich. 1996. "Pharmacotherapy for Obesity: Do the Benefits Outweigh the Risks?" *The New England Journal of Medicine* 335 (9): 659–60.

Morris, J. A., Jr., E. J. MacKenzie, and S. L. Edelstein. 1990. "The Effect of Preexisting Conditions on Mortality in Trauma Patients." *Journal of the American Medical Association* 263 (14): 1942–46.

Newcomb, P. A., B. E. Storer, M. P. Longnecker, R. Mittendorf, E. R. Greenberg, R. W. Clapp, K. P. Burke, W. C. Willett, and B. MacMahon. 1994. "Lactation and a Reduced Risk of Premenopausal Breast Cancer." *The New England Journal of Medicine* 330 (2): 81–87.

Norell, S. E. 1995. "Workbook of Epidemiology." New York: Oxford University Press.

Pershagen, G., G. Akerblom, O. Axelson, B. Clavensjo, L. Damber, G. Desai, A. Enflo, F. Lagarde, H. Mellander, M. Svartengren, and G. A. Swedjemark. 1994. "Residential Radon Exposure and Lung Cancer in Sweden." *The New England Journal of Medicine* 330 (3): 159–64.

Perneger, T. V., P. K. Whelton, and M. J. Klag. 1994. "Risk of Kidney Failure Associated with the Use of Acetaminophen, Aspirin, and Nonsteroidal Anti-inflammatory Drugs." *The New England Journal of Medicine* 331 (25): 1675–79.

Pettiti, D. B., S. Sidney, A. Bernstein, S. Wolf, C. Quesenberry, and H. K. Ziel. 1996. "Stroke in Users of Low-Dose Oral Contraceptives." *The New England Journal of Medicine* 335 (1): 8–15.

Rookus, M. A., and F. E. van Leeuwen. 1996. "Induced Abortion and Risk for Breast Cancer: Reporting Recall Bias in a Dutch Base-Control Study." *Journal of the National Cancer Institute* 88 (23): 1759–64.

Rosenberg, L., R. S. Rao, J. R. Palmer, B. L. Strom, P. D. Stolley, A. G. Zauber, M. E. Warshauer, and S. Shapiro. 1998. "Calcium Channel Blockers and the Risk of Cancer." *Journal of the American Medical Association* 279 (13): 1000–1004.

Slattery, M. L., and R. A. Kerber. 1993. "A Comprehensive Evaluation of Family History and Breast Cancer Risk. The Utah Population Database." *Journal of the American Medical Association* 270 (13): 1563–68.

Swanson, C. A., R. J. Coates, J. B. Schoenberg, K. E. Malone, M. D. Gammon, J. L. Stanford, I. J. Shorr, N. A. Potischman, and L. A. Brinton. 1996. "Body Size and Breast Cancer Risk Among Women Under Age 45 Years." *American Journal of Epidemiology* 143 (7): 698–706.

Thompson, W. D. 1994. "Statistical Analysis of Case-Control Studies." *Epidemiologic Reviews* 16 (1): 33–50.

Timmreck, T. C. 1998. *An Introduction to Epidemiology, 2nd ed.* Sudbury, MA: Jones and Bartlett Publishers.

World Health Organization. 1996. http://www.who.ch/psa/toh/Alert/apr96/gifs/table3.gif

COHORT STUDIES

John N. Lewis and Steven T. Fleming

Introduction

Chapter 4 details the retrospective case control study. A very different approach to epidemiologic research is the **cohort study**, which is usually conducted prospectively. A cohort is defined formally by The American Heritage Dictionary, Second College Edition, as "*n*. 1. One of the ten divisions of a Roman legion, consisting of 300 to 600 men. 2. A group or band united in a struggle." Epidemiologists use this word to identify a group of people who are identified at the beginning of a study and followed prospectively for a period of time to observe what happens to them. Unusual variations on this theme are cohorts that acquire new members over time and cohorts that are identified retrospectively (Mantel 1973).

Cohort studies may be contrasted graphically to case control studies by comparing Figures 5.1 and 5.2 to Figure 4.1 in Chapter 4. The cohort is observed to have exposed members and unexposed members. These groups may be referred to as the exposed cohort and the unexposed cohort.

A classic example is the Framingham Study (Haider et al. 1999; Truett, Cornfield, and Kannel, 1967). Framingham is a town to the west of Boston, at the starting point of the Boston Marathon. In the late 1940s, a large sample of

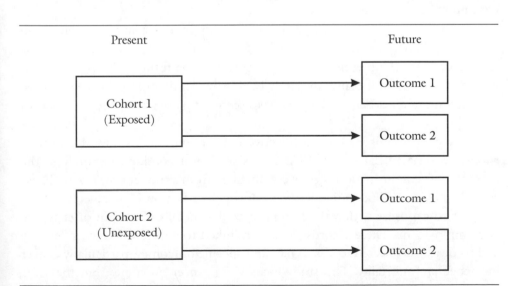

FIGURE 5.1
Schematic for Prospective Cohort Studies

FIGURE 5.2

Schematic for
Retrospective
Cohort Studies

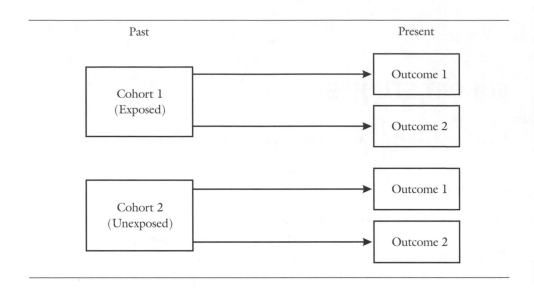

the adult population of Framingham was recruited into the study. They received complete medical examinations and identified factors such as blood pressure, smoking, cholesterol, and other characteristics thought to be relevant to risk of cardiovascular disease. Over many years (the study is still going on), members of the cohort have been examined regularly with changes in relevant findings noted. Comprehensive records of medical events and deaths are meticulously collected. This large cohort study provided the definitive early findings on the relationship of cardiovascular risk factors to cardiovascular outcomes, including mortality and incidence of atherosclerotic disease, myocardial infarction, and stroke, among others. The Framingham Study has been able to change with time, adding new members to the cohort and producing answers to important new questions that continue to be generated.

The less common retrospective cohort study is displayed graphically in Figure 5.2. Variations can be extended even further by designing a cohort study that looks from the present to both the past and the future. The arrows point from past to present, because the study begins by identifying a cohort in the past and then it examines data in the present to see what has happened to members of the cohort.

A good example of a retrospective cohort study is a study of cancer in rubber workers (Delzell et al. 1981). This study was conducted entirely in the present. Past employment records were obtained from a rubber tire factory. These records provided worker identification information data on jobs/tasks that were relevant to exposure within the factory as well as details on length of exposure and employment. These records were then linked to a statewide cancer registry and to death certificate records to measure specific outcomes, particularly cancer incidence and mortality. This study focused on cancer outcomes, but the same cohort data could also have been used to examine outcomes such as heart or lung disease had some sort of reliable disease registry been available for that purpose. Of course, as in the Framingham Study, the individual workers could have been tracked down and their outcomes examined over time, but this approach would have been far more expensive, in terms of time and resources, than the one used.

To compare and contrast retrospective cohort studies with case control studies, consider how the relationship between rubber work and cancer could have been examined in a case control study (Table 5.1). The same cancer registry could have been used to select persons with incident cancer or death attributed to cancer. These could have been matched to controls (e.g., persons of the same age, gender, and residence) who did not have cancer. The investigators could then have obtained and examined data that identified cases and controls who had past exposure as employees in rubber factories.

The retrospective cohort study of rubber workers used available exposure data to subdivide the cohort based on duration of work in the rubber factory, job descriptions in making rubber tires, and the like. Other desirable data, such as tobacco smoking history, were not available. Approached as a case control study, such research could easily have looked at a variety of other past exposures as well (e.g., smoking, asbestos work, diet, alcohol consumption, genetic history, etc.), so long as those data were available.

Each study method has advantages and disadvantages. If the intention is to focus on a particular population or on persons with particular exposures, the retrospective cohort design is preferable. (The rubber workers study was supported by the rubber industry and rubber workers' union, and it could have been expanded to look at outcomes other than cancer for rubber workers.) If, on the other hand, the focus is on a particular disease, then case control design has advantages. A cancer study with that design can examine exposures of much wider scope than that of just the rubber industry.

Even when a cohort design might be a desirable choice, putting together the needed resources may be difficult and expensive. Prospective cohort studies usually require a long-term commitment and are very costly. In a retrospective cohort study, on the other hand, it may be difficult or impossible to obtain sufficiently

Order of Tasks	Tasks	
	Retrospective Cohort Study	Case Control Study
First	Identify past rubber workers	Identify cancer cases
Second	Determine past exposure history	Identify controls (persons without cancer)
Third	Determine cancer incidence	Determine past exposure history (rubber work, etc.)
Fourth	Analyze relationship of exposures to outcomes	Analyze relationship of exposures to outcomes

TABLE 5.1
Comparison of a Retrospective Cohort Study and a Case-Control Study of Cancer in Rubber Workers

comprehensive information from the past. Such studies need to be designed carefully and constructed based on the availability of complete retrospective cohort data (defining the cohort and its exposures) and the availability of appropriate outcomes data to which the cohort data can be linked. An important strength of the cohort design is the researcher's ability to directly measure relative and attributable risk.

The availability of good outcomes data (such as a cancer registry) can make case control design a good choice. This is especially true if an outcome being measured is not common (e.g., an uncommon cancer). In such situations the case control design is highly efficient, because the study of a relatively small number of cases and controls together with the availability of appropriate exposure information can lead to important results not easily detected in cohort studies.

A difficulty inherent in case control studies is the need to choose controls very carefully. An unexpected link that may exist between the controls and the exposure being studied can bias the results and compromise the value of the study. One example is an unsuccessful study of the relationship of carbon dioxide exposure to myocardial infarction (heart attacks) in the workplace (Lewis 1975). Cases—workers who had the onset of myocardial infarction (worker's compensation data)—were matched with controls—workers who had worker's compensation claims for skin conditions. It was assumed incorrectly that no link existed between the skin conditions and the exposure being studied, carbon monoxide in the workplace. The data showed that workers with skin conditions were more likely to be exposed to carbon monoxide than workers with myocardial infarction. The unexpected association that upset this study was that skin conditions in the workplace were frequently caused by oils and other environmental exposures in "dirty" industries, whereas myocardial infarctions were common among all workers, most of whom work in "clean" environments. The poor choice of controls made a sensitive analysis of a relationship between carbon monoxide and myocardial infarction impossible. A better choice of controls might have been workers randomly selected from all workplaces. Fortunately, this study was done quickly and at low cost, features that are advantages of case control studies compared with cohort studies.

Just as the ability to *directly measure* relative and attributable risk is a strength of cohort studies, the need to *estimate* the same rates is a weakness of case control studies. Many examples have been found in which a case control study has been a cost-effective way to gain preliminary support of a hypothesis, leading to a cohort study or an intervention study, or both, performed at greater expense to provide more definitive evidence.

Selection of Cohorts

Cohort studies begin with the selection of a group or population that will be traced to particular outcomes at later times. Details are gathered about different exposures and/or risk categories of the cohort. When data on outcomes have been collected, the original cohort is usually divided in the analysis into different cohorts based on exposure or risk category. Some examples of cohort selection follow:

1. "A private census of the population of Beaver Dam, Wisconsin, was performed from September 15, 1987 to May 4, 1998 to identify all residents in the city or township of Beaver Dam who were aged 43–84 years. Of the 5,927 eligible individuals, 4,926 participated in the baseline examination" (Klein, Klein, and Moss 1998)
2. "All boys with a Canadian Institute for Health Information entry code of NB (newborn) born to residents of Ontario in fiscal year 1993 were included. Two cohorts of male infants were identified—circumcised . . . and uncircumcised" (To et al. 1998).
3. "In June 1976, questionnaires were sent to all married, female, registered nurses born between 1921 and 1946 and living in eleven U.S. states . . . . Of the 172,413 who were sent this questionnaire, 120,557 completed information about whether they had used permanent hair dyes or smoked cigarettes" (Hennekens et al. 1979)
4. "In 1975, at baseline, 7,925 healthy men and 7,977 healthy women of the Finnish Twin Cohort aged 25 to 64 years . . . responded to a questionnaire on physical activity habits and known predictors of mortality." (Kujala et al. 1998).

As these examples show, characteristics of the cohort must be defined carefully. Usually the population from which the cohort is determined is larger than the cohort. In the Beaver Dam study, for example (Klein, Klein, and Moss 1998), the eligible population of 5,924 was reduced to a cohort of 4,926. Not included were 998 individuals because some died prior to the baseline examination, some declined participation, and other exclusions, carefully detailed in the text, occurred.

The eligible population in the hair dyes and cancer study (Hennekens et al. 1979) was the same as that in another study of coffee consumption and coronary heart disease (Willett et al. 1996). The cohort selection and size in the two studies are slightly different because of differences in completeness of the data for the different exposure/risk categories.

Exposure

Exposure measures in case control studies and the relationship between "exposure" and "risk factor" are discussed in Chapter 4. We defined exposure as something that increased or decreased the probability of disease. Cohort studies frequently include fine detail in the definition and an evaluation of exposures. Exposures may be external agents (infectious and otherwise), behaviors (both protective and malevolent), and other risk factors such as genetic predisposition.

It is also important to conceptualize the "active agent," which is hypothesized to be the cause of disease, and the best construct of "dose," which captures intensity, frequency, and duration (White, Hunt, and Casso 1998). Moreover, one should distinguish between past and present exposures, and deal with exposures that change over the course of the cohort study. If the literature suggests an "etiologically relevant time window" during which exposure is most relevant, then it is important to measure exposures only during this time period; otherwise, exposure measurement error will occur (White, Hunt, and Casso 1998). The etiology of cancer, for instance, is rather complicated and may include an initial exposure stage followed by a promotion stage during which time the cancer progresses. In this case, a particular window of time may be open when the initial exposure is causally related to disease. Consider the relationship between sun exposure and skin cancer, for instance. The active agent has been recast recently to include both ultraviolet (UV) A and B radiation. The dose can be conceptualized to include intensity (early morning, midday, or afternoon sun exposure), frequency (daily, weekends, or once a year), and duration (summer months versus all year round). We can assess current and past sun exposures and determine if an etiologically relevant time window appears during which time sun exposure is causally related to skin cancer—early childhood, for instance.

To elaborate further the complexities of exposure definition and assessment, consider the following examples of exposure in cohort studies:

1. Hu et al. (1999) carefully measured levels of egg consumption and factors such as the presence of diabetes and other known risk factors for cardiovascular disease. They assessed the relationship of egg consumption to cardiovascular disease outcomes.
2. In the Framingham Study, chronic cough was found to be associated with risk of myocardial infarction (Haider et al. 1999).
3. Following the bombing of Hiroshima and Nagasaki, epidemiologists used careful measurements of radiation exposure to evaluate the relationship to long-term survival and cancer incidence (Schull 1995).
4. Studies of prostate cancer in cohorts of men have examined various characteristics of the men and of laboratory tests performed prior to cancer incidence in an effort to determine predictive factors for cancer outcomes (Gann, Hennekens, and Stampfer 1995; Johansson et al. 1997; Rodriguez et al. 1997).

Before the study by Hu et al. (1999) of the association of egg consumption (exposure) to cardiovascular disease incidence (outcome), there was a popular assumption that cholesterol in eggs increased the risk of cardiovascular disease (CD). Other cohort studies had demonstrated a strong association between elevated serum cholesterol and cardiovascular outcomes. The findings of Hu et al. were a surprise, as the study demonstrated no association in most persons between egg consumption and CD incidence. An exception was an association observed between egg consumption and CD incidence in persons with diabetes. This is a good example of the ability of cohort studies to provide fresh insight.

Hu et al. (1999) also demonstrate ways in which complex exposure information can be gathered and analyzed in cohort studies to produce precise results that relate a specific exposure (eating eggs) to the outcome being studied (incidence of cardiovascular disease). This report was based on two prospective cohort studies, the Health Professionals Follow-up Study of men (1986–1994) and the Nurses Health Study of women (1980–1994) (Colditz, Manson, and Hankinson 1997). Comparable exposure data had been collected that included details on more than 30 exposure types or risk factors known or suspected to be associated with cardiovascular disease incidence. Participants were asked how many eggs they had eaten in the past year, using nine options: from never to six or more per day. In the analysis they were divided into five levels of egg exposure. Questionnaires were completed by participants at the beginning and at regular intervals throughout the studies. If exposure for an individual was different in different questionnaires, the exposure levels were averaged based on the length of time for each exposure. Participants with diabetes were analyzed separately from the others. The diabetic participants had a significantly elevated incidence of cardiovascular disease in the highest egg consumption category compared to the lowest, and a significant trend was traced as well. Other participants had no significant association between egg exposure and disease incidence. The analysis adjusted for more than ten variables known to affect or to be associated with disease risk, including smoking history, hypertension, age, body mass index, menopausal status, and physical activity. As with egg exposure, many of the other exposures were measured using multiple possible levels. The ability to design a study with this extent of exhaustive exposure data is a major advantage of prospective cohort studies. Retrospective cohort studies and case control studies cannot usually include exposure data in this much detail, as those studies are usually designed after the exposures have occurred.

The report by Haider et al. (1999) detailed a positive **association** between chronic cough and the incidence rate of myocardial infarction. The word "association" is appropriate to most epidemiologic studies. Conclusions about **cause and effect**, on the other hand, are rarely justified by the data and should be speculated on only in the discussion section.

Two possible ways for chronic cough to be considered an **exposure** in this study are:

1. The cough relates directly to heart disease, perhaps an early symptom of heart failure; and
2. The cough is an **intervening variable**. It is a pulmonary symptom of tobacco smoking, which is an important risk factor for myocardial infarction. If tobacco smoking history were not adequately measured in the study, then tobacco smoking would be a **confounding factor** (confounding is discussed in detail in Chapter 4).

A simpler example of **confounding** would be an association between yellow fingers and lung cancer. Cigarette smoking is the **confounding factor**, as it is closely associated with both yellow fingers and lung cancer.

Schull (1995) reported extensive studies of radiation exposure in the bombing of Hiroshima and of the outcomes of exposed residents who were followed over a long period of time. The persons in this cohort were the survivors of the nuclear explosion. The various radiation exposures and other factors such as the effects of fire were studied in great detail. Much of this detailed exposure information was not measured directly but was estimated after the fact through modeling of the event using detailed knowledge of the radiation produced by an atomic bomb. Much of this knowledge was based on measurements made of other bombs long after the bombing of Hiroshima had occurred. Comparably detailed information was gathered on the lives, disease incidence, and deaths of the survivors, some of whom are still alive today. Cancer incidence was the outcome of greatest interest. In addition to detailed available information and estimates of radiation *exposure* of individual survivors, it was possible to analyze *risk factors* such as age, gender, and genetic differences. This prospective cohort study was, in fact, the combination of many studies in a variety of fields, including physics, clinical medicine, and epidemiology. The scope of this work was so great and it took so long to complete that an appropriate overview required a book published 50 years after the exposure occurred (50 years after the diverse studies began).

The prostate cancer cohort studies cited earlier (Gann, Hennekens, and Stampfer 1995; Johansson et al. 1997; Rodriguez et al. 1997) explore the important unknown areas of the usefulness of a screening test in predicting cancer outcomes, the role of family history as a risk factor, and other observations of "exposure" that may cast new light on the very difficult management of this disease. Gann and colleagues conducted a retrospective cohort study based on an ongoing randomized double-blind intervention study of aspirin and beta carotene (Steering Committee of the Physician's Health Study Research Group 1989). Participants had provided a blood sample in 1982 that was frozen and saved. These samples had a prostate-specific antigen (PSA) test performed retrospectively, and occurrence of prostate cancer in the participants was examined retrospectively for a ten-year period that began in 1982. A **nested case control design** was used in the analysis. With this type of design one compares the exposure(s) of subjects who develop the disease (cases) to a sample of subjects who do not (controls). The case control study is nested into the cohort study in the sense that one can conduct a retrospective analysis once a sufficient number of cases of disease emerge from the cohort study. The "exposures" of interest were the PSA levels and the duration of observation, ending in the diagnosis of prostate cancer. An elevated PSA could be considered a *risk factor* for prostate cancer or an indicator of pre-clinical cancer. Exposures were measured as a specific PSA level at the beginning of the cohort study and through the length of exposure (duration of observation). The study concluded that "a single PSA measurement had a relatively high sensitivity and specificity for detection of prostate cancers that arose within 4 years."

Johansson et al. (1997) followed a group of men in a county in Sweden who were diagnosed with prostate cancer between 1977 and 1984. Measurement of outcomes (deaths) was complete through 1994. "Exposures" were the presence at enrollment (diagnosis) of cancer of different stages and the presence of either treatment or no treatment. The findings of greatest interest were that "patients with localized prostate cancer have a favorable outlook following watchful waiting" and that treatment of localized cancer with surgery, radiation, or hormonal therapy had no advantage over watchful waiting. As expected, cancers that were more advanced at diagnosis had worse outcomes.

Many cohort studies have reported the association of tobacco exposure with cancer incidence and other outcomes (Cornuz et al. 1999; Klein, Klein, and Moss 1998). Such studies emphasize the importance of defining exposure in great detail. Such detail includes the route of exposure and the variety of tobacco products (smoking, chewing, cigarettes, cigars, mainstream smoke, sidestream smoke, "smokeless tobacco"); the variation of active substances that are not uniform (nicotine, tars, carbon monoxide, etc.); and dose (the duration and amount of exposure). The term pack-years of exposure to cigarettes has frequently been used as a dose indicator, years of exposure multiplied by packs smoked per day. This provides a cumulative dose, but it has also been shown that years of exposure and daily dose at any point in time may have independent effects on outcomes. The situation is further complicated by current thinking about carcinogens, in which some exposures may be necessary to initiate a long interval of cancer development, while other exposures may function independently as facilitators, so that their effects may appear quickly. As in the study of eggs by Hu et al. (1999), cohort studies, and particularly prospective cohort studies, provide the best methods to include for measuring exposure in great detail.

Relative Risk in a Cohort Study

The cohort study design is illustrated in Figure 5.3, where the incidence of disease in the exposed cohort is $a/(a + b)$, and the incidence of disease in the unexposed cohort is $c/(c + d)$. Unlike the case control study (which uses the odds ratio as an estimate of relative risk), the incidence of disease in the exposed and unexposed group can be calculated directly because cohorts are defined from the onset of the study. Thus, the *relative risk* is simply the ratio of the exposed and unexposed incidence: $a/(a + b) \div c/(c + d)$.

For example, suppose a prospective cohort study were designed to test the association of smoking to coronary heart disease (CHD). Of the 1,000 men who smoked, 40 developed coronary heart disease; of the 2,000 nonsmoking (or unexposed) members, 50 developed CHD. Figure 5.4 summarizes the results, including the relative risk of 1.6, indicating that smokers are 1.6 times as likely to develop CHD as nonsmokers.

FIGURE 5.3
Cohort Study
Design

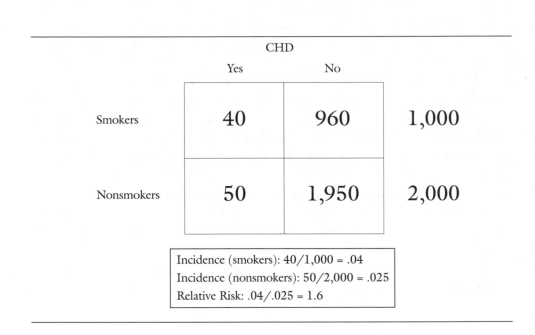

FIGURE 5.4
Smoking and
Coronary Heart
Disease (CHD)

Attributable Fraction

As described in the previous chapter, attributable fraction is the proportion of disease that is attributed to a particular risk factor. In case control studies the odds ratio is used to estimate the attributable fraction because risk (the rate of an outcome) is not measured directly in a known population. In a cohort study the risk in a known population (the cohort) is measured directly. Further, the cohort may be an entire population or a random sample of a larger population. For a cohort study the attributable fraction formula is the same as that for the case control study except that relative risk (RR) is used instead of the odds ratio. In this case p is the proportion of the population with the risk factor and RR is the relative risk:

$$\text{Attributable Fraction } (AF) = \frac{p\,(RR-1)}{p\,(RR-1)+1} \times 100\%$$

The attributable fraction for the earlier CHD and smoking example can be calculated as follows if one assumes that 25 percent of the population smokes:

$$\frac{0.25\,(1.6-1)}{[0.25\,(1.6-1)]+1} \times 100 = 13\%$$

The attributable fraction points out one of the strengths of a cohort study. If the cohorts are representative of the general population, then the incidence of disease in the exposed and unexposed groups is also representative. The CHD and smoking study would enable us to conclude that 13 percent of all heart disease is attributable to smoking. This is a critical conclusion in planning how best to expend resources to prevent heart disease.

Another value of attributable fraction concerns exposures that are highly associated with bad outcomes (high relative risk) but are themselves uncommon or rare. For example, vinyl chloride exposure as a risk factor for cancer has a high relative risk. In fact, the relative risk is even greater than that of tobacco smoking. But very few people in the general population are exposed to vinyl chloride. So the attributable fraction of cancer risk associated with vinyl chloride is very low. Eliminating vinyl chloride exposure would likely have a very small effect on cancer outcomes in the general population. Eliminating tobacco exposure, by contrast, would likely have a very large effect.

The attributable risk is a measure of the potential savings to be gained by eliminating the risk factor in a population; it is calculated as the difference between the incidence of disease in the exposed group minus the incidence of disease in the unexposed group. Referring to Figure 5.3, the attributable risk would be calculated as:

$$\text{Attributable Risk } = a/(a+b) - c/(c+d)$$

In the case of the preceding smoking and CHD example, this would be 0.04−0.025 or 0.015. In other words, 1.5 out of 100 cases of CHD can be attributed to smoking.

Measuring Incidence

The simplest way of calculating an incidence rate is to divide the number of subjects who develop a disease by the number of subjects in the cohort. Thus, 40 smokers out of a cohort of 1,000 developed CHD in the preceding example, for an incidence rate of 40 per 1,000 or 0.04. A related, but somewhat more complicated method of calculating incidence, is with incidence density. Most prospective cohort studies span multiple years, during which time the cohorts change in size as subjects enter or drop out of the study. Subjects may become disengaged from the research due to death, lack of interest, side effects, or many other reasons collectively referred to as loss to follow-up. One solution to this problem is to calculate incidence in terms of density, such as person-years or person-months of exposure.

Consider the following hypothetical case, as illustrated in Figures 5.5 and 5.6: a five-year study with five subjects in each group. Note that of the five exposed subjects (Figure 5.5), three develop the condition, say, coronary heart disease. Subject one finishes the study; subject two dies (D) after two years without developing CHD; subject three gets the disease after two years (X); subject four gets CHD and dies in year 3 (XD); subject five gets CHD in year 1 and dies in year 4. Of the unexposed subjects (Figure 5.6), subject one finishes the study, while subject two is lost to follow-up in year 4. Subjects three and five both get CHD in year 4, but only one dies at the end of the

FIGURE 5.5
Cumulative
Incidence vs.
Incidence
Density—Exposed

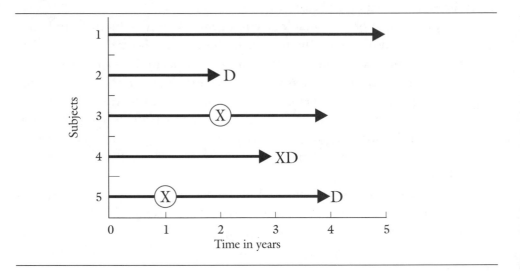

FIGURE 5.6
Cumulative
Incidence vs.
Incidence
Density–Unexposed

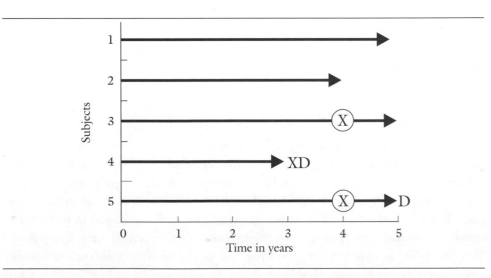

study. Subject four gets CHD and dies in year 3. The cumulative incidence over five years would be 3/5 = 60 percent for each group. Incidence density, on the other hand takes into consideration both loss to follow-up and disease onset. In other words, the "at-risk" period would end if the subject were to drop out of the study, develop the disease, or die. Thus, there are 13 person-years of exposure for the exposed group and 20 person-years of exposure for the unexposed group. The incidence density for the unexposed group would be 3/13, or three cases of CHD for every 13 person-years of exposure. For the unexposed group, the incidence density would be 3/20, or three cases of CHD for every 20 person-years of exposure. Relative risk with cumulative incidence would be 3/5 ÷ 3/5 = 1.0, indicating no increased risk of CHD with exposure. With incidence density, the relative risk would be 3/13 ÷ 3/20 = 1.54, indicating that one is 1.54 times as likely to develop CHD with an exposure.

Survey Methodology

Surveys are used to sample populations in a variety of ways. These include opinion polls, marketing surveys, and the U.S. Census (intended, so far, to be a 100 percent sample). Surveys may be used for epidemiologic purposes, one of which is to support cohort studies. Selection of a cohort through use of a questionnaire is a specialized survey. Members of a population or of a sample of a population may be sent a questionnaire asking them to submit information in support of a study. In the Finnish Twin Cohort study, participants were members of the Twin Cohort who responded to a mailed questionnaire "that included items on physical activity, occupation, body weight, height, alcohol use, smoking, and physician-diagnosed diseases" (Kujala et al. 1998). In a study of smoking and the risk of hip fracture, women were mailed a questionnaire biennially over a period of up to 12 years (Cornuz et al. 1999). When survey methodology is used in this way, either as a 100 percent sample or as a smaller random sample of a cohort, it is critical that the response rate be high. Further, failure to collect data for nonresponders may bias the results of the study.

Another use of surveys is the regular assessment of a population's health and risk factor status, which is done by interviewing a random sample of the population. The Centers for Disease Control and Prevention (CDC) works with each state to conduct a regular survey of the state's population in the Behavioral Risk Factor Surveillance System (BRFSS Coordinators 1998). This is a random-digit dialing survey, sampled by state, of all adults in the United States who have telephones. Information is obtained about a variety of indicators of health status, risk factors such as smoking, and preventive behavior such as immunizations. The survey is repeated annually or biennially using a new random sample of the state. The BRFSS provides useful data for public health management on progress within states and comparisons among states.

Cohort Study Advantages and Disadvantages

The cohort study has a number of advantages over the case control study. While the case control design "inherently acknowledges time," the cohort study "explicitly incorporates the passage of time" (Samet and Muñoz 1998). Moreover, one can calculate incidence and relative risk directly rather than by estimate. Determining causality is less of an issue because exposure(s) precede the onset of disease by virtue of the study design. Misclassification bias, particularly recall bias, is less of a problem since exposure(s) are systematically and regularly documented during follow-up activities. Finally, the cohort design can be used to study multiple outcomes, such as diseases, or multiple exposures as long as these variables are measured. On the other hand, the cohort study is expensive, time-consuming, and potentially biased by attrition as subjects are lost to follow-up. Moreover, it may be difficult to model changes in exposure(s) over time or crossovers (subjects who give up smoking, for instance). With the cohort study, it is nearly impossible to study rare diseases.

Summary

Cohort studies begin with a defined population (cohort); measure baseline information about exposures (personal characteristics, health status, behavior, and risk factors); may measure interim modifications of these exposures; and measure outcomes of interest (morbidity and mortality). Although typically the cohort is followed prospectively, the cohort may be defined and the exposures measured retrospectively, with outcomes measured in the present. Retrospective cohort studies differ from case control studies. In the former, the study begins with the measurement of exposures and traces the cohort forward in time until outcomes occur. In the latter, the study begins by choosing cases based on outcomes and controls with different outcomes, and traces backward in time to measure past exposures of the cases and controls. The prospective cohort study is usually the most elegant study and allows extremely detailed and exact measurement of exposures, but it is usually expensive in terms of resources and the time required. Case control studies and retrospective cohort studies may provide a more efficient, less expensive way to obtain tentative conclusions. Both case control studies and all forms of cohort studies can show an association between exposure and disease, but they do not establish a causal relationship. To determine a causal relationship between exposure and disease, one must use an experimental study design such as a randomized clinical trial, which is the topic of Chapter 6.

Case Study 5.1

You have been motivated by the recent tobacco company settlements to design yet another cohort study that will test the hypothesis that both active and passive smoking causes heart disease and lung cancer. You want this study to be as valid as possible and to be practically flawless in terms of bias and confounding.

1. What are the outcomes of this study and how will they be measured?
2. How will you minimize misclassification bias of disease (see Chapter 4)?
3. What would be the advantages and disadvantages of retrospective and prospective study designs?
4. You would like to confirm a dose-response relationship. How will you conceptualize the "active agent" and measure dose in terms of intensity, frequency, and duration?
5. Does the concept of dose differ for active versus passive smoking?
6. What are the confounding variables that you need to measure?
7. What are the sources of misclassification bias of exposure?
8. How will you minimize selection bias?
9. How will you deal with dropouts?

Assume that you design a prospective cohort study to test the effect of active smoking only on CHD. You have assembled two groups of middle-aged adults—2,000 smokers and 2,000 nonsmokers—and follow them for ten years. You measure heart disease by an exercise treadmill test, followed by cardiac catheterization. The cumulative ten-year incidence of CHD for the various cohorts is given in the table. Exposure is defined as average packs per day for the period of observation, while person-years of exposure is accumulated during the ten-year observation period only:

Exposure	No. of Subjects	Incidence	Person-Years
Nonsmoker	2,000	50/1,000	18,000
<1 pack	1,000	70/1,000	7,000
1–2 packs	500	80/1,000	6,000
>2 packs	500	100/1,000	3,000

10. What is the relative risk of CHD for various levels of smoking using cumulative incidence?
11. Is there a dose-response relationship?
12. What is the attributable fraction if approximately 30 percent of the population are smokers?
13. A number of subjects dropped out of the study by the end of ten years, many of whom were smokers who quit or reduced their level of smoking activity. Using the incidence density approach, what is the relative risk of CHD for various levels of smoking activity?

Case Study 5.2

The Scottish Health Heart Study is a large cohort study that evaluated the relation-ship between dietary factors, cardiovascular disease incidence, and all-causes mortality (Todd et al. 1999). In that study the relationship of dietary fiber to outcomes in men was displayed (Table 5.2). Todd and colleagues concluded that dietary "fiber will impact on both CHD risk and the general health of the population."

1. Does dietary fiber appear to be more protective against CHD risk or against non-CHD death?
2. The authors do not detail the causes of "non-CHD death." Speculate about what those causes could be and what they might have to do with dietary fiber.
3. If the 95 percent confidence interval for "CHD case" were (8.1, 9.0) instead of (8.1, 8.6), how would it affect the conclusions?

TABLE 5.2
Relationship of Dietary Fiber to Coronary Heart Disease Outcomes

	Number	Fiber (g/4.18 MJ)
No Event	5,076	8.8 (8.7, 8.9)[*]
CHD[**] Case	454	8.4 (8.1, 8.6) $p = .002$[***]
No-CHD Death	224	7.7 (7.3, 8.0) $p < .001$

[*]Numbers in parenthesis, 95% confidence inerval.
[**]CHD, coronary heart disease.
[***]p-values are presented for comparisons of mean values with that of the no-event group.
Source: Todd, S., M. Woodward, H. Tunstall-Pedoe, and C. Bolton-Smith. "Dietary Antioxidant Vitamins and Fiber in the Etiology of Cardiovascular Disease and All-Causes Mortality: Results from the Scottish Heart Health Study." Copyright © 1999, *American Journal of Epidemiology*, 150 (10): 1073–80. Adapted by permission.

Case Study 5.3

The following table (Table 5.3) displays data from an "unknown cohort study" with a high mortality rate. All of the subjects experienced life-threatening exposures, although risk varied by class, employment, age, and gender.

TABLE 5.3
Data for an Unknown Cohort Study with a High Mortality Rate

	Male			Female			Total		
	No. in Group	No. Died	Mortality	No. in Group	No. Died	Mortality	No. in Group	No. Died	Mortality
Upper Class									
Adult	175	118	67%	144	4	3%	319	122	38%
Child	5	0	0%	1	0	0%	6	0	0%
Middle Class									
Adult	168	154	92%	93	13	14%	261	167	64%
Child	11	0	0%	13	0	0%	24	0	0%
Lower Class									
Adult	462	387	84%	165	89	54%	627	476	76%
Child	48	35	73%	31	17	55%	79	52	66%
Employees									
Adult	862	670	78%	23	3	13%	885	673	76%
Child	0	0		0	0		0	0	

Source: Great Britain, Parliament (1999).

1. What was the size of the cohort, the number with a bad outcome, and the mortality rate?
2. Was it more protective to be upper class or to be a female?
3. Compared to upper-class adult females, what was the relative risk for lower-class adult males? What was the attributable risk using the same comparison?
4. You are probably familiar with this event. Draw conclusions about its characteristics. Can you guess what actually happened?

References

Behavioral Risk Factor Surveillance System (BRFSS) Coordinators. 1998. "Influenza and Pneumococcal Vaccination Levels Among Adults Aged ≥ 65 Years—United States, 1997." *Morbidity and Mortality Weekly Report* (2 October, no. 47): 797–802.

Colditz, G. A., J. E. Manson, and S. E. Hankinson. 1997. "The Nurses' Health Study: 20–Year Contribution to the Understanding of Health Among Women." *Journal of Women's Health* 6 (1): 49–62.

Cornuz, J., D. Feskanich, W. C. Willett, and G. A. Colditz. 1999. "Smoking, Smoking Cessation, and the Risk of Hip Fracture in Women." *The American Journal of Medicine* 106 (March): 311–14.

Delzell, E., C. Louik, J. N. Lewis, and R. R. Monson. 1981. "Mortality and Cancer Morbidity Among Workers in the Rubber Tire Industry." *American Journal of Industrial Medicine* 2 (3): 209–216.

Gann, P. H., C. H. Hennekens, and M. J. Stampfer. 1995. "A Prospective Evaluation of Plasma Prostate-Specific Antigen for Detection of Prostatic Cancer." *Journal of the American Medical Association* 273 (4): 289–94.

Great Britain, Parliament. 1998. *Report on The Loss of The S.S. Titanic.* New York: St. Martin's Press.

Haider, A. W., M. G. Larson, C. J. O'Donnell, J. C. Evans, P. W. F. Wilson, and D. Levy. 1999. "The Association of Chronic Cough with the Risk of Myocardial Infarction: The Framingham Heart Study." *The American Journal of Medicine* 106 (March): 279–84.

Hennekens, C. H., F. E. Speizer, B. Rosner, C. J. Bain, C. Belanger, and R. Peto. 1979. "Use of Permanent Hair Dyes and Cancer Among Registered Nurses." *Lancet* (30 June): 1390–993.

Hu, F. B., M. J. Stampfer, E. B. Rimm, J. E. Manson, A. Ascherio, G. A. Colditz, B. A. Rosner, D. Spiegelman, F. E. Speizer, F. M. Sacks, C. H. Hennekens, and W. C. Willett. 1999. "A Prospective Study of Egg Consumption and Risk of Cardiovascular Disease in Men and Women." *Journal of the American Medical Association* 281 (15): 1387–94.

Johansson, J-E., L. Holmberg, S. Johansson, R. Bergström, and H-O. Adami. 1997. "Fifteen-year Survival in Prostate Cancer: A Prospective, Population-based Study in Sweden." *Journal of the American Medical Association* 277 (6): 467–71.

Klein, R., B. E. K. Klein, and S. E. Moss. 1998. "Relation of Smoking to the Incidence of Age-related Maculopathy: The Beaver Dam Eye Study." *American Journal of Epidemiology* 147 (2): 103–10.

Kujala, U. M., J. Kaprio, S. Sarna, and M. Koskenvuo. 1998. "Relationship of Leisure-Time Physical Activity and Mortality." *Journal of the American Medical Association* 279 (6): 440–44.

Lewis, J. N. 1975. Unpublished study on Massachusetts workplaces.

Mantel, N. 1973. "Synthetic Retrospective Studies and Related Topics." *Biometrics* 29 (3): 479–86.

Rodríguez, C., E. E. Calle, H. L. Miracle-McMahill, L. M. Tatham, P. A. Wingo, M. J. Thun, and C. W. Heath, Jr. 1997. "Family History and Risk of Fatal Prostate Cancer." *Epidemiology* 8 (6): 653–57.

Samet, J. M., and A. Muñoz. 1998. "Evolution of the Cohort Study." *Epidemiologic Reviews* 20 (1): 1–14.

Schull, W. J. 1995. *Effects of Atomic Radiation: A Half-Century of Studies from Hiroshima and Nagasaki.* New York: Wiley-Liss.

Steering Committee of the Physicians' Health Study Research Group. 1989. "Final Report on the Aspirin Component of the Ongoing Physicians' Health Study." *The New England Journal of Medicine* 321 (3): 129–35.

To, T., M. Agha, P. T. Dick, and W. Feldman. 1998. "Cohort Study on Circumcision of Newborn Boys and Subsequent Risk of Urinary-Tract Infection." *Lancet* (352): 1813–16.

Todd, S., M. Woodward, H. Tunstall-Pedoe, and C. Bolton-Smith. 1999. "Dietary Antioxidant Vitamins and Fiber in the Etiology of Cardiovascular Disease and All-Causes Mortality: Results from the Scottish Heart Health Study." *American Journal of Epidemiology* 150 (10): 1073–80.

Truett, J., J. Cornfield, and W. Kannel. 1967. "A Multivariate Analysis of the Risk of Coronary Heart Disease in Framingham." *Journal of Chronic Disease* 20 (7): 511–24.

White, E., J. R. Hunt, and D. Casso. 1998. "Exposure Measurement in Cohort Studies: The Challenges of Prospective Data Collection." *Epidemiologic Reviews* 20 (1): 43–56.

Willett, W. C., M. J. Stampfer, J. E. Manson, G. A. Colditz, B. A. Rosner, F. E. Speizer, and C. H. Hennekens. 1996. "Coffee Consumption and Coronary Heart Disease in Women." *Journal of the American Medical Association* 275 (14 February): 458–62.

RANDOMIZED CLINICAL TRIALS

Steven T. Fleming

Introduction

The gold standard of epidemiological research is the **randomized clinical trial (RCT)**, also referred to as the **randomized controlled trial**. The RCT is a true experimental study design, in the sense that the researcher can maintain some control over the conditions of the study and, more importantly, over the assignment of subjects to experimental and control groups. The random assignment of subjects to experimental (i.e., treatment) and control groups is the critical structure of the RCT study design, the purpose of which is to ensure that the two groups are alike in all characteristics other than the treatment under study. With observational studies, like the case control study, for instance, one must make inferences based on comparing two groups of patients who may differ in important ways, other than whether or not they receive a particular treatment. Moreover, the RCT usually follows a formally articulated **protocol,** with stated objectives and specific procedures for selecting patients, executing treatments, and measuring outcomes. This chapter examines the importance of the randomization process, the various types of RCTs, methods associated with RCTs, and problems and issues related to RCTs.

In Chapter 4, we mentioned that most epidemiological studies compare one group to another to determine the effect of risk factors (i.e., exposures) or treatments (i.e., interventions) on the incidence or course of disease. The studies are classified based on when the disease identified, when the exposure or treatment is recognized, and when the analysis is conducted. Figure 6.1 illustrates this paradigm for the randomized controlled trial. Subjects are randomly assigned to either the experimental or control groups in the present. Experimental groups will receive some kind of exposure, controls will not. The two groups will be followed prospectively over a defined time interval and observed. At some point in the future, the researcher will classify subjects in each group into two or more outcome categories. For example, suppose one is examining whether or not tamoxifen can prevent recurrence of breast cancer (Group 1992). Patients would be randomly assigned to either the experimental group (which receives tamoxifen) or control group (which does not receive tamoxifen). The two groups would be followed prospectively, and at some designated time patients in each group would be classified as having suffered a recurrence of breast cancer (outcome 1) or not (outcome 2).

FIGURE 6.1
Schematic for
Randomized
Clinical Trials

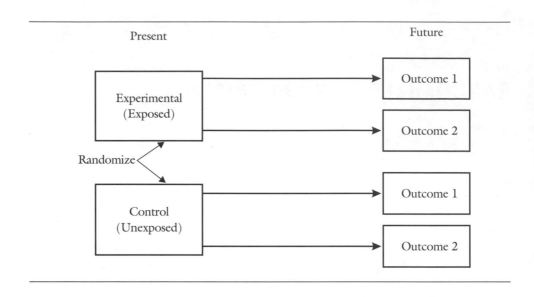

Lilienfeld distinguishes between three types of RCTs: **therapeutic trials, intervention trials,** and **preventive trials** (Lilienfeld and Stolley 1994). With therapeutic trials, a particular agent or procedure is purported to change the disease process either in terms of survival, severity, or cure. With intervention trials, one is attempting to prevent the onset of disease, typically through the manipulation of risk factors. Preventive trials involve agents or procedures, such as vaccines, that can prevent disease from occurring. The medical literature is full of studies that test the efficacy of therapeutic agents or procedures, such as high-dose chemotherapy for breast cancer (Gradishar et al. 1996), zidovudine for HIV disease (Ioannidis et al. 1995), or angioplasty versus thrombolytic therapy for acute myocardial infarction (Weaver et al. 1997). We can turn to the health services research literature for examples of intervention trials—for example, whether vouchers improve breast cancer screening rates (Stoner et al. 1998), or if capitation affects the health of the chronically mentally ill (Lurie et al. 1992), or if comprehensive geriatric assessment affects survival and functional status in the elderly (Reuben et al. 1995). Preventive trials may include agents such as vaccines, or preventive strategies such as education, each of which is focused typically on primary prevention— curtailing the onset of disease. Intervention and therapeutic trials deal primarily with secondary or tertiary prevention. For example, mammography screening is a secondary prevention intervention designed to detect early-stage breast cancer; lumpectomy or simple mastectomy, on the other hand, is a tertiary prevention intervention designed to halt the spread of the disease.

Randomization

Quite simply, a randomized clinical trial is designed to determine whether or not a particular agent or intervention works. To isolate the effect of the intervention from all other factors (one or more of which may affect the outcome as well), the experimental and control groups should be virtually the same in all respects. In other words, the groups should not differ in ways that may affect the outcome of the study. Randomization is the process that is used to avoid confounding (refer to the discussion of confounding in Chapter 4). If the two groups are not identical in all respects, the effect of a particular intervention cannot be distinguished from the effects of other factors or characteristics of the group. In short, the results of the study become confounded or difficult to disentangle and interpret. Moreover, the results of the study may be biased if the degree to which the intervention is efficacious is either under- or overestimated. The underlying premise behind the theory of random assignment to experimental and control groups is that subjects cannot be given a choice of treatment or control because selection into these two groups would then be based on physical, medical, social, and/or cultural characteristics that could affect the outcomes of the study, apart from the treatment or intervention being evaluated.

Suppose, for example, that seriously ill subjects (or their physicians) would be more likely to choose experimental treatment if they had a choice and were not randomly assigned to either treatment or control groups. Their selection into the experimental treatment group might be based on a preference for aggressive treatment as a last hope to improve chances of survival. If the experimental treatment did indeed improve survival, this effect would be underestimated inasmuch as the more seriously ill patients would be more likely to die with or without the treatment. The experimental group would have proportionately more seriously ill patients. Alternatively, the less seriously ill patients (or their physicians) might be more likely to choose experimental therapy if it is perceived to be aggressive and not well tolerated by the seriously ill. In this case, the treatment effect would be overestimated, with improved survival attributable both to treatment and to healthier patients. In short, the results would be confounded and difficult to disentangle. Randomization avoids this problem by preventing the selection of patients into treatment and control groups based on characteristics (such as severity of illness) that might affect the outcomes.

The unit of randomization depends on the study design and may be the individual patient, group practice, or geographic area such as zip code or census district. The following studies are illustrative. Notice that the control group may receive some treatment (or the usual treatment) rather than no treatment, which may be ethically unacceptable:

1. "There were four experimental group practices . . . and four control practices" (Palmer et al. 1996).
2. "Beneficiaries were randomly assigned to prepaid care in one of seven capitated health plans compared with fee-for-service care"(Lurie et al. 1994).
3. "A cohort of 419 mother-infant pairs were randomized to an intervention . . . or control group" (Wood et al. 1998).

4. "Patients were randomly assigned to the intervention . . . or to usual care" (Pilote et al. 1992).

A number of different techniques may be used to implement randomization. Suppose that you have a list of 90 subjects who are eligible to participate in a study in which you want treatment and control groups of ten each. Randomization assumes that each subject in the sample has an equal probability of being selected. Thus, you could not simply select the first ten for the treatment group and the last ten for the controls, nor could you select every other subject since those at the top of the list would more likely be selected. Those at the top of the list might be healthier, or smarter, or live next to a toxic waste dump—and the sample would be biased. One simple approach is with a random number table. Table 6.1 below was generated from a SAS random number function (also refer to the random number table in Chapter 3).

To use the table, simply look at the number of digits corresponding to the size of the eligible universe of subjects. Since there are 90 eligible subjects in the universe, only the last two digits of each random number need to be examined. Move either vertically or horizontally across the table to select the samples. Thus, the treatment group would consist of the following ten subjects on the list: #68, #25, #2, #23, #66, #18, #61, #83, #15, #59. Notice that 13 random numbers were examined to select ten subjects, because subjects #95 and #96 were not on the list. If a subject is repeated, another random number is examined.

One must also define the universe of subjects eligible for participation in the randomization process. This means that one must clearly define the hypotheses regarding the individuals, physician groups, hospitals, or other units of randomization on whom the treatment or agent is supposed to have an effect. For example, in the study by DeBusk and colleagues (1994), the question was whether coronary risk factors could be modified by a case management system. The eligible universe of subjects in this case were patients who had suffered an acute myocardial infarction; other studies may involve only patients with breast cancer, for example, (Group 1992) or lung cancer (Pritchard and Anthony 1996). In addition there may be other organizational or geographic constraints that limit the parameters of a study to a particular state or county, or set of hospitals, clinics, or group practices. The universe of eligible patients, excerpted here from the Pilote study, for instance, is limited to (a) hospitalized patients, (b) during a particular time frame, (c) with a defined medical condition, (d) assigned to a coronary care unit, and (e) in one of four specific hospitals:

TABLE 6.1
Table of Random Numbers

782468	934325	708702	134495	436096
274523	789866	307818	878496	488261
016483	954515	942359	617472	171822
234612	487090	070291	562403	364472
872116	843552	954017	758833	144873

1. "Patients were enrolled from selected primary care clinics of Group Health Cooperative (GHC) of Puget Sound" (Simon et al. 1996).
2. "Twelve breast cancer clinics participated in the study, and eligible breast cancer patients were randomized between January 1, 1985, and December 31, 1986" (Rosselli-Del-Turco et al. 1994).
3. "From 31 July 1987 to 31 December 1989, 902 patients hospitalized for an acute myocardial infarction were assessed for eligibility. These patients were treated in the coronary care units of four San Francisco Bay area Kaiser-Foundation Medical Centers." (Pilote et al. 1992).

As mentioned earlier, the concept of randomization is based on probability theory, with each subject in the eligible universe having an equal probability of selection into either the treatment or control group. Elwood (1998) points out the benefits and limitations of this approach. Presumably, randomization of a large number of subjects (say 100 in each group) will ensure that treatment and control groups will be similar in terms of known (and unknown) characteristics that may be potential confounders. The probability of significant differences being present in any of these characteristics (attributable to chance alone) increases with a smaller sample size. It is common practice for researchers to describe the characteristics of each group to ensure the reader that the process of randomization did indeed result in groups with similar characteristics. For example, Stoner and colleagues (1998) studied whether vouchers for free mammograms improved cancer screening rates. They compared treatment and control groups in terms of potentially confounding characteristics such as the subject's perceived risk of breast cancer, family history of breast cancer, and distance to the nearest mammography unit (each of which could independently affect cancer screening rates, apart from the "treatment" of receiving a voucher).

Historical Controls and Crossover Studies

Under some circumstances, it is inappropriate to assign a group of patients to conventional therapy, particularly if the usual therapy is ineffective. In this case, the experimental group of patients serves as **historical controls**; that is, the patients' response to some form of treatment in the past is compared to their response with the experimental intervention. Although this type of study may seem to be in the best interest of the patient, it is not a particularly strong design; that is, the results may be disputed.

The **crossover study**, a more rigorous approach to using historical controls, has become an important part of pharmaceutical research (Senn 1995). With this type of study, patients are randomly assigned to treatment and control groups, but at some point in time they switch groups. In other words, controls are given the experimental intervention and vice versa. Measurements are taken at the end of each phase. There are obvious limitations with this approach: the residual effects of treatment may persist even after patients switch from one group to the other, in which case, the treatment is "contaminated." This is clearly the case with surgical interventions (one cannot undo a surgical operation), and it may be true of many pharmaceuticals as well. "In short, crossover studies should not be abandoned; they should be used intelligently" (Senn 1995).

Methods of Randomized Clinical Trials

The purpose of conducting an RCT is to determine whether or not a particular treatment, agent, or program has a significant effect on the onset of the disease, course of illness or, in the case of health services research, other outcomes, such as utilization of services. The change in measurable outcome between the treatment and control groups is referred to as the **treatment effect**. In the medical literature, treatment effects would typically include survival (Fisher et al. 1995; Pritchard and Anthony 1996), general health or functional status (Lurie et al. 1994), or some change in the course of illness. Ioannidis and colleagues, for instance, in their analysis of ten studies that examined the effect of zidovudine on AIDs used specific clinical "endpoints" defined in each study, obviously related to the progression of the disease (1995). Other treatment effects would include mammography screening rates (Stoner et al. 1998) and immunization rates (Wood et al. 1998).

A variety of statistical techniques can be used to assess whether or not the treatment effect is statistically significant. One can determine if a statistically significant difference is found in survival curves (Rosselli-Del-Turco et al. 1994), for instance. There is also a test for calculating the statistical significance of differences in proportions, such as smoking cessation (DeBusk et al. 1994); immunization rates (Wood et al. 1998); or amounts, such as average total charges (Simmer et al. 1991). The size of the treatment effect is another factor. The effect may be statistically significant, but not practically or clinically significant.

Some studies, for instance, report the odds ratio (Group 1995; Weaver et al. 1997) or relative risk, which quantifies the number of times more likely that a particular outcome is probable, given exposure to the treatment. Other studies simply report the difference between outcomes and whether or not the difference is statistically significant (Lurie et al. 1994) or the reduction in the odds of an undesirable outcome such as death (Group 1995).

Sample Size

One of the more difficult decisions to make in designing an RCT is how big the trial sample should be. These studies are clearly the most expensive type of epidemiological inquiry, and the cost is directly dependent on the size of the sample. The precision with which one can discern a difference between treatment and control groups that is statistically significant, however, depends on sample size. One can detect smaller differences with a larger sample. And therein lies the tradeoff between cost and precision. The concepts of Type I and Type II error, statistical power, and determination of sample size are discussed next.

FIGURE 6.2
Conclusions of an
RCT versus Reality

RCT	Reality	
	Effective	Not Effective
Effective	Correct	Type I error False Positive
Not Effective	Type II error False Negative	Correct

Source: Adapted from D. E. Lilienfeld and P. D. Stolley, *Foundations of Epidemiology.* Copyright © 1994, Oxford University Press, New York, NY. Used by permission.

Figure 6.2, adapted from Lilienfeld and Stolley (1994), illustrates the concept of Type I and Type II error by a simple typology. Randomized clinical trails are designed to conclude that a treatment is either effective or not effective in terms of its ability to delay the onset or progression of disease, improve survival, increase utilization, or whatever. The conclusion is based on both the size of the sample and the size of the treatment effect. In fact, we can never know whether the treatment truly works, but the RCT is the best and most sophisticated attempt that we have to discern reality. Suppose the results of the RCT suggest that the treatment, agent, or program—collectively referred to as the exposure—is effective, and, in fact, it is. This means that reality and the study are congruent. If the study proves that the treatment is not effective, and it truly is not, then reality and study are also congruent. Both of these scenarios deserve our heartfelt celebration, although one can never actually know for sure—ponder the prolonged debate over whether smoking causes lung cancer, for instance. If the study suggests that the treatment is effective when it really is not, this is referred to as **Type I** or **α-error**. It is called a false positive, because we have incorrectly asserted that a treatment is efficacious. If the study leads to the conclusion that the treatment is not effective when, in fact, it is effective, this is referred to as **Type II** or **β-error**. It is a false negative because we have incorrectly concluded that the treatment is not effective, when it actually is. Types I and II error are inversely related. If we assume that no change takes place in sample size, as the likelihood of reporting a false positive result increases, the likelihood of not reporting a treatment effective increases, and vice versa.

Clearly one would want to minimize both Type I and Type II error. Each type of error can have negative consequences to the medical community. False negatives may thwart the future investigation of potentially promising drugs or procedures—or the results of the study may not even be published in the literature. False positives may result in the premature dissemination of a technology or agent that simply is not efficacious. The only way to decrease both Types I and II error, and thus to improve the validity with which one can make inferences based on randomized trials, is to increase the sample size or increase the minimum effect size. Typically, researchers want Type I error to be 5 percent or less, which means a 5 percent probability or less that the conclusion that the treatment was effective was false and due to chance alone. Type II error should be 20 percent or less. The **power** of the study is $1 - p(Type\ II\ error)$. Thus if Type II error is 20 percent, the power of the study is 80 percent, meaning that there is an 80 percent probability that the finding of "no effect" is, in fact, accurate.

The minimum sample size can be estimated by using a different formula for RCT, cohort, and case control studies (Elwood 1998). In general, the size depends on (1) the minimum Types I and II error that the researcher is willing to accept and (2) the minimum treatment effect. Sample size decreases if one is willing to tolerate proportionately more false positive and negative results. Size also decreases if one requires a larger treatment effect before concluding that the treatment is efficacious. In other words, precision, in terms of either lower Types I and II error or smaller treatment effects requires the cost and magnitude of a larger sample size.

The formula for calculating sample size for a cohort or trial design with equal groups is (Elwood 1998):

$$n = \frac{(p_1 q_1 + p_2 q_2) \times K}{(p_1 - p_2)^2}$$

where p_1 and p_2 are the proportion of patients with a particular outcome in groups 1 and 2, q_1 and q_2 the proportion of patients with the other outcome in groups 1 and 2, and K is a constant that reflects the Types I and II error that the researcher is willing to tolerate. For instance, $K = 6.2$ when the Type I error = 5% (one-sided) and the Type II error is 20% (power = 80%), whereas $K = 17.8$ with a Type I error = 1% and a power = 95%.

Recently, clodronate was found to have a dramatic effect on reducing new metastases in breast cancer (Diel et al. 1998): the rate of new metastases was 13 percent for women who took the drug and 29 percent for those who did not. If the study was to be replicated looking for the same kind of effect, how big should the sample size be? With p_1 and p_2 set at .13 and .29, respectively, q_1 and q_2 = 0.87 and 0.71. Assume a one-sided Type I error = 5% and a power of 80%, so $K = 6.2$. Sample size, n, should be at least 77 in each group. Note that with a lower tolerance for error, say Type I = 1% and power = 95%, $K = 17.8$ and the sample size should be at least 222 subjects in each group.

Duration and Masking

Since all RCTs are prospective by design, subjects are followed over a period of time to determine the effect of treatment on specific identified outcomes, such as mortality. The length of time necessary to make valid inferences from the study depends on the particular hypothesis in question and on the size of the expected treatment effect. The concern is the lapse in time and the extent to which the exposure in question will have an effect in that time on measurable outcomes.

Some exposures, particularly in preventive trials or in those involving risk factor modification, may demonstrate a beneficial effect on outcomes many years in the future. Although the initial RCT design may have to be lengthened (or shortened) after the commencement of the study, constraints, such as cost and the recruitment of eligible subjects, may be problematic.

The purpose of randomization is to allocate subjects into treatment and control groups so that selection bias is not introduced, since subjects with risk factors or other confounding characteristics may be more likely to self-select one group or the other. Furthermore, many clinical trials do not make either the patient or others involved with the study aware of group assignment—in effect, they are **blinded**. This is also referred to as **masking**. The concept of masking is based on the premise that patients, clinicians, and researchers ought not to be aware of whether a patient is receiving an experimental agent, treatment, or program because that could change behaviors in a way that would bias outcomes.

Single masking means that subjects (i.e., patients) have no idea whether or not they are receiving an experimental treatment, although they would have consented to participation in the study. This requires that the researcher design bogus or placebo exposures. With drugs, for instance, it is convenient to give control subjects pills devoid of pharmacological benefit (placebo). This becomes more difficult if side effects to the medication are anticipated. A fully executed informed consent would require making subjects aware of potential side effects should they be assigned to the treatment group. The onset of side effects could easily unravel single masking. The idea behind single masking is that subjects may change behaviors in a way that could compromise the study if they are aware of group assignment. For example, control subjects may seek alternative therapies or modify risk factors if they know that they are not receiving an experimental treatment. To the extent that this "compensation" has a favorable effect on outcomes, the observed treatment effect will be underestimated. It is somewhat more difficult or even impossible, of course, to develop bogus options for surgical procedures or programs.

Double masking refers to blinding both the subject and the subject's observer with regard to group assignment. The observer is anyone who is measuring outcomes, such as a clinician performing a physical exam, or an interviewer supervising an oral or written interview. Double masking is necessary to prevent the observer from changing the structure or thoroughness of the observation in a way that could bias the measured outcome. Byar and colleagues exemplify this point in a discussion of the utility of blinding in AIDs trials:

> Blinding is especially desirable when subjective end points, such as pain, functional status, or quality of life, are studied, because such evaluations are open to substantial bias. Likewise, without blinding, evaluation of the incidence of opportunistic infections may be biased, because knowledge of the treatment could affect the frequency or thoroughness of surveillance. (Byar et al. 1990)

With **triple blinding**, the subject, observer, and reviewer of the data are not aware of group assignment. Triple blinding assumes that the researchers or statistical analysts can introduce bias into the process of manipulating or interpreting the data to the extent that they have preconceived notions about the efficacy of the treatment.

Integrity of the Randomization

Given a sufficient number of subjects, randomization increases the likelihood, over all other study designs, that both known and unknown characteristics are equally distributed into treatment and control groups. Although this may not always be the case, the researchers should report whether the difference in each measurable characteristic is statistically significant. If so, stratification of the analyses may be appropriate, where one can compare the treatment effects for the characteristic (e.g., gender) where there is a statistically significant difference between the treatment and control group. Another alternative is to block-randomize at the very beginning of the study, that is, randomize within subgroups (gender, age, race) of the eligible population to ensure that the treatment and control groups are identical.

If the randomization is successful, treatment and control group should be similar *as originally configured*. Several opportunities arise during the design and execution of the study for the composition of the treatment and control groups to change in such a way that the integrity of the study is jeopardized. Eligible subjects may refuse to participate in the study or drop out at some point in time, or they may cross over to the other study group. The **refusals**, **dropouts**, or **crossovers** may bias the results of the study to the extent that the treatment and control groups no longer have similar characteristics.

Eligible subjects may refuse to participate in the study before they are randomized, in which case the randomized group of subjects may no longer be representative of some universe of patients. Suppose the more seriously ill patients refuse to be involved in the study because of transportation problems. The randomized group of subjects would be somewhat healthier, but unrepresentative, of the true population. A somewhat thornier problem exists if subjects refuse to participate after they are randomized to either the treatment or control group, although blinding patients to group assignment should reduce the likelihood that this would occur. In this situation, the composition of the treatment and control group may be dissimilar to the extent that the refusals are nonrandom, related to patient characteristics, and based on patient preferences for experimental treatment or conventional therapy. For example, suppose in an unblinded randomized study proportionately more seriously ill patients refuse conventional therapy. The result would be a "control" group of somewhat less seriously ill patients. If the outcome that is measured (e.g., mortality) is related to severity of illness, the treatment effect may be underestimated, because the group receiving the experimental treatment is composed of more seriously ill patients. The researcher may decide to reduce the likelihood of refusals by enlisting volunteers, a policy not without risk, because volunteers may differ in significant ways from the population they are intended to represent, that is, they may be healthier, smarter, or more motivated.

Dropouts pose similar problems. Some subjects are simply lost to follow-up, while others choose to discontinue, perhaps because they cannot tolerate the side effects of the experimental medication. The loss of subjects in a study may be nonrandom if dropouts from the experimental and control groups have different characteristics. For example, suppose that dropouts from the experimental group tended to be somewhat sicker, because they could not tolerate the medication. Control group dropouts tended to be somewhat healthier because they were not well-motivated. The result would be an experimental and control group dissimilar on the basis of severity of illness. The treatment effect would probably be underestimated since the experimental group might now be composed of patients for whom the treatment may not be as efficacious (i.e., if intolerance is related to efficacy). The burden of proof is on the researcher to demonstrate that neither refusals nor dropouts differ from the study participants in terms of characteristics or factors that may influence the outcomes of the study.

Another troubling problem occurs when patients cross over or change from the experimental treatment group to the control or conventional therapy group, or vice versa. This may occur, for instance, if patients cannot tolerate the side effects of the new treatment, or if the more seriously ill patients in the control group require the experimental intervention. The critical question is not necessarily whether to allow patients to cross over—clinical judgment should supercede the purity of experimental design—but how to classify these patients once they have changed treatment.

The classic example of this crossover problem involves those studies that have compared medical versus surgical treatment for heart disease. The surgical intervention is typically coronary artery bypass graft surgery. Some of the larger studies have reported crossover rates that range from 25 percent to 38 percent (Weinstein and Levin 1989), which means that a substantial number of subjects originally assigned to the medical control group had to undergo surgical intervention. Should these patients continue to participate in the study, and if so, how? Weinstein and Levin (1989) summarize the possibilities: (1) drop the crossovers, (2) switch the crossover group assignment at the time of the crossover, (3) use the "intention to treat" principle, or (4) discard the study. The first two possibilities would clearly change the composition of the two groups to the extent that control patients who cross over to the surgical intervention group are typically more seriously ill. Regardless of whether the crossovers are dropped or whether they change groups, the presumed similarity of the treatment and control groups brought about by randomization is destroyed. The "intention to treat" principle would preserve the original classification despite crossover to a different treatment. But although the original composition of the two groups is maintained with this approach, the purity of treatment received by each group is clearly contaminated. The crossovers are really receiving a different kind of treatment than the other patients in the control group.

The crossover problem may also arise if preliminary results of the study indicate an extremely promising treatment effect, as, for instance, in some of the studies of antiretroviral therapy for HIV infection (Volberding and Graham 1994). In one study, patients were assigned to either "immediate" or "deferred" treatment with zidovudine (an antiretroviral drug), with the deferred group supposedly not receiving the drug until the onset of symptoms. One-third of this group, however, crossed over and received the drug prematurely.

The integrity of randomization is also compromised if the character of the treatment(s) changes. In part, this is an issue of compliance. Subjects in a study may fail to comply with the treatment (e.g., they do not take the pills or take only some of the pills). To avoid (or at least measure) this problem, researchers provide patients with too many pills and ask them to return the unused ones. Lack of compliance, or partial compliance, changes the character of the treatment and affects the outcomes of the study. The treatment may also be affected by "dilution" or "contamination." This means that some subjects in the control group are "influenced" by their participation in the study even though they are not assigned to receive the intervention. Elwood (1998) discusses this phenomenon in his mention of the Multiple Risk Factor Intervention Trial (Group 1982), where subjects were randomized to received a special intervention to reduce risk factors for coronary artery disease. The control group reduced risk factors as well (although not as much), despite not receiving the special intervention. Presumably, control subjects were influenced by being participants in the study and adjusted their risk factors as a result of feedback from their physicians. In effect, an alternative (and only somewhat inferior) treatment was configured ad hoc by control subjects and their physicians. This resulted in a dilution or contamination of the original study design.

Ethical Considerations

The special relationship between a patient and his physician is grounded in trust, based on a long history of physician dedication to focusing their considerable skills on the care of individual patients, guided by the Hippocratic oath to "do no harm." Despite this sacred trust, physicians regularly face ethical dilemmas, such as when their view of what is best for the patient is challenged by others (third party payers, for instance). The randomized clinical trial leads them into a particularly difficult ethical quagmire. Physicians are called on to engage their patients in a process that may provide less than optimal treatment in the interest of some larger social good—the advancement of knowledge. Hellman and Hellman reflect on this dilemma:

> The randomized clinical trial routinely asks physicians to sacrifice the interests of their particular patients for the sake of the study and that of the information that it will make available for the benefit of society. This practice is ethically problematic. . . . If the physician has no preference for either treatment (is in a state of equipoise), then randomization is acceptable. If, however, he or she believes that the new treatment may be either more or less

successful or more or less toxic, the use of randomization is not consistent with fidelity to the patient (Hellman and Hellman 1991).

The legal doctrine of informed consent requires that patients be made aware of the risks and benefits of treatment and that they provide a formal consent. However, the principles of randomization and masking, discussed earlier, make informed consent somewhat more difficult. Patients are not given the choice, or perhaps even the knowledge, of which strategy of care they are receiving— experimental treatment, conventional treatment, or no treatment. The experimental treatment may carry some unknown risks with the promise of additional benefits. The calculus of weighing benefits and costs makes it unlikely that both patient and clinician are neutral to the choice of experimental or conventional treatment. Baum (1993) gives a cogent summary of this argument:

> One of the wittiest and most scholarly men that I know once explained to me, with irrefutable logic, that randomised controlled trials are ethically impossible. For a patient to be recruited, the clinician must be in perfect equipose about either of the two treatments being evaluated, and that has to be a rare event. Moreover, the patient, having been provided with and understanding perfect information about the trial, must also express perfect equipose—another extremely rare event. The likelihood of these rarities coexisting reaches an astronomically small probability number.

A tension exists between wanting to use the RCT to demonstrate therapeutic benefit and knowing when it is ethically unacceptable to randomly assign some patients to inferior care. No rational patient would choose less than optimal treatment in the interest of science, particularly when no alternatives exist. The double-blind placebo-controlled study of the efficacy of AZT in the treatment of patients with AIDS and AIDS-related complex is a classic example (Fischl et al. 1987). No other conventional therapy for AIDS existed at that time. The study had to be ended prematurely once a significant difference in mortality was demonstrated. In some instances, uncontrolled clinical trials may be the recommended study design if patients with a poor prognosis have no other alternatives and the experimental treatment is expected to have no significant side effects (Byar et al. 1990). Furthermore, it may be difficult to justify an RCT to support a growing body of evidence from other less-sophisticated studies when the preponderance of evidence supports a causal relationship between a particular exposure and outcome. For instance, some would argue that we have not conclusively proven that smoking causes cancer, yet few would be willing to support a randomized clinical trial in which subjects were randomly assigned to smoking and nonsmoking groups and followed over a lifetime.

Randomized Clinical Trials and Hospital Firms

One efficient method of conducting a randomized clinical trial is through the use of **hospital firms**. According to Neuhauser (1991), the three underlying concepts of firm research are (1) parallel providers, (2) ongoing random assignment, and (3) continuous/efficient evaluation and improvement. Basically, hospitals configure parallel and presumably similar systems of care (called "firms") to which patients are randomly assigned, and the outcomes of which can be routinely evaluated and improved. Hospital firms become de facto laboratories for controlled trial research, inasmuch as patients can be randomly assigned to the parallel firms as either the experimental intervention group or the control group. The hospital firm is an attractive idea, to the extent that these organizations are interested in being sites for clinical research. The costly and cumbersome process of developing an approach and structure for randomization is present and ongoing in hospital firms.

A number of hospitals have developed firms since the 1980s, and Metro-Health Medical Center (MCC) in Cleveland is only one example (Cebul 1991). In MCC, the large department of medicine was split into three parallel group practices. Faculty are randomly assigned to one of three groups, stratified by subspecialty. Residents are randomly assigned when they enter the training program. Nurses, paramedical staff, and clerical staff are dedicated solely to each firm, which is assigned a specific inpatient unit. Patients are assigned to firms using block randomization, which basically means that patients are distributed in randomized blocks of three. With block "231," for instance, the first patient would be assigned to firm 2, the next to firm 3, and the third to firm 1. The Metrohealth firm system was used in a recent study (Curley et al. 1998) to test the efficacy of interdisciplinary hospital rounds as compared with traditional rounds (MDs only). The interdisciplinary rounds, which brought together the MDs, RN, pharmacist, nutritionist, and social worker, were associated with a shorter mean length of stay, lower mean total charges, and similar outcomes in terms of hospital mortality rates.

Firms are specifically designed to accommodate at least three types of controlled trials: (1) clinical trials, (2) education trials, and (3) health services research or quality improvement (QI) (Cebul 1991). With clinical trials, the firms are randomly assigned to the new treatment modality or conventional therapy. Education trials can be designed to compare different teaching approaches, with one or more firms assigned to receive the special intervention. Hospital firms are ideally configured to conduct health services research or QI research, where the issues are modes of delivery, treatment strategies, and outcomes of care.

The design and execution of firm research is not without some concerns (Cebul 1991). The randomization process cannot guarantee that each firm will have patients and providers with similar characteristics. In fact, the randomization protocol within firms should prevent clever schemes to circumvent the process, such as allowing residents to choose "interesting" patients (Dawson 1991). The burden is on the researcher to demonstrate the equivalence of each firm at the beginning of the controlled trial. Indeed, the definition of equivalence may vary depending on the research (Cebul 1991). There is also the question of unit of analysis: patient, provider, or some larger group. The threat of contamination may be even more of a concern with hospital firms than with other kinds of controlled trials, given the "proximity" of competing units, particularly if providers are not blinded (Cebul 1991). Finally, one must face the ethical issues that emerge from placing patients in an "experimental" environment in which they might be exposed to some risks. According to Goldberg and McGough:

> In a sense, firm-system patients are not simply being asked to participate in this or that class of research activity, but rather whether or not they are interested in joining a clinical community whose routine practice has been redefined to include some level of minimal-risk experimentation (Goldberg and McGough 1991).

Meta-Analysis

Frequently, a review of the literature will reveal a number of studies, some randomized, some not, that have examined the efficacy of a particular treatment or agent. Many of these studies are based on small samples, with low statistical power, and nonsignificant or conflicting treatment effects. Researchers, clinicians, and other decision makers then face the challenge of making sense out of the many worthy efforts that have already taken place, perhaps before a large-scale and more conclusive RCT can be funded. The term meta-analysis refers to a set of complex statistical techniques that have been developed to pool the results of multiple studies and to derive aggregate treatment effects. Meta-analysis is supposed to answer four fundamental questions (Lau and Ioannidis 1998): (1) Do different studies have similar results? (2) What is the best estimate of the treatment effect? (3) To what extent is this estimate precise and robust? and (4) Why are there differences among the studies? The purpose of meta-analysis is to increase statistical power, resolve disagreements among multiple studies, improve effect size estimates, and pose new questions (Sacks et al. 1987).

Horwitz compares meta-analysis to the single center and multicenter RCT (Horwitz 1995). With the **single center RCT**, data are collected from multiple subjects according to an established protocol for selecting and randomizing patients, administering treatments, and measuring outcomes. The **multicenter RCT** is the "logical extension," where researchers use the same research protocol albeit at different sites. One might be tempted to draw a "methodologic analogy" between meta-analysis and the multicenter RCT, in the sense that the purpose of both is to combine the results from multiple and somewhat independent sources of inquiry. The major difference, however, is the lack of a common protocol, which leads to heterogeneity—different patients, different treatments, and different outcomes.

The first challenge with meta-analysis is to identify which studies to include. This involves the difficult chore of searching the literature (both published and unpublished) for relevant studies, while recognizing that a publication bias exists against small studies and those without a statistically significant treatment effect. Even more difficult, perhaps, is determining the degree of heterogeneity that can be tolerated in terms of different kinds of patients, protocols, treatments, and outcomes. "Apples and oranges" should not be combined, but one might derive meaningful results by combining "McIntosh" and "Rome" apples.

The actual statistical techniques that have been formulated to combine the results of multiple studies are beyond the scope of this book. By way of summary, the simplest approach is to calculate an average "effect size" (ES), where the ES for each study is the difference between control and treatment group means divided by the standard deviation of the control group (Wortman 1983). The ES is weighted by the degree of uncertainty associated with the results. Other sophisticated approaches have been developed when treatment effects are reported as a risk ratio, odds ratio, risk difference, or incidence rate. Consider Weaver and colleagues (1997), for example, who were interested in comparing primary coronary angioplasty (PTCA) with intravenous thrombolytic therapy ("Lytic") for acute myocardial infarction. They identified ten randomized studies that met the criteria for inclusion in the meta-analysis. The measured outcome is mortality, and the treatment effect is measured in terms of an odds ratio: the number of times more likely a PTCA patient is to die than one treated with thrombolytics. Confidence intervals are presented around each estimate, indicating the degree of uncertainty, and a total treatment effect is estimated using meta-analytical techniques.

Although meta-analysis provides a reasonable and quantitative approach to aggregating the fruit of scientific inquiry, it is not without problems, limitations, and severe criticism (Spitzer 1995). Generally, meta-analysis should not be used to contrive statistical significance from a collection of small, insignificant studies, although there may be occasions when this is appropriate, particularly when small treatment effects are relevant (Victor 1995). Meta-analysis is a reasonable approach for dealing with contradictory studies, for reaching urgent consensus, or when the opportunity to conduct a large-scale RCT is gone (Friedman et al. 1996).

Heterogeneity is the Achilles heel of meta-analysis, the vulnerable underbelly at which most critics take aim. Clearly, the credibility of aggregating multiple studies into one large pool depends on demonstrating that all of the studies are reasonably similar in terms of protocol. Some would argue that this is the exception rather than the rule or that, in fact, the observed differences among these "somewhat" similar studies may be clinically relevant. In other words, the process of combining results to obtain some global effect may obscure meaningful differences among the studies related to patients or protocol (Horwitz 1995). Feinstein goes so far as to describe meta-analysis as "statistical alchemy for the 21st century," which uses a "mixed salad principle" (i.e., combining apples with oranges) to try to get something from nothing "while simultaneously ignoring established scientific principles" (1995). While the jury may still be out regarding the conceptual validity of the meta-analytic approach, it should be justified empirically as well. This may be difficult; for example, Lelorier and colleagues compared 19 meta-analyses with 12 large and subsequent randomized controlled trials and reported a large measure of disagreement. The authors concluded that "the meta-analysis would have led to the adoption of an inefficient treatment in 32 percent of cases . . . and to the rejection of a useful treatment in 33 percent of cases (1997)." One hopes that other efforts to validate meta-analysis will be more encouraging.

Community Trials

It may be more appropriate for certain kinds of interventions to increase the unit of analysis from the individual subject or patient to a larger "community" unit, such as city, town, region, or census tract. These studies are referred to in the literature as "community trials," and they may or may not be randomized designs. This kind of study is especially appropriate for interventions that are easier or less costly to deliver through some common venue, for example, over the radio or television, or in the water supply, or when it may be difficult to prevent treatment "contamination" as discussed earlier.

The design of a community trial is similar in many ways to the more traditional randomized controlled trial. A protocol should be articulated that specifies the procedures for recruiting and selecting communities, delivering the experimental intervention, and measuring the specific effects. Sample size may be even more of a constraint due to the cost and logistics of recruiting multiple communities. If possible, the communities should be similar in terms of size, economies, and ethnicities (Lilienfeld and Stolley 1994), with stable populations and medical care systems that are self-contained (Kessler and Levin 1972).

The execution of the community trial is also similar to the more traditional RCT. The process of recruiting communities to participate in the study is analogous to obtaining informed consent. Local community leaders and elected officials must be convinced of the merit of participating in the study and must formally consent as representative of the many residents who will be affected by the intervention. Baseline measurements of the outcome(s) that should be affected by the intervention (e.g., neonatal mortality rates) are collected for each of the eligible communities that have agreed to participate. The communities are then randomly assigned to either treatment or control groups and followed for a defined period of time. The difference between end-of-study and baseline outcome(s) is calculated and compared for treatment and control communities to determine if the treatment effect is statistically significant.

Two examples of community trials are the Stanford Five City Project (Farquhar et al. 1985, 1990) and the Minnesota Heart Health Program (Luepker et al. 1996). Both studies involved individual and community-wide health education efforts, and both used a relatively small number of communities (five for Stanford and six for Minnesota). Both were designed to decrease the rate of cardiovascular disease through prevention. The Stanford study measured physiological risk factors such as blood pressure, weight, and cholesterol, whereas the Minnesota study was aimed at the incidence of coronary heart disease and stroke.

With other studies the unit of analysis may be smaller. In one study, for instance, 450 Indonesian villages were randomized into a vitamin A treatment group and a control group that did not get the supplementation (Abdeljaber et al.

1991). In another, an AIDS education program was tested in Tanzania where 18 public primary schools were randomly assigned to an educational intervention designed to promote risk reduction (Klepp et al. 1997). In a third, 296 households in Tecumseh, Michigan were stratified by size and were randomized into a treatment group that received virucidal nasal tissues and a group of controls (Longini and Monto 1988). The question was whether or not these tissues were effective in reducing the transmission of influenza across family members.

The choice of whether to design a community trial vis-à-vis the more traditional RCT depends on the nature and complexity of the intervention, as well as the size of the population on which the intervention must focus (Blackburn 1983; Kottke et al. 1985; Farquhar et al. 1990; Lilienfeld and Stolley 1994). Interventions dealing with risk factor modification and behavioral change, for instance, may be delivered more effectively through some community vehicle, such as education programs in the mass media (Syme 1978). In addition, in cases involving complex interventions, it may be easier to adjust and manipulate the environment with a community trial. If the targeted disease is highly prevalent in certain communities, or if the population to be studied must be necessarily large, it may be more efficient to orchestrate a community trial rather than to incur the expense of recruiting many individual subjects (Lilienfeld and Stolley 1994).

Conclusion

Neuhauser (1991) pointed to the biblical account of Daniel (before his deliverance from the lion's den) as one of the first clinical trials. The question was whether a diet of vegetables was as efficacious as Babylonian cuisine in terms of "countenance." The conclusion that was reached after a ten-day trial period was that "their countenances appeared fairer and fatter in flesh than all the children which did eat the portion of the king's meat" (Daniel 1:15, KJV). This was an interesting observation, though the study was clearly not randomized, nor was it free of confounding factors, given the history of divine intervention on the part of the Lord God of Israel. The randomized clinical trial of today has enjoyed the reputation of being the exalted, gold standard of research to which all other modes of inquiry must bow. Clearly this distinction rests on the laurels of the randomization, as it should, since potentially confounding factors should be equally allocated to treatment and control groups. The authority of the noble RCT can be challenged, however, by threats to validity in the form of refusals, dropouts, crossovers, and contaminated treatments. The RCT is an elegant research design, but not a flawless one.

Case Study 6.1

Simmer and colleagues report on a randomized controlled trial at Henry Ford Hospital in Detroit, Michigan (1991) that compares clinical and financial outcomes on two different inpatient staffing models. The General Internal Medicine inpatient nursing unit was the site of the study in which patients were randomly assigned to either a resident (teaching) or staff (nonteaching) service. The resident service provided patient care with the more traditional resident team consisting of a supervising resident, two interns, and a number of third- and fourth-year medical students. The staff service consisted of two senior-level physicians, a physician assistant, and a medical assistant. All patients had an attending physician. Table 6.2 (Simmer et al. 1991, from Tables 3 and 4) summarizes the results of the study.

1. Exactly what is the experimental "treatment" here? How might differences in the composition of the two services be expected to affect outcomes?
2. What other factors might explain the significant differences in financial and clinical outcomes?
3. Describe the integrity of the randomization process and the potential for bias in this study.

	Resident	Staff	Significance
Length of stay	7.58	9.21	$p < 0.005$
Total charges	$6,908	$8,588	$p < 0.010$
Laboratory charges	$820	$1,170	$p < 0.001$
Pharmacy	$592	$814	$p < 0.005$
Radiology	$495	$479	NS
Readmissions within 15 days	7.8%	6.8%	NS
In-hospital mortality	5.2%	8.2%	$p < 0.54$
Eight-month mortality	12.5%	14.0%	NS

TABLE 6.2

Clinical and Financial Outcomes for Two Staffing Models

Source: Simmer, T. L., D. R. Nerenz. "A Randomized, Controlled Trial of an Attending Staff Services in General Internal Medicine." Copyright © 1991, *Medical Care*. Adapted by permission.

Case Study 6.2

The RAND Health Insurance Experiment was probably the largest controlled trial designed to improve health financing policy, particularly with regard to the issue of cost sharing (Newhouse 1991). Between November 1974 and February 1977, 7,691 families were enrolled in the study in six different sites: Dayton, Ohio; Seattle, Washington; Fitchburg/Leominster, Massachusetts; Charleston, South Carolina; Franklin County, Massachusetts; and Georgetown County, South Carolina. The sites were supposed to represent the major census regions; northern and southern rural sites; and a range in city sizes, waiting times to appointments, and physicians per capita. Each family was randomly assigned to one of 14 different fee-for-service plans or a prepaid group practice—Group Health Cooperative (GHC) in Seattle. A comparison group of patients from GHC was also evaluated (Fischl et al., 1987; Friedman et al. 1996). The plans varied by coinsurance rate (0, 25 percent, 50 percent, or 95 percent) and by maximum dollar expenditure (MDE), with an MDE of $1,000 for most families, but 5, 10, or 15 percent of income (or $1,000, whichever was less) for low-income families. The families were

TABLE 6.3
Health Insurance
Experiment:
Utilization by
Insurance Plan

	No. Visits	Outpatient Expenses	No. Admissions	Hospital Expenses	Rate/100 Persons	Hospital Days/100 Persons	Face-to-Face Visits	Preventive Visits
Free	4.55	$340	0.128	$409	13.8	83	4.2	0.41
25%	3.33	$260	0.105	$373	10.0	87	3.5	0.32
50%	3.03	$224	0.092	$450	10.5	46	2.9	0.29
95%	2.73	$203	0.099	$315	8.8	28	3.3	0.27
GHC					8.4	49	4.3	0.55
GHC control					8.3	38	4.7	0.60

Source: Adapted from J. P. Newhouse, "Controlled Experimentation as Research Policy," in *Health Services Research: Key to Health Policy*, edited by E. Ginsberg, Tables 7-3 and 7-7. Copyright © 1991, Harvard University Press, Cambridge, MA. Used by permission. Adapted from tables 7-3, 7-7.

followed for either three or five years. Table 6.3 presents some of the major results of the study.

1. What kinds of factors is the randomization process likely to control for in this study?
2. How do you interpret the results of this study with regard to the effect of cost sharing on utilization?
3. Was it possible to use "blinding" in this study? Why or why not?
4. Describe any ethical concerns with this study.
5. Why would this RCT design be better than a cohort study of groups with different coinsurance rates?
6. How might a change in the environment affect the results of the study?

References

Abdeljaber, M. H., A. S. Monto, R. L. Tilden, M. A. Schork, and I. Tarwotojo. 1991. "The Impact of Vitamin A Supplementation on Morbidity: A Randomized Community Intervention Trial." *American Journal of Public Health* 81 (12): 1654–56.

Baum, M. 1993. "New Approach for Recruitment into Randomised Controlled Trials [see comments]." *Lancet* 341 (8,848): 812–13.

Blackburn, H. 1983. "Research and Demonstration Projects in Community Cardiovascular Disease Prevention" *Journal of Public Health Policy* 4 (4): 398–421.

Byar, D. P., D. A. Schoenfeld, S. B. Green, D. A. Amato, R. Davis, V. DeGruttola, D. M. Finkelstein, C. Gutsonis, R. D. Gelber, S. Lagakos, M. Lefkopoulou, A. A. Tsiatis, M. Zelen, J. Peto, L. S. Freedman, M. Gail, R. Simon, S. S. Ellenberg, J. R. Anderson, R. Collins, R. Peto, F. Peto. 1990. "Design Considerations for AIDS Trials." *The New England Journal of Medicine* 323 (19): 1343–48.

Cebul, R. D. 1991. "Randomized, Controlled Trials Using the Metro Firm System." *Medical Care* 29 (7, Supplement): JS9–JS18.

Curley, C., J. E. McEachern, T. Speroff. 1998. "A Firm Trial of Interdisciplinary Rounds on the Inpatient Medical Wards: An Intervention Designed Using Continuous Quality Improvement." *Medical Care* 36 (8, Supplement): AS4–AS12.

Dawson, N. V. 1991. "Organizing the Metro Firm System for Research." *Medical Care* 29 (7, Supplement): JS19–JS25.

DeBusk, R. F., N. H. Miller, H. R. Superko, C. A. Dennis, R. J. Thomas, H. T. Lew, W. E. Berger, R. S. Heller, J. Rompf, D. Gee, H. C. Kraemer, A. Bandura, G. Ghandour, M. Clark, R. V. Shah, L. Fisher, B. Taylor. 1994. "A Case-Management System for Coronary Risk Factor Modification After Acute Myocardial Infarction." *Annals of Internal Medicine* 120 (9): 721–29.

Diel, I. J., E. Solomayer, S. D. Costa, C. Gollan, R. Goerner, D. Wallwiener, M. Kaufmann, G. Bastert. 1998. "Reduction in New Metastases in Breast Cancer with Adjuvant Clodronate Treatment." *The New England Journal of Medicine* 339 (6): 357–63.

Elwood, M. 1998. *Critical Appraisel of Epidemiological Studies and Clinical Trials.* New York: Oxford University Press.

Farquhar, J. W., S. P. Fortmann, J. A. Flora, C. B. Taylor, W. L. Haskell, P. J. Williams, N. Maccoby, P. D. Wood. 1990. "Effects of Communitywide Education on Cardiovascular Disease Risk Factors: The Stanford Five-City Project." *Journal of the American Medical Association* 264 (3): 359–65.

Farquhar, J. W., S. P. Fortmann, N. Maccoby, W. L. Haskell, P. T. Williams, J. A. Flora, C. B. Taylor, B. W. Brown Jr., D. S. Solomon, S. B. Holley. 1985. "The Stanford Five-City Project: Design and Methods." *American Journal of Epidemiology* 264: 359–365.

Feinstein, A. R. 1995. "Meta-Analysis: Statistical Alchemy for the 21st Century." *Journal of Clinical Epidemiology* 48 (1): 71–79.

Fischl, M. A., D. D. Richman, M. H. Grieco, M. S. Gottlieb, P. A. Volberling, O. L. Laskin, J. M. Leedom, J. E. Groopman, D. Mildvan, R. T. Schooley. 1987. "The Efficacy of Azidothymidine (AZT) in the Treatment of Patients with AIDS and AIDS-Related Complex." *The New England Journal of Medicine* 317 (4): 185–91.

Fisher, B., S. Anderson, C. K. Redmond, N. Wolmark, D. L. Wickerham, W. M. Cronin. 1995. "Reanalysis and Results After 12 Years of Follow-up in a Randomized Clinical Trial comparing total mastectomy with lumpectomy with or without irradiation in the treatment of breast cancer." *The New England Journal of Medicine* 333 (22): 1456–61.

Friedman, L. M., C. D. Furberg, and D. L. DeMets. 1996. *Fundamentals of Clinical Trials.* St. Louis, MO: Mosby.

Goldberg, H. I., and H. McGough. 1991. "The Ethics of Ongoing Randomization Trials." *Medical Care* 29 (7, Supplement): JS41–JS48.

Gradishar, W. J., M. S. Tallman, and J. S. Abrams. 1996. "High-Dose Chemotherapy for Breast Cancer [see comments]." *Annals of Internal Medicine* 125 (7): 599–604.

Group, E. B. C. T. C. 1992. "Systemic Treatment of Early Breast Cancer by Hormonal, Cytotoxic, or Immune Therapy." *Lancet* 339 (8,785): 71–85.

Group, E. B. C. T. C. 1995. "Effects of Radiotherapy and Surgery in Early Breast Cancer: An Overview of the Randomized Trials." *The New England Journal of Medicine* 333 (22): 1444–55.

Group, M. R. F. I. T. R. 1982. "Multiple Risk Factor Intervention Trial: Risk Factor Changes and Mortality Results." *Journal of the American Medical Association* 248 (12): 1465–77.

Hellman, S., and D. S. Hellman. 1991. "Of Mice but Not Men: Problems of the Randomized Clinical Trial [see comments]." *The New England Journal of Medicine* 324 (22): 1585–89.

Horwitz, R. I. 1995. "Large-Scale Randomized Evidence: Large Simple Trials and Overviews of Trials. Discussion: A Clinician's Perspective on Meta-Analysis." *Journal of Clinical Epidemiology* 48 (1): 41–44.

Ioannidis, J. P., J. C. Cappelleri, J. Lau, P. R. Skolnik, B. Melville, T. C. Chalmers, H. S. Sacks. 1995. "Early or Deferred Zidovudine Therapy in HIV-Infected Patients Without an AIDS-Defining Illness." *Annals of Internal Medicine* 122 (11): 856–66.

Kessler, I. I., and M. L. Levin. 1972. *The Community as an Epidemiological Laboratory.* Baltimore, MD: Johns Hopkins University Press.

Klepp, K. I., S. S. Ndeki, M. T. Leshabari, P. J. Hannan, B. A. Lyimo. 1997. "AIDS Education in Tanzania: Promoting Risk Reduction Among Primary School Children." *American Journal of Public Health* 87 (12): 1931–36.

Kottke, T. E., P. Puska, J. T. Salonen, J. Tuomilehto, A. Nissinen. 1985. "Projected Effects of High-Risk Versus Population-Based Prevention Strategies in Coronary Heart Disease." *American Journal of Epidemiology* 121 (5): 697–704.

Lau, J., and J. P. A. Ioannidis. 1998. "Quantitative Synthesis in Systemic Reviews." In *Systemic Reviews: Synthesis of Best Evidence for Health Care Decisions*, 91–101. Philadelphia, PA: American College of Physicians.

Lilienfeld, D. E., and P. D. Stolley. 1994. *Foundations of Epidemiology.* New York: Oxford University Press.

Longini, I. M., and A. S. Monto. 1988. "Efficacy of Virucidal Nasal Tissues in Interrupting Familial Transmission of Respiratory Agents: A Field Trial in Tecumseh, Michigan." *American Journal of Epidemiology* 128 (3): 639–44.

Luepker, R. V., L. Rastam, P. J. Hannan, D. M. Murray, C. Gray, W. L. Baker, R. Crow, D. R. Jackobs Jr., P. L. Pirie, S. R. Mascioli, M. B. Mittelmark, H. Blackburn. 1996. "Community Education for Cardiovascular Disease Prevention: Morbidity and Mortality Results from the Minnesota Heart Health Program." *American Journal of Epidemiology* 144 (4): 351–62.

Lurie, N., J. Christianson, I Moscovice. 1994. "The Effects of Capitation on Health and Functional Status of the Medicaid Elderly: A." *Annals of Internal Medicine* 120 (6): 506–11.

Lurie, N., I. S. Moscovice, M. Finch, J. B. Christianson. 1992. "Does Capitation Affect the Health of the Chronically Mentally Ill? Results from A." *Journal of the American Medical Association* 267 (24): 3300–3304.

Neuhauser, D. 1991. "Parallel Providers, Ongoing Randomization, and Continuous Improvement." *Medical Care* 29 (7, Supplement): JS5–JS8.

Newhouse, J. P. 1991. "Controlled Experimentation as Research Policy," in *Health Services Research: Key to Health Policy*, edited by E. Ginzberg, 397. Cambridge, MA: Harvard University Press.

Palmer, R. H., T. A. Louis, H. F. Peterson, J. K. Rothrock, R. Strain, E. A. Wright. 1996. "What Makes Quality Assurance Effective? Results from a Randomized, Controlled Trial in 16 Primary Care Group Practices." *Medical Care* 34 (9 Supplement): SS29–S39.

Pilote, L., R. J. Thomas, C. Dennis, P. Goins, N. Houston-Miller, H. Kraemer, C. Leong,

W. E. Berger, H. Lew, R. S. Heller, J. Rompf, R. F. DeBusk. 1992. "Return to Work After Uncomplicated Myocardial Infarction: A Trial of Practice Guidelines in the Community." *Annals of Internal Medicine* 117 (5): 383–89.

Pritchard, R. S., and S. P. Anthony. 1996. "Chemotherapy Plus Radiotherapy Compared with Radiotherapy Alone in the Treatment of Lung Cancer." *Annals of Internal Medicine* 125 (9): 723–29.

Reuben, D. B., G. M. Borok, G. Wolde-Tsadik, D. H. Ershoff, L. K. Fishman, V. L. Ambrosini, Y. Liu, L. Z. Rubenstein, J. C. Beck. 1995. "A Randomized Trial of Comprehensive Geriatric Assessment in the Care of Hospitalized Patients." *The New England Journal of Medicine* 332 (20): 1345–50.

Rosselli-Del-Turco, M., D. Palli, A. Cariddi, S. Ciatto, P. Pacini, V. Distante. 1994. "Intensive Diagnostic Follow-up, After Treatment of Primary Breast Cancer: A Randomized Trial." *Journal of the American Medial Association* 271 (20): 1593–7.

Sacks, H. S., J. Berrier, D. Reitman, V. A. Ancona-Berk, T. C. Chalmers. 1987. "Meta-Analysis of Randomized Controlled Trials." *The New England Journal of Medicine* 316 (8): 450–55.

Senn, S. 1995. "A Personal View of Some Controversies in Allocating Treatment to Patients in Clinical Trials." *Statistics in Medicine* 14 (24): 2661–74.

Simmer, T. L., D. R. Nerenz, et al. 1991. "A Randomized, Controlled Trial of an Attending Staff Service in General Internal Medicine." *Medical Care* 29 (7, Supplement): JS31–JS40.

Simon, G. E., M. VonKorff, J. H. Heiligenstein, D. A. Revicki, L. Grothaus, W. Katon, E. H. Wagner. 1996. "Initial Antidepressant Choice in Primary Care: Effectiveness and Cost of Fluoxetine vs. Tricyclic Antidepressants." *Journal of the American Medical Association* 275 (24): 1897–902.

Spitzer, W. O. 1995. "The Challenge of Meta-Analysis." *Journal of Clinical Epidemiology* 48 (1): 1–4.

Stoner, T. J., B. Dowd, W. P. Carr, G. Maldonado, T. R. Church, J. Mandel. 1998. "Do Vouchers Improve Breast Cancer Screening Rates? Results from a Randomized Trial." *Health Services Research* 33 (1): 11–28.

Syme, S. L. 1978. "Life Style Intervention in Clinic-Based Trials." *American Journal of Epidemiology* 108 (1): 87–91.

Victor, N. 1995. "The Challenge of Meta-Analysis": Discussion, Indications and Contra-indications for Meta-Analysis." *Journal of Clinical Epidemiology* 48 (1): 5–8.

Volberding, P. A., and N. M. Graham. 1994. "Initiation of Antiretroviral Therapy in HIV Infection: A Review of Interstudy Consistencies." *Journal of Acquired Immune Deficiency Syndromes* 7 (Supplement 2): S12–S23.

Weaver, W. D., R. J. Simes, A. Betriu, C. Grines, F. Zijlstra, E. Garcia, L. Grinfeld, R. Gibbons, E. Ribeiro, M. DeWood, F. Ribichini. 1997. "Comparison of Primary Coronary Angioplasty and Intravenous Thrombolytic Therapy for Acute Myocardial Infarction: A Quantatative Review." *Journal of the American Medical Association* 278 (23): 2093–98.

Weinstein, G. S., and B. Levin. 1989. "Effect of Crossover on the Statistical Power of Randomized Studies." *Annals of Thoracic Surgery* 48 (4): 490–95.

Wood, D., N. Halfon, C. Donald-Sherbourne, R. M. Mazel, M. Schuster, J. S. Hamlin, M. Pereyra, P. Camp, M. Grabowsky, N. Duan. 1998. "Increasing Immunization

Rates Among Inner-city, African American Children: A Randomized Trial of Case Management." *Journal of the American Medical Association* 279 (1): 29–34.

Wortman, P. M. 1983. "Meta-Analysis: A Validity Perspective." In *Evaluation Studies Review Annual*, edited by R. J. Light, vol. 8, 157–66. Beverly Hills, CA: Sage Publications.

PART

II

Application of Managerial Epidemiology to Health Services Management

Epidemiology and the Planning Function

F. Douglas Scutchfield, Joel M. Lee, and Steven T. Fleming

> *Ms. Findcare, the head of social services, sends a memo to Mr. Jones in which she reports a number of complaints regarding the coordination of care for the elderly population, particularly those with Alzheimer's disease. She questions whether the ongoing strategic plan is addressing the current or future needs of Medicare enrollees. What kinds of epidemiologic data need to be collected to assess the needs and services required by both current and potential elderly enrollees?*

Although most individuals have personal plans, and most organizations have formal planning documents, the commonplace use of the term "planning" focuses on an informal concept. A variety of explanations exist for the professional construct of planning, which is described as:

- making current decisions in light of their future effects;
- a means to assess the future and make provision for it;
- making current choices to influence the future;
- guidance of change;
- deciding in advance what to do, how to do it, when to do it, and who is to do it;
- the design of a desired future and of effective ways of bringing it about;
- the ability to control the future consequences of present actions; and
- a process that involves making and evaluating each of a set of interrelated decisions before action is required.

The healthcare organization should include epidemiologic measurement in the planning process, regardless of which of these descriptions is embraced. Decisions about where the organization is going, how to guide the organization through change, and the design of a desired future, must include an assessment of healthcare markets, specifically in terms of the kinds of morbidity that customers have in the present or will have in the future. The purpose of this chapter is to describe ways to incorporate epidemiologic concepts and measurement into the process of community and institutional planning. We discuss the history of health planning in section one, distinguish among various types of health planning in section two, and consider community health planning in the third section, with a particular focus on the tools and benchmarks of planning, such as *Healthy*

People 2000. Section four deals with institutional planning, and a strategic planning model is elaborated in section five. In the final section of this chapter we describe healthcare marketing, relate the marketing and planning processes, and discuss the prominent role that epidemiology should play in both processes.

History of Health Planning

Planning in healthcare has a reasonably long history. Early planning efforts focused on hospital bed need with various models, dating back to the 1920s, based on beds per 1,000 population in a service area. The evolution of hospital bed planning is useful as an example of the increased sensitivity of the resource planning method over time. In 1921, Hoge (1958) developed a model for bed ratio per 25 percent of estimated prevalence of illness. However, he did not address hospital occupancy rate or geographic location. By the late 1920s, additional models were developed to address differences in hospital service areas, including variation in urban/rural populations, contagious disease, pediatrics, maternity, chronic illness, and convalescent care. In 1933, the Committee on the Cost of Medical Care and Lee and Jones (1933) reported estimated illness incidence and prevalence figures by medical diagnostic category, using U.S. Public Health Service and industrial data. Expert physician judgment was used to estimate resource requirements based on past experience, not on future demand. The subsequent evolution of bed planning included the designation of service centers or "areas of study" hospitals and the use of population death ratios as measures of bed need.

When the Second World War ended, the inadequacy of total hospital beds in the United Sates became a pressing concern. In light of this, the Hill-Burton Hospital Survey and Construction Act of 1946 was enacted into federal law to inventory bed supply requirements and to promote hospital construction. The legislation was designed to (1) address the need for additional rural hospital beds, (2) coordinate public and private health services, (3) increase efficiency of the system through the control of new equipment and facilities where use would be insufficient, and (4) establish regionalized service areas. The Hill-Burton Act provided funding for construction costs for short-term general hospital beds, with service area population density and current bed occupancy as criteria for project funding. Hill-Burton also included policies to address the setting of priorities by states, prohibition of discrimination in facility access and use, and the provision of services at no cost to indigent patients. As a part of that legislation, states were required to develop a hospital plan that delineated how and where hospitals were to be constructed. At that time, total estimates indicated a need for 165,000 additional hospital beds in the United States. In 1964, amendments to the Hill-Burton act dropped uniform beds-per-1,000 population rates and directed states to address community context in setting priorities for funding. Under Hill-Burton, the connection between epidemiologic measures and resource use was done at the macro level with population density as the measure of need, rather than morbidity profiles, as was the case in the earlier Lee and Jones (1933) report.

Federally mandated health services planning continued in the establishment of the Regional Medical Program in 1966 to address cancer, heart disease, and stroke through the establishment of regionalized programs covering the entire United States. The Partnership for Health Act of 1967 (Comprehensive Health Planning) established regional health plans and reviewed funded projects for appropriateness. The Social Security Amendments of 1972, section 1122, provided state agency review of proposals to use federal funds for projects with a cost greater than $100,000. The National Health Planning and Resources Development Act of 1974 consolidated the Hill-Burton, Regional Medical Program, Comprehensive Health Planning, and Section 1122 legislation and authorized a $1 billion, three-year program for health planning and resource development. This legislation was very ambitious: it created an administrative and voluntary board that represented consumers, health providers, and payers at the state level and in health service areas across the United States. In exchange for federal financial support, states were required to establish state health planning laws, including certificate-of-need laws. The regional Health Systems Agencies (HSAs) were responsible for the development of a long-range health plan for their area, the health system plan (HSP), and annual plans to implement the HSP called the annual implementation plan (AIP). They were also responsible for initial certificate-of-need review for the states and for the approval of local federal grants designed to improve or change the healthcare system. Funding for the federal legislation was phased out in the early 1980s, although some HSAs continued to operate for a period of time as local support and private contributions for their operation attempted to replace the federal funding. Certificate-of-need legislation has also been revised or repealed in many states. The proximate causes of the demise of this most ambitious law was underfunding of specific aspects of the law, questions about efficacy, and—most significantly—the notion that the healthcare system should be deregulated to respond to market forces.

The idea of health planning, however, did not entirely disappear with the departure of the National Health Planning and Resource Development Act. During this period of transition, many healthcare organizations, in an effort to comply with legislative mandates, created positions for planners. The need for organizations to plan still existed. Not even the collapse of certificate-of-need legislation, for example, could affect the needs of hospitals to respond to consumer demand for new services. Many hospitals recognized the usefulness of planning and retained their planners after the federal and state mandates ended. It appears that hospitals found value in planning activities and redefined the responsibilities of staff to include the functions of planning and marketing in a competitive environment. Interest in planning has also been promoted by the recent focus by managers on total or continuous quality improvement, as evidenced by the recent establishment of Baldrige National Quality Awards in Health Care and the

Ernest D. Codman Quality Award of the Joint Commission on Accreditation of Health Care Organizations. Nevertheless, the planning function in health organizations retains many of the health planning methods and functions that were used by Health Systems Agencies and other legislatively mandated public planning organizations. In fact, most large American hospitals will have some administrator with the notion of planning in his or her title, such as vice president for development and planning.

It should be clear that, to some degree, each of these planning programs embraced epidemiologic concepts and measurement. Even the early Hoge model (1958) was based on an estimate of the prevalence of disease, as was the Lee-Jones report (1933). The Regional Medical Program focused specifically on the top three causes of mortality: heart disease, cancer, and stroke. The health services agencies funded by the National Health Planning and Resources Development Act were steeped in epidemiologic data as they developed the long-range health plans for their local areas.

In assessing the efficacy of these formalized planning efforts, we need to address a variety of questions. Was the construction or purchase of unneeded services prevented? Do healthcare organizations currently make decisions in accordance with plans? Is the public better served by the healthcare system? Has money been saved? It is difficult to evaluate these questions because we have no way of measuring the number of projects that were considered and then dropped after conscientious internal review. Other public programs with active planning components have included examination of the Graduate National Medical Advisory Commission and the *Healthy People* series.

Planning: Definitions and Distinctions

Peddecord (1998) has defined planning as "a future-oriented systematic process of determining a direction, setting a goal and taking actions to achieve that goal." Planning is essential to all managerial functions, and perhaps it is one of the most important activities in which those who are responsible for a healthcare program or activity engage. A plan sets a course of action. It describes the direction that an organization is pursuing and the ways in which it will go about the process of achieving positive outcomes. Without a plan the manager will not know what to do in pursuit of an objective, how to accomplish results along the way, and when the final objective has been achieved.

Most planning proceeds from the model of planning, implementation, and evaluation, and leads to further planning. Many of the components of implementation, such as the directing and controlling function (Chapters 8 and 9), are spelled out elsewhere in this book. Planning involves not only the technical aspects that form the major focus of this chapter, but also the social processes that drive it forward. Planning is rarely done by an individual; it most often is done in organizations or communities of individuals and organizations with an interest—as stakeholders—in the work and in the results of that organization.

Typically a plan consist of five components, although the order may vary:

1. *Ends:* specification of outcomes in goals and objectives;
2. *Means:* selection of policies, programs, procedures, and practices by which objectives and goals are to be pursued;
3. *Resources:* determination of the types and amounts of resources required, the ways in which they will be generated or acquired, and their allocation to activities;
4. *Implementation:* design and organization of decision-making procedures so that the plan can be carried out; and
5. *Control:* design of a procedure for anticipating or detecting errors in the plan, or plan failures, and for preventing or correcting problems on a continuing basis.

A major distinction in planning is whether the planning is being carried out at the institutional level or the community level. **Institutional planning** is in some ways easier given the institution's hierarchical structure. And, theoretically, all are looking out for the institution's best interest. On the other hand, **community health planning** involves many institutions and organizations, each with its own vested interest and agenda. The major effort in community health planning is to recognize that each organization has its own agenda. The challenge is to harmonize plans so that all are accommodated to one final outcome. Table 7.1 illustrates the major distinctions between community and institutional planning.

Whether health planning is community or institution based, five significant categories or levels of planning exist. Strategic, operational, and tactical planning all focus on the organization as it defines its future direction and implementation. The first and most general of these three categories is **strategic planning**, which has a comprehensive scope and a long-range time line; it is the most relevant for application, as in defining the future structure of the organization. Strategic planning is usually done at the upper levels of the organization's governing body and senior staff, and frequently has a three- to five-year time line. A strategic plan normally will include four components that prescribe all aspects of planning:

Vision: clear identification of the most successful view of the organization in the very long run;

Mission: encapsulated purpose of the organization and its reasons for existing;

Goals: broad statements of the achievements required for fulfillment of the organzation's mission; and

Objectives: specific measurable outcomes linked to the goal statements.

Clearly, an organization should incorporate epidemiologic concepts and measurement into the strategic planning process. Suppose the vision of a healthcare organization is to be recognized for excellence in patient care, education, and

TABLE 7.1

Institutional vs. Community Planning

Selected Characteristics, Attributes, or Steps in a Planning Process	Institutional	Community-Based
Main focus or reason for planning	Furthering that organization's goals: profit, survival, improving services to the market that is served	Concerned with the health and welfare of an entire defined population (e.g., cross-institutional planning, safety net planning)
Who does planning? Which organizations or groups?	All organizations, both public and private, must plan for institutional success or survival	Health and public welfare agencies, public school districts, community-based organizations with broad mandates
Are strategic issues (issues that relate to the core concerns or values of the business or community) addressed?	Yes, but only within the context of the organization's goals	Yes, but terms such as *community* or *health system* may be used
Short time frame (months)	Yes	Community planning may need to be rapid; some planning goes on for years
Long time frame (years)	Yes	Yes
Need for political savvy	Essential in large organizations—many factions must be reconciled	Essential—many groups must be satisfied or dealt with; self interest of groups may make consensus difficult or impossible
Information needs and use	Information from inside and outside the organization is needed	Information may be complex and from many sources—difficult to find information for some concerns
Examples of management science or planning techniques used	Budgets, operations research, cost analysis, models, statistical process control may be useful for program or operational plans	Group management techniques and nominal group process may be useful
Assessment of needs	Usually termed "marketing" or "market research" in an institution situation	Often done in a community context: which services are needed and by whom, and so forth

continued

Implementation: operational planning and program planning	Most planning done at this level by supervisors, workers	Not an emphasis— institutions that have resources usually do implementation
Results or outputs of the planning process	Organizations develop action plans, business plans, or program plans to implement programs, finance operations, raise money	Community-based planning groups may not have an organizational base or resources but may provide recommendations to policymakers and organizations that provide services
Emphasis on written documents	May be little emphasis on the written plan per se—more emphasis on policies, procedures, action plans, budgets, or business plans that implement the agreed-upon strategy	Well-detailed plans may be needed to communicate to those who can influence public policy or implement action

Source: Peddecord, K. M. 1998. "Public Health Management Tools Planning." In *Maxcy-Rosenau-Last: Public Health and Preventive Medicine, 14th ed.*, edited by R. B. Wallace and B. N. Doebbeling. Stamford, CT: Appleton & Lang.

research. "Excellence" in patient care is an undefined benchmark for which there are some epidemiologic measures, such as case-fatality rates or risk-adjusted mortality measures. Alternatively, the vision statement may envision assisting "people in taking responsibility for their own health by actively promoting wellness and facilitating healing" (Duncan, Ginter, and Swayne 1995). The foundation here for wellness, obviously, is the vast body of epidemiologic literature that identifies risk factors such as diet, smoking, and other wellness-enhancing or disease-promoting behaviors. Suppose the mission statement claims an interest in health status improvement for people in a defined geographic area. The mission statement presumes that one can measure health status improvement in a geographic region through epidemiologic measures such as mortality and morbidity rates. Goals and objectives can be defined specifically in epidemiologic terms such as reducing neonatal mortality, the rates of nosocomial infection, risk-adjusted surgical mortality rates for cardiovascular disease (see Chapter 9), early- versus late-stage diagnosis of cancer, and so on.

A second level of planning is **operational planning**, which has a functional scope. Although its time range is shorter and more functional, operational planning continues to address the organization's broadest levels of operation, such as financial planning. Other levels of planning are more functional. Tactical or operational planning is normally conducted at the unit level and has a much shorter time range. Its application focuses on the more routine activities of a department, such as the scheduling of staff to accommodate seasonal variations in demand. **Tactical planning** is generally carried out throughout the organization and concerns itself with the achievement of mission, vision, goals, and objectives on a day-to-day basis. It usually has a much shorter time horizon than strategic plans and is concerned with the nuts and bolts of running an organization.

Two additional levels of planning—project/program planning and contingency planning—address more specific aspects of organizational operation. **Project** or **program planning** addresses very specific activities of the organization. Its application is the design and management of a specific activity of the organization, such as construction of a new facility or service. The scope and time frame for this type of planning varies with the activity and is sometimes managed by an external construction company. A final category of planning is **contingency planning**. A contingency plan addresses the possible but not certain occurrence of a specific future event such as a disaster, unplanned weather, a union strike, or an epidemic. Scope varies, and the time line of the event is normally short, but decisions must be made immediately if the event occurs. As a result, contingency plans are developed in advance to ensure preparedness for these events. A recent problem with healthcare planning has been that of a turbulent and uncertain environment, which has made it difficult to plan a number of years into the future while, at the same time, many operational tasks require a great deal of time to complete. Rapid environmental change makes it difficult to plan for the evolution of managed care. An example would be limiting a strategic plan time horizon to a few years while implementation of an operational plan, such as a marketing strategy, may require just as many years to achieve the enrollment critical to self-sufficiency. Despite these limitations, planning remains essential, and each level of planning has an individual and specific function in healthcare. These functions are complementary: the performance of each planning function is required to maximize organizational performance.

Regardless of whether planning is done on the community or institutional level, and regardless of the level of planning that involves the professionals, the first step in developing an effective plan is to collect and analyze data regarding the present situation and the future. These data can be quantitative or qualitative, or both. For example, in addressing tuberculosis, quantitative data for planning might include the number of patients in the community who have active tuberculosis or the population at risk. These data are usually statistical in nature and can be manipulated through use of the epidemiological and biostatistical tools at the planner's disposal to address trends or conduct comparisons to other areas. Qualitative data, on the other hand, is not necessarily statistical. For example, the results of a focus group that has considered a question cannot be statistically manipulated. These results, however, are very useful data with an important role in planning; they can provide important insights to the planning process. Another type of qualitative data is key informant surveys, which are generally open-end discussions with major community leaders or stakeholders. Again, key informants are not a "random sample," and this type of survey does not lend itself to the usual epidemiological and statistical techniques available to the health planner. Again, this does not diminish the value of the data, it just limits their manipulation.

Community Health Planning Tools and Benchmarks

It is important in any planning process to have benchmarks. One of the most frequently used tools in community health planning is the Healthy People series. In 1979, *Healthy People*, the surgeon general's report on health promotion and disease prevention, was released. This monograph did several things: first, it established a series of goals that we, as a nation, should achieve in the year 1990. These goals were related to decreased mortality, by age group, for those up to 65 years of age, and they related to morbidity for those over 65:

Life Stage	1990 Target
Infants	35% lower death rate/9 deaths per 1,000 live births
Children	20% lower death rate/34 per 100,000
Adolescents/Young Adults	20% lower death rate/93 per 100,000
Adults	25% lower death rate/400 per 100,000
Older Adults	20% fewer days of restricted activity

The monograph also identified 15 priority programs, under the rubrics of health promotion, preventive services, and health protection.

Immediately following the release of this report, the Centers for Disease Control and Prevention, along with the federal Office of Disease Prevention and Health Promotion, convened a series of working groups. These groups had the charge to create specific objectives tied to the 15 priority areas that would help track our ability to achieve the life stage goals. Their report, published in 1980, was titled *Promoting Health/Preventing Disease; Objectives for the Nation* and presents materials in the following standard format:

- Nature and extent of the problem
- Prevention and promotion measures
- Specific national objectives for
    - Improved health status
    - Reduced risk factors
    - Improved public/professional awareness
    - Improved services/protection
    - Improved surveillance
- Principal assumptions underlying the objective
- Data necessary for tracking the objective

The process worked well, and as 1990 approached, the U.S. Department of Health and Human Services created a working group to establish objectives for the year 2000. In 1990, the next in the series of prevention benchmarks was published, *Healthy People 2000*, which had three major goals:

- Increase the span of healthy life for all Americans
- Reduce health disparities among Americans
- Achieve access to preventive services for all Americans

As with the 1990 objectives, the priority areas were grouped into a series of three principal areas (health promotion, health protection, and preventive services), each with health status objectives, risk reduction objectives and service/protection objectives. To illustrate, here are examples from one priority area, tobacco.

Health status objective: Reduce coronary heart disease deaths to no more than 100 per 100,000 people.

Risk reduction objective: Reduce cigarette smoking to a prevalence of no more than 15 percent among those aged 20 and older.

Service and protection objectives: Increase to at least 75 percent the proportion of worksites with a formal smoking policy that prohibits or severely restricts smoking in the workplace.

A logical question is, How well are we doing with these measures? Table 7.2 shows the 1977 baseline level on life stage objectives, the 1980 targets, where we finally ended up in 1990, the 1987 baseline, 2000 targets, and the status in a midcourse review done in 1992. Apparently, we were successful in exceeding the target in children, and we met the target in infants and adults; we were unsuccessful, however, in meeting the target for young people. We appeared to be doing very well with children again in this last decade as we nearly met the target for this age group only two years into the 1990s. Table 7.2 also shows how we were doing, in the midcourse 1995 review, in meeting the objectives target and the targets for minority populations.

TABLE 7.2
Progress on
Life-Stage
Objectives, 1995

Age Group	Year 1990 Targets*			Year 2000 Targets*		
	1977 Baseline	1990 Target	1990 Final	1987 Baseline	2000 Target	1992 Status
Infants (age <1)	1,412	900	908	1,008	700	852
Children (age 1–14)	42.3	34	30.1	33.7	28	28.8
Young people (age 15–24)	114.8	93	104.1	97.8	85	95.6
Adults (age 25–64)	532.9	400	400.4	426.9	340	394.7

*Deaths per 100,000 population
Source: Adapted from U.S. Department of Health and Human Services, Public Health Service. 1996. *Healthy People 2000: Midcourse Review and 1995 Revisions*. Washington DC: Government Printing Office.

The objectives for the year 2010 were released in January 2000. They are available on the web at http://web.health.gov/healthypeople. Table 7.3 compares priority areas for each of the three *Healthy People* series. Although new areas of interest are included in the more recent series (e.g., HIV disease), many of the priority areas remain the same: tobacco use, sexually transmitted diseases, nutrition, and so on.

It is obvious with this discussion that data systems must be designed and developed to track the objectives in the various reports. Such systems usually include vital statistics tracking systems. They may include special studies, such as the Behavioral Risk Factor Survey (BRFS) surveillance system that the CDC and the states use to track the various risk factors for disease. With all of its data sources, the major way that data are presented and reported has to do with both incidence and prevalence. In addition, traditional descriptive epidemiology is used to define the time, place, and person variables associated with the various objectives.

Several planning tools have been developed for use in community health planning activities. One of the most used tools—the one most linked to *Healthy People 2000*—is *Healthy Communities 2000: Model Standards.* This tool has been developed by the American Public Health Association (APHA) in conjunction with the CDC and several national public health organizations (1991). Table 7.4 shows how *Healthy Communities* can be used to tie local benchmarks to the national benchmarks contained in *Healthy People 2000* for tobacco use. The elimination of tobacco is one of eight model standard goals under health promotion. This goal can be accomplished by health status, risk reduction, and services/protection objectives that allow local communities to target dates for completion of each objective, and by indicators to measure success. According to Table 7.4, each community specifies a time (with year 2000 as the target) when tobacco-related mortality and morbidity, CHD, lung cancer, and COPD mortality rates will meet *Healthy People 2000* objectives. Moreover, a number of risk reduction objectives can be targeted, such as the prevalence rates of smoking and smoking cessation, as indicated in the table. *Healthy Communities 2000: Model Standards* encourages a consensus process to involve community leaders in the development of local goals, outcome and process objectives, and implementation plans to achieve the agreed-on objectives.

Another more recent tool, the *Healthy People 2010 Toolkit*, has been developed by the Public Health Foundation. Like *Healthy People 2010*, the tool kit is available on the World Wide Web at http://www.health.gov/healthypeople/state/toolkit. It identifies seven action areas:

- Building the foundation: leadership and structure
- Identifying and securing resources
- Identifying and engaging community partners
- Setting health priorities and establishing objectives

TABLE 7.3
Priority Areas for *Healthy People*

Category	1990	2000	2010
Health Promotion (1990; 2000) / Promote Healthy Behaviors (2010)	Smoking cessation; Misuse of alcohol/drugs; Improved nutrition; Exercise and fitness; Stress control	Tobacco; Alcohol and other drugs; Nutrition; Physical activity/Fitness; Family planning; Mental health/Disorders; Violent/Abusive behavior; Education/Community programs	Tobacco use; Nutrition and overweight; Physical activity/Fitness
Health Protection (1990; 2000) / Promote Health and Safe Communities (2010)	Toxic agent control; Occupational safety/Health; Accidental injury control; Infectious agent control	Food and drug safety; Occupational safety/Health; Unintentional injuries; Environmental health; Oral health	Education and Community-based programs; Food safety; Occupational safety and Health; Injury/Violence protection; Environmental health; Oral health
Preventive Services (1990; 2000) / Prevent and Reduce Diseases/Disorders (2010)	Immunizations; Family planning; Pregnancy and infant care; Sexually transmitted diseases; High blood pressure control	Immunization and Infectious diseases; Maternal and infant health; Sexually transmitted diseases; HIV infection; Heart disease and stroke; Cancer; Diabetes and chronic disabling conditions	Immunization and Infectious diseases; Sexually transmitted diseases; HIV; Heart disease and stroke; Cancer; Diabetes; Chronic kidney disease; Disability and secondary conditions; Mental health and mental disorders; Respiratory diseases; Substance abuse; Arthritis, osteoporosis, and chronic back conditions
Improved Systems for Personal and Public Health (2010)			Medical product safety; Family planning; Public health infrastructure; Maternal/Infant/Child health; Access to quality health services; Health communication; Vision and hearing

Source: U.S. Department of Health and Human Services. 1991. *Healthy People 2000: National Health Promotion and Disease Prevention Objectives.* Pub. No. (PHS) 91–50212. Washington, DC: Government Printing Office.; *Healthy People.* 1979. Pub. No. (PHS) 79-55071. Washington, DC: Government Printing Office; http://web.health.gov/healthypeople/prevagenda/focus.htm.

Category	Objectives	Indicator
Tobacco-Related Mortality	By ———reduce deaths due to tobacco-related diseases to no more than ———per 100,000 people *Model standards note*: Tobacco-related deaths include 20 diseases based on the Surgeon General's Report	Tobacco-related diseases death rate
Tobacco-Related Morbidity	By ———reduce morbidity due to tobacco-related diseases to no more than ———per 100,000 people *Model standards note*: Tobacco-related deaths include 20 diseases based on the surgeon general's report	a. Hospital days b. Disability days c. Costs
Deaths from Coronary Heart Disease	By ———(2000) reduce coronary heart disease deaths to no more than ———(100) per 100,000 people. (Age-adjusted baseline: 135 per 100,000 in 1987)	CHD death rate
Deaths from Lung Cancer	By ———(2000) slow the rise in lung cancer deaths to achieve a rate of no more than ———(42) per 100,000 people. (Age-adjusted baseline: 37.9 per 100,000 in 1987) *Model standards note*: Because this objective as stated is to slow the rise in deaths, the target rate is higher than the baseline rate.	Lung cancer death rate
Deaths from Chronic Obstructive Pulmonary Disease	By ———(2000) slow the rise in deaths from chronic obstructive pulmonary disease to achieve a rate of no more than ———(25) per 100,000 people. (Age-adjusted baseline: 18.7 per 100,000 in 1987)	COPD death rate
Prevalence of Cigarette Smoking	By ———(2000) reduce cigarette smoking to a prevalence of no more than ———(15) percent among people age 20 and older. (Baseline: 29 percent in 1987, 32 percent for men and 27 percent for women)	Percent smoking cigarettes
Smoking Cessation During Pregnancy	By ———(2000) increase smoking cessation during pregnancy so that at least ———(60) percent of women who are cigarette smokers at the time they became pregnant quit smoking early in pregnancy and maintain abstinence for the remainder of their pregnancy. (Baseline: 39 percent of white women ages 20–44 quit at any time during pregnancy in 1985)	Percent who quit smoking during pregnancy

TABLE 7.4
Model Standards
Objectives and
Indicators for Some
Tobacco-Related
Health Status and
Risk-Reduction
Objectives

Source: Adapted from American Public Health Association. 1991. *Healthy Communities 2000 Model Standards: Guidelines for Community Attainment of the Year 2000 National Health Objectives.* Washington, DC: American Public Health Association.

- Obtaining baseline measures, setting targets, and measuring progress
- Managing and sustaining the process
- Communicating health goals and objectives

Each of these seven areas includes

- a brief explanation and rationale;
- a checklist of major activities;
- tips for success;
- national and state examples to illustrate *Healthy People* processes in action;
- recommended "Hot Picks" of resources for more information; and
- planning tools easily adapted to state or local needs.

Obviously, epidemiology becomes important in the areas related to setting priorities and objectives and in obtaining baseline data and tracking progress. Again, it is traditional descriptive epidemiology and the concepts of disease prevalence and incidence that form the base of this community health planning process.

Another useful health planning tool is the Planned Approach to Community Health (PATCH). Developed by the CDC to focus on issues of chronic disease prevention, this model proceeds through a series of phases as well:

- Community mobilization
- Data collection and organization
- Health priorities selection
- Interventions
- Evaluation

An important point regarding PATCH is its explicit inclusion of evaluation in its methodology. As was pointed out at the beginning of this chapter, planning is part of a circular process that includes planning, implementation, and evaluation, and the sum of the process, in turn, leads to further planning.

The final model for discussion here is the Assessment Protocol for Excellence in Public Health (APEX/PH). This model was developed by the National Association for City and County Health Officers to assist local health departments in effectively planning, implementing, and evaluating programs designed to improve the health status of their communities. Health departments, however, are not the only settings in which the model has been used. APEX consists of three components:

- Organization capacity assessment
- Community process
- Completing the cycle

The organizational capacity assessment is designed to identify strengths and weaknesses in the health department's capacity to carry out the programs that will be identified by the community to improve health status. The health department director and senior staff carry out the assessment. This first APEX component looks at issues such as a program's authority to operate and manage major administrative areas such as finance and human resources.

The second component involves the creation of a community group to identify health problems, set priorities, and establish the health status objectives they wish to achieve. Generally the local group's objectives can follow the national objectives set out in *Healthy People 2000*, or the group can use *Healthy Communities 2000* to develop objectives. The major output of this process is the creation of a community health plan that is data driven and that represents the concerns of the community.

Finally, completing the cycle describes the implementation of that community health plan. This involves putting the results of the organizational assessment and the community health plan together and implementing the program. It allows the health department to better manage itself as the department contributes to the improvement of the community's health status. The steps in APEX/PH are outlined in Figure 7.1.

Effective planning is essential to organizational success. It is imperative to give clear direction about where the organization or community is headed. The goals and objectives must be clear and, in the case of health programs, accurate knowledge must be present to identify and describe the major community health problems that need to be addressed. This is true whether you are discussing health planning for the community or your institution's health planning. It is imperative that the tools of descriptive epidemiology play a part in identifying major health problems, and the use of time, place, and person descriptors of these health problems allows for the most effective planning. The ability to set priorities is influenced substantially by the burden of disease and its impact on the community: again, questions for epidemiology. Finally, it is important to remember that planning is part of the plan-implement-evaluate cycle: epidemiology is useful in the evaluation effort, as well.

- Prepare for organizational capacity assessment
- Score indicators for importance and current status
- Identify strengths and weaknesses
- Analyze and report strengths
- Analyze weaknesses
- Rank problems in order of priority
- Develop and implement action plans
- Institutionalize the assessment process

FIGURE 7.1
Assessment Protocol for Excellence in Public Health (APEX/PH) Steps

---

Source: Centers for Disease Control and Prevention (CDC). 1991. *APEX(PH) Assessment Protocol for Excellence in Public Health*. Bethesda, MD: CDC.

A number of health planning tools exist that can assist managers in the planning effort. These tools are well proven and many are experienced in their use. The successful planner will be familiar with them and their use in a variety of settings.

Institutional Planning

In healthcare organizations, planning tends to be done the way it has always been done. This is a consequence of several factors: staff do what they know and what they have experience doing, and they do what they are told to do, frequently by people who have similar previous work experiences. As a result, planning is frequently limited. In ways similar to theories of management, many proponents have advocated "one best way to plan," rather than recognizing that planning is situational. Issues of planning can be addressed on a positive or a normative basis. **Positive theory**, descriptive about what currently exists, makes predictions based on precedent, whereas **normative theory** addresses values and questions of future possibilities. There are four basic models of planning theory: rational/comprehensive, mixed scanning, incremental, and radical planning (Berry 1974).

Rational/Comprehensive planning seeks to consider the broadest view of the environment and its complexity. Basically the method identifies all opportunities for possible action by decision makers, identifies each consequence of each possible action, and selects the action that should result in the preferred set of consequences. The method seeks to consider data concerning all resources for technical decisions, and it works well if the future is stable, clear trends exist, values are implicit, and efficiency is the highest goal. Rational/Comprehensive planning is relevant to issues such as the development of a long-range master plan or the definition of specific health services in a particular community.

Incremental planning, a second method, involves conducting successive comparisons of options where the means to achieve outcomes are not considered. Incremental planning is most appropriate in addressing applied problems such as scarce resources, where there is an emphasis on workability and agreement on policy, and where conflicting values exist or compromise is important. Incremental planning is relevant to issues such as long-term situations where change is gradual, such as budget. A third method is **mixed scanning**, which creates a situational blend of the first two strategies using incremental decisions that lead to a fundamental issue. Mixed scanning permits a detailed examination of some aspects of a plan, along with limited detail in other areas; it is particularly applicable in a rapidly changing environment, where decision making requires flexibility. Mixed scanning is appropriate for issues such as the operation of a complex medical center. The fourth planning strategy, **radical planning**, emphasizes innovation and spontaneity and considers experimentation as a component of the learning process to achieve innovation. Radical planning may be most applicable to the resolution of an issue such as establishment of a new type of health program.

A Strategic Planning Model

A strategic plan is a useful and necessary tool in corporate strategy development— but it is not (nor should it be) the end objective. Strategic planning seeks to define the organization and its future with an emphasis on designing and bringing about a desired future rather than designing and implementing programs to achieve specific objectives.

Although a variety of approaches to strategic planning exist, they are all based on a generalized concept. This can be illustrated by Figure 7.2, from the accounting firm of Coopers & Lybrand. This model seeks to divide the strategic planning process into four sets of activities that answer four specific questions:

- Where are we now?
- Where should we be going?
- How should we get there?
- Are we getting there?

These questions focus on the activities of planning. For example, to answer the question "Where are we now?" a situational analysis is required where participants must collect and assemble data that address the organization's environment and operations. This leads to an assessment, such as a strengths/weaknesses/opportunities/threats (SWOT) analysis, and concludes with the establishment of a set of issues and challenges for the organization. The question "Where should

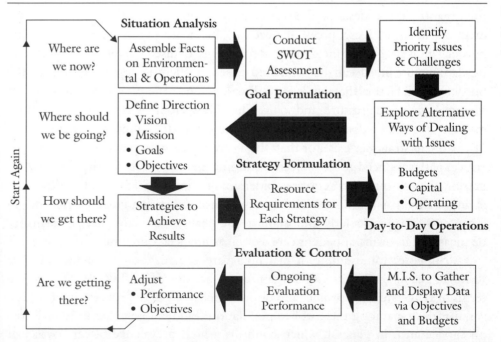

FIGURE 7.2
Strategic Planning Model

Source: Adapted from Keck, R. K., Jr. 1986. "Strategic Planning in the Health Care Industry: Concentrate on the Basics." *Health Care Issues* (September), reprinted in *Handbook of Business Strategy 1985/1986 Yearbook,* Coopers & Lybrand.

we be going?" can be answered with goal formulation, including an exploration of alternative strategies, and the development of organizational direction in the form of statements of vision, mission, goals, and objectives. Strategy formulation answers the question "How should we get there?" The exercise includes development of strategies or actions to achieve goals and an assessment of the resources needed to achieve each strategy goal (including budgets). Following the strategic implementation of operations, planners address evaluation and control through the final question, "Are we getting there?" The monitoring that this entails requires the collection and analysis of data, followed by the use of this performance feedback to adjust the organization's goals—and the management of operations to achieve these outcomes. This continuous process then is repeated from the beginning, using evaluation data as input for the next situational analysis and further refinement of the strategic planning process. This model breaks down a complex process of decision making into workable segments, but it requires a great deal of time and effort nevertheless. One must bear in mind, throughout the process, that in developing such a plan, the objective is not to write a plan, but to get something accomplished—to take action now regarding the future direction and profitability of the organization

All of these activities are informed by the collection of epidemiologic data. Morbidity profiles, for instance, describe the "Where are we now?" question. For a hospital, this might include case-mix measures or a breakdown of patients by DRGs. Physician practices could characterize patient mix by Current Procedure Terminology (CPT) code or the Resource-Based Relative Value Scale (RBRVS), in the case of Medicare Patients. The "Where should we be?" question requires the organization to describe the service population (both current and potential) in terms of need. Descriptors of need would include both current morbidity burden (measured by the incidence and prevalence of disease) and future morbidity burden. Future need can be estimated based on demographics, as well as the burden of risk factors that can lead to disease, such as the prevalence of smoking, obesity, high blood pressure, and so on. The "How should we get there?" question may also require epidemiologic input, to the extent that alternative patient care or treatment strategies exist, or that "best care" strategies, practice guidelines, or critical pathways need to be collected and implemented. Obviously, the "Are we getting there?" question requires epidemiologic input. Such input is described in more detail in the discussion of surveillance and risk-adjusted outcomes in Chapter 9. It is particularly important in the healthcare sector that performance be measured in terms of patient care as well as financial outcomes.

Suppose, for example, a managed care organization is engaged in the strategic planning process. The organization has described "where they are" in terms of DRG and CPT profiles and notices a relatively high proportion of cardiovascular disease among the enrolled population. Epidemiologic data are collected on service area, in general, which confirms a high prevalence of cardiovascular disease, as well as cardiovascular risk factors such as smoking and obesity. The organization decides to address the "Where should we be?" question by focusing specifically on cardiovascular disease, among other things. The question of how to get there is somewhat more complex; it involves many decisions, such as whether or not to promote prevention through smoking cessation and weight reduction programs. Epidemiologic studies may provide useful insight into this decision-making process.

Marketing

An organization's most precious asset is its relationship with customers as defined in terms of quality, service, and price. Although many view marketing as advertising, it is a far more complex set of activities. At the most basic level, marketing can be defined as an exchange between two parties to satisfy the needs of both: in the case of healthcare, an exchange of health services for appropriate compensation. Traditional marketing can be described by the **four Ps** of marketing: product, place, price, and promotion. **Product** or service defines the activity of the organization and can be described, for healthcare, as the set of activities focused on particular diagnoses, such as acute myocardial infarction. Alternatively, product/service can be described as the benefits the service provides to the patient, such as relief from pain or anxiety or help in achieving a longer life.

Place or location refers to how the product or service will be delivered to the patient. This marketing concept refers not simply to location, but to other factors such as operating hours, referral mechanisms, and enablers and barriers to access based on both external market segmentation and internal operational factors. The third measure, **price** or fees, addresses not only the charge for the service (which usually is not paid by the patient), but everything that the organization requires the patient to go through to use the service. Price links revenue and consumer satisfaction, as it controls a potential conflict of interest between providing the highest-quality product and increasing revenue. **Promotion** includes activities to acquaint the prospective patient with the organization and the services it offers. Promotion is a matter of communicating information between an organization and a market; it describes the means by which the patient becomes aware of the services offered and develops an interest in using one or more of the services. Strategic concepts in marketing include product differentiation, price competition, market segmentation by socioeconomic variables, product segmentation for different populations, and mass marketing/advertising. A subcategory of marketing, with a direct relationship to healthcare, is known as social marketing, which focuses on behavior (e.g., on changing health behaviors such as smoking or diet).

Although planning and marketing are closely related both conceptually and operationally (MacStravic 1977), it is the former that has received more considerable attention in terms of governmental policy: note the litany of health planning legislation reviewed earlier in the chapter (Lee 1989). "Planning presents a method for design and management of change, while marketing offers design and management of exchange relations with important publics" (Lee 1989). Clearly, both planning and marketing are informed by epidemiologic measures. A critical stage of planning is environmental assessment (or needs assessment), in which the organization or agency attempts to characterize the needs of the population served. In the case of healthcare, this must involve morbidity profiles, described specifically in terms of the incidence and prevalence rates of acute and chronic disease. Marketing strategies should also incorporate epidemiologic measures. Product definition, for instance, depends to some degree on descriptions of need. The development of a women's health "product" should be defined on the basis of dimensions of need in this area, much of which is epidemiologically derived—the prevalence of breast and ovarian cancer, for instance. Strategies with regard to place include an assessment of barriers to access. These barriers may be recognized, to some degree, on the basis of epidemiologic measures, the high incidence of cervical cancer among women in eastern Kentucky, for example. Promotional activities may include motivational messages, based in part on epidemiologic studies. Primary prevention, such as cancer screening, can be promoted by encouraging clients to consider the advantages of early- versus late-stage diagnosis in terms of survival studies. Social marketing has clear epidemiologic roots to the extent that behaviors, such as smoking, diet, and sexual behaviors, have been epidemiologically linked to morbidity.

Conclusion

Earlier we described planning as making assessments and provision for the future, or as making current choices to influence the future, which may involve guiding the process of change. We have demonstrated the need and the means by which both community and institutional planning should be intimately acquainted with epidemiologic measures. *Healthy People 2000* for example, groups objectives in terms of health status objectives (measured in terms of disease-specific mortality rates, for instance) and risk reduction objectives (measured in terms of reducing the prevalence of a risk factor among the population). With institutional planning, questions regarding the current and future position or role within a health service market require both internal and external assessment processes that thrive on valid epidemiologic measures. Finally, to the extent that planning and marketing are flip-sides of the same coin, organizations would benefit by using epidemiology to describe the morbidity and risk factor burden of current and potential markets, and by using epidemiologic studies to facilitate the promotion of healthcare products to the consumer.

Case Study 7.1

Eastern Kentucky Health

Eastern Kentucky Health (EKH) is a fictitious IPA model health maintenance organization that serves patients in a number of counties in southeastern Kentucky. EKH has entered into partnership with several local communities to meet *Healthy*

People 2000 objectives, but it is struggling with a number of priority areas dealing with tobacco use, obesity, hypertension, and related mortality (refer to Table 7.5):

1. What are the kinds and sources of data that need to be collected to make rational planning decisions?
2. What kinds of interventions should EKH consider to address the key priority areas?
3. How might EKH market these programs to the enrolled population?

Case Study 7.2

Poudre Valley

Poudre Valley is a profitable hospital in Fort Collins, Colorado with a 90 percent market share and a 7 percent operating margin, according to a report by Fitch IBCA, a New York-based credit rating agency. Lower Medicare reimbursement under the balanced budget act is likely to continue to eat away at those earnings, according to Fitch. But Stacey, Poudre Valley Health System CEO, says planning for the new campus began three years ago, and that the lower reimbursement isn't a reason to back out of the plan. "We've known for some time that rates are going down. It's important for us to be as diversified as possible and have opportunities in outpatient medicine," he says.

Construction on the building is already under way. The facility will include a catheter lab, an ambulatory surgery center, a radiology diagnostic center, and an oncology diagnostic center. Total costs will run to $55 million, Stacey says.

The physicians are equity partners in each of these joint ventures and will pay between one-third and half the cost of the new project. That lessens the capital strain on the hospital, but also cuts into its profits, which are divided according to ownership, but Stacey says the tradeoff is well worth it.

"It really ties (the doctors) into cost containment," he says. (*Preemptive strike*: Part of what drove the deals, according to Stacey, was the knowledge that if the hospital didn't partner with the doctors and help build them new facilities, the doctors could build competing facilities.) Stacey adds, "We think this strategy allows us to maintain access to revenue streams that we otherwise might have lost." (Saphir 1999).

1. Describe the kinds of planning activity that preceded the decision to invest $55 million in the new facilities.
2. What kinds of epidemiologic data should have been collected to inform this decision-making process?
3. What are the advantages and disadvantages of having physicians as equity partners?
4. To what extent should physicians be a source of epidemiologic data?
5. What other sources of epidemiologic data could be collected?

TABLE 7-5
Mortality Rates, Smoking, and Obesity

Category	Baseline (1987)	Kentucky (1998)**	United States (1998)**	2000 Goal
Cigarette Smoking				
High school education, adults	34%	36%	23%	20%
Blue collar workers, adults	36%	40%	29%	20%
White, adults		31%	23%	
Blacks, adults	34%	26%	23%	18%
Women of reproductive age*	29%	28% (women)	21% (women)	12%
Pregnant women‡	25%	28% (women)	21% (women)	10%
Obesity		36%	32%	
Adolescents	15%†			15%
Adults	26%†			20%
Low-income women	37%†			25%
Black women	44%†			30%
Reduce coronary heart disease mortality (per 100,000)	135			100
Slow the rise in lung cancer mortality (per 100,000)§	47.9			53
Slow the rise in COPD mortality (per 100,000)§	18.7			25

*Baseline for women 18–44; †Baseline is 1976–1980; ‡1985 baseline.

§The objective is to slow the rise; the rate in 2000 is projected to be higher than the goal.

** Behavioral Risk Factor Surveillance System.

Source: American Public Health Association. 1991. *Healthy Communities 2000 Model Standards: Guidelines for Community Attainment for the Year 2000 National Health Objectives.* Washington, DC: APHA.

References

American Public Health Association (APHA). 1991. *Healthy Communities 2000 Model Standards: Guidelines for Community Attainment of the Year 2000 National Health Objectives.* Washington, DC: APHA.

Berry, D. E. 1974. "The Transfer of Planning Theories to Health Planning Practice." *Policy Sciences* 5: 343–61.

Centers for Disease Control and Prevention (CDC). 1991. *APEX(PH) Assessment Protocol for Excellence in Public Health.* Bethesda, MD: CDC.

Duncan, W. J., P. M. Ginter, and L. E. Swayne. 1995. *Strategic Management of Health Care Organizations.* Malden, MA: Blackwell Publishers.

Hoge, V. M. 1958. "Hospital Bed Needs: A Review of Developments in the United States." *Canadian Journal of Public Health* 49 (1): 1–8.

Keck, R. K., Jr. 1986. "Strategic Planning in the Health Care Industry: Concentrate on the Basics." *Health Care Issues* (September), reprinted in *Handbook of Business Strategy 1985/1986 Yearbook*, Coopers & Lybrand.

Lee, J. M. 1989. "Marketing in Health Services Administration." In *Handbook of Human Services Administration*, edited by J. Rabin and M. Steinhauser. New York: Marcel Decker.

Lee, R. I., and L. W. Jones. 1933. *The Fundamentals of Good Medical Care.* Publication of the Committee on the Costs of Medical Care, No. 22. Chicago: University of Chicago Press.

MacStravic, R. E. 1977. *Marketing Health Care.* Germantown, MD: Aspen Systems.

Peddecord, K. M. 1998. "Public Health Management Tools Planning." In *Maxcy-Rosenau-Last: Public Health and Preventive Medicine, 14th ed.*, edited by R. B. Wallace and B. N. Doebbeling, Stamford, CT: Appleton & Lang.

Saphir, A. 1999. "Erector Set." *Modern Healthcare* 29 (49): 50.

U.S. Department of Health and Human Services, Public Health Service. 1996. *Healthy People 2000: Midcourse Review and 1995 Revisions.* Washington, DC: Government Printing Office.

U.S. Department of Health and Human Services. 1991. *Healthy People 2000: National Health Promotion and Disease Prevention Objectives.* Pub. No. (PHS) 91–50212. Washington, DC: Government Printing Office.

———. 1980. *Promoting Health/Preventing Disease: Objectives for the Nation.* Washington, DC: Government Printing Office.

———. 1979. *Healthy People.* Pub. No. (PHS) 79-55071. Washington, DC: Government Printing Office.

Epidemiology and the Directing Function

Kevin C. Lomax and Steven T. Fleming

> *Mr. Jones needs to discuss with the medical staff of Group Health East a new incentive and performance appraisal system that will link both quality of care and utilization to capitation contracts. Jones needs to demonstrate leadership in this area and wants to be a credible supporter of this plan. How might he use epidemiology to bolster his arguments in favor of this plan?*

The purpose of this chapter is to describe how healthcare managers can incorporate epidemiologic concepts and principles into the directing function. Rakich, Longest, and Darr (1992) describe direction as "activities [that] include motivating, leading, and communicating, as well as other activities that influence employee behavior." In fact, they devote separate chapters to motivation, leadership, and communication. Doubtless all of these activities relate to directing, a crucial function and perhaps the most preeminent role of a manager. Our goal for this chapter is not to convince the reader that epidemiologic principles should wax prominent in each and every directing decision that the executive makes. Rather, we suggest that a fundamental understanding of epidemiology, including the notions of risk, burden of disease, and various kinds of epidemiologic inquiry, may elucidate some decisions, and can become a source of power and credibility for the healthcare executive.

In this chapter, we discuss how epidemiology can be used to motivate people and whether the use of epidemiologic principles is consistent with theories X, Y, and Z of management. We articulate a theory of leadership, differentiate between managers and leaders, and discuss the application of epidemiologic concepts and methods to each of these roles. Finally, we describe ways in which epidemiology can improve communication within the organization.

Theory of Motivation

A number of theories postulate approaches for motivating people to behave in ways that are consistent with organizational goals (Rakish, Longest, and Darr 1992). These theories can be categorized by their relationship to content or process. The content theories focus on particular needs that motivate human behavior, such as the need for esteem. The process theories focus on the expectations and preferences that individuals have for outcomes related to their performance.

Figure 8.1 illustrates an integrative model for motivation that assimilates both the content and the process theory. Notice that performance is determined in part by the effort exerted by workers subject to the constraints of ability (such as skills and training) and particular situations (e.g, budgetary constraints). The degree to which workers enjoy satisfaction with the job is related to the intrinsic and extrinsic rewards they receive, which then motivates continued or increased effort. Workers also have expectations (expectancy) regarding their performance, according to Vroom (1964), either in terms of rewards (such as more money) or other intrinsic kinds or satisfaction—"a job well done" or "patient gratitude" at the very least.

Epidemiology and Motivation

The directing function of a manager involves motivating people; thus the challenge here is to maximize performance over the long term, through a system of rewards leading to satisfaction. The manager can integrate epidemiology into the calculus of motivation at several stages in the model. The translation of effort into performance depends, to a significant degree, on ability. It is the manager's responsibility to ensure that subordinates possess the necessary knowledge and skills to effectively complete their tasks. We suggest that epidemiology is one of these competencies for many healthcare workers.

Consider the following scenario, for instance. Suppose that you are the administrator of a large nursing home and have a desire to maximize the performance of the nurses aides. In order for their efforts to be translated into effective performance, some physical and mental skills are necessary, such as proper body mechanics in moving patients. A fundamental knowledge of risk factors and disease would be helpful so that these workers could understand the rationale behind their

FIGURE 8.1

Integrative Model of Motivation

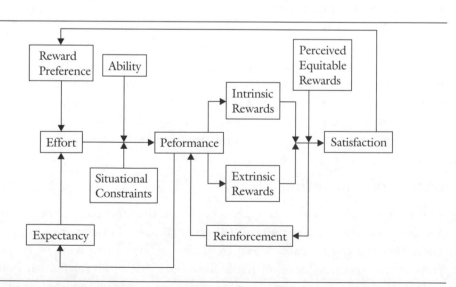

Source: Rakich, J. S., B. B. Longest, and K. Darr. 1996. *Managing Health Services Organizations*. Baltimore, MD: Health Professions Press.

behavior, such as the prevalence of bedsores in nursing home patients caused by lack of mobility and the relative risk of infection and hospitalization associated with these adverse outcomes.

The purpose of integrating epidemiologic theory is to elucidate, provide rationales for behavior, and thereby motivate. Consider the following illustrations in the hospital setting:

Housekeeping. Your job at keeping this place clean is important to patient welfare. Did you know that the kind of microbes that live around here tend to be resistant to the antibiotics that we currently have available? It's so easy for patients to get really sick if they are exposed to these microbes, particularly if they just had surgery. That's why we spend so much time scrubbing the operating rooms.

Dietary. Proper nutrition is so important for patient satisfaction and recovery. It's really important to wash our hands regularly before handling food since the really nasty bacteria that grow around here could infect the food we feed patients. That food could then become a source of food poisoning for our patients.

RN. I really appreciate that you are using proper infection control techniques with the Foley catheters. Do you have any idea how many of these patients end up with urinary track infections? The risk of kidney infections with a UTI is another caution, particularly for the patients who are immuno-compromised.

Performance may also lead to satisfaction to the extent that workers receive either intrinsic or extrinsic rewards. Extrinsic rewards, such as bonuses or other forms of recognition, may be tied directly to patient outcomes that will, one hopes, be risk-adjusted to some degree (see Chapter 9). For example, nurses aides may be individually rewarded to the degree that their patients remain free of bedsores. The aides who care for the immobile patients who are at higher risk of bedsores ought not to be penalized if their patients get bedsores despite careful attention. Intrinsic rewards would include knowing that one's efforts are worthwhile, useful, or appreciated. This should involve a process of communicating to healthcare workers, in epidemiologic terms, the burden of illness in the population that is served, the kinds of treatment that are effective in reducing that burden, and the roles that are played specifically by each worker in reaching those goals. Nurses should know, for instance, the incidence of nosocomial infections in most large medical centers, the increasing incidence of drug-resistant strains of some common pathogens, and the critical connection between aseptic technique and infection control.

Performance and effort are also related by the factor of "expectancy." Vroom suggests that people make choices to fulfill needs (in any employment situation, for instance), but they must believe that their performance will lead to some desired outcome or reward (1964). Moreover, they must value the outcome. Expectancy is "what individuals perceive to be the probability that their efforts will lead to a desired level of performance" (Rakich, Longest, and Darr 1992).

In a sense, this is a feedback loop to the extent that workers evaluate their own performance, weigh it against expectations, and modify their effort accordingly. Managers can use epidemiologic input as a tool to convince healthcare workers that their efforts will lead to patient improvement.

Consider the following example. Mr. Smith is a 76-year-old patient recovering from esophageal cancer. He had major surgery to remove the tumor one year ago, but it recently spread to the brain. The series of radiation therapy treatments to treat the brain cancer has left him immobile, depressed, and unwilling to eat. According to the integrative model of motivation suggested in Figure 8.1, the effort expended by nurses to ambulate Mr. Smith, cheer him up, and get him to eat depends to some degree on expectations regarding the utility (or futility) of their work. Do the nurses think that their efforts will be useful and make a positive contribution toward patient recovery? If nursing managers were to communicate the context of Mr. Smith's illness in epidemiologic terms, they might get more effort on the part of the nurses. For example, they would want to communicate the probability of survival for an esophageal cancer patient with metastases to the brain, the importance of ambulation in this kind of case, and whether or not this kind of depression is typically a treatable illness.

It may also be necessary to healthcare workers to motivate patients. If one accepts the supposition that motivation is simple because behavior is goal-directed (Rakich, Longest, and Darr 1992), this applies to patients as well as employees and is grounded in the basic tenets of epidemiology. For example, the underlying premise behind what Pearce (1996) refers to as "modern epidemiology" is the shift in unit of analysis from populations to individuals, and thus the move is to discovery and delineation of individual risk factors of disease. The purpose of this knowledge clearly is goal directed to the extent that these risk factors can be modified. Why does one need to know that a high-fat diet can lead to heart disease? Presumably so that one can be motivated to modify one's diet in a way that can reduce that risk. Managers need to communicate the basics of epidemiology to workers, particularly those who deal directly with patients, so that workers can understand the rationale behind therapeutic services or efforts to modify patient behavior. For example, a post-surgical cancer patient would be more motivated to practice breathing exercises if he or she knew that these exercises decreased the chances of developing pneumonia.

Theories of Management and Motivation

Management research over the past few decades has been based on three theories of management. Two of the three are McGregor's bipolar management views of Theory X and Theory Y. The third, Theory Z, was developed by Ouchi (1981) as an extension of McGregor's postulates. Theory X proposes an autocratic management style that probably should not be embraced by the healthcare industry, because the basic assumptions of the theory are not consistent with the service orientation of healthcare organizations. Healthcare organizations are simply about people. Therefore, positive healthcare outcomes cannot be realized without the effort and ability of people within the organization. If people are viewed as objects to be used at the sole discretion of the organization, positive outcomes through genuine service are not going to materialize.

The Theory Y model of management, which is participative in nature, is more directly related to healthcare organization because of the inherent nature of "serving" in the healthcare field. This distinction in managerial attitudes about employees is critical in a healthcare setting, because healthcare delivery is founded on the premise of service and on the assumption that individuals enter a healthcare profession for more than monetary reward. Thus, healthcare workers should be entering their field highly motivated and with a positive work attitude. However, this may be more common among healthcare professionals, such as physicians, nurses, and skilled technicians, and not among low-level workers, such as nurses aides or housekeepers. This divergence of motivation and attitudes between higher- and lower-level employees could perhaps be reduced by in-service training on the basics of epidemiology for all levels of employees. The ultimate purpose of such training would be to establish a connection between routine low-level tasks (such as housekeeping) and patient outcomes.

According to Theory Z, the overarching goal of the organization should be to create an organizational culture that involves workers as critical participants (Shortell 1982). Part of this "empowerment" process may include the cultivation of an "epidemiologic perspective" among managers and employees. Although such a perspective is laudable, it may be difficult to attain or afford in the present-day healthcare environment. Furthermore, the five components of Theory Z management, as espoused by Ouchi (1981), are not consistently applied in the healthcare industry: (1) **Lifetime employment** is almost nonexistent in American business, healthcare organizations included, given the current atmosphere of merger, acquisition, and cost reduction. In addition, many healthcare organizations are burdened with severe financial constraints, thus creating a "temporary employee" mentality. Many healthcare organizations are finding it difficult, if not impossible, to (2) **invest in skills development,** such as epidemiologic training. Information technology, such as electronic patient records will one day make it possible to (3) **balance implicit and explicit decision-making criteria**. While the former would include culture and philosophy, the latter could include not just financial ratios, but also epidemiologic measures such as morbidity, mortality, and the relative risk of protective and malicious behaviors. Epidemiologic training could facilitate (4) **participatory decision making** to the extent that such knowledge improves communication within and among different levels of the organization. Finally, Theory Z organizations are supposed to have a (5) **holistic view of employees**, with less emphasis on superior-subordinate relationships among people in the organization (Rakich, Longest, and Darr 1992). Clearly, total quality management (TQM) is a step in the right direction in this regard, as would be the nurture of an epidemiologic way of thinking about the business and practice of healthcare.

Performance, according to Figure 8.1, is also a function of the type of reinforcement an employee receives. Reinforcement theory was proposed by behavioral psychologist B. F. Skinner. The basic premise of reinforcement theory is that people are conditioned by the outcomes of their past situational responses (Skinner 1953). Some researchers have argued, however, that this predetermined view of behavior restricts free choice in each situation. There are four managerial options for applying reinforcement theory to management practice and motivating employees: (1) positive reinforcement, (2) negative reinforcement, (3) extinction, and (4) punishment (Skinner 1953). Positive reinforcement refers to providing desirable consequences for specific behavior. In the case of nurses aides, providing concert tickets or paid time off for having attained specific epidemiologic goals in the organization would be an example of positive reinforcement. Conversely, negative reinforcement is the application of negative consequences to the same behavior. If the specific outcomes were not reached, the aides could be assigned weekend duty, for instance. The third component of reinforcement theory, extinction, refers to the weakening of a specific behavior by failing to respond to it in any way. Finally, punishment is the weakening of a behavior by administering an undesirable consequence such as suspension. Temporarily suspending a nurses aide for the specific violation of an organization policy, or for failure to follow published hygiene directions regarding patients for an extended period of time would be an example of this fourth component of reinforcement theory.

As this section has noted in detail, motivation is the key to performance in the organization, and an understanding of epidemiology may itself be a motivator. The next section deals with leadership, more specifically, ways in which epidemiologic concepts and principles can be used to develop leadership skills, become a source of power, and influence leadership behavior.

Epidemiology and Leadership Behavior

The literature on leadership can be segmented into two camps: managership and leadership. Research on managership, conducted primarily by psychologists, examines the role of middle- and lower-level supervisors. These studies focus on various elements of the supervisor-subordinate relationship (e.g., supervisory styles, behaviors, situational characteristics, subordinate perceptions, and attributions) and their impact on employee satisfaction and productivity. The studies of leadership conducted primarily by organizational theorists analyze the role of top administration. These studies focus on the relationship of top executives to the people and the systems they direct as well as to the external environment in which they operate. The key executive activities include strategies to mobilize internal and external support, efforts to develop employees, decisions regarding the purpose and direction of the organization, assessment of external threats and opportunities, and responses to those threats and opportunities. These activities are viewed as critical to the organization's survival, legitimacy, and goal attainment (Hersey and Blanchard 1977).

Rakich and colleagues (1992) present an integrative model of leadership (Figure 8.2) that suggests that leadership behavior is determined by traits, skills, power, situations, and intervening variables such as resources and teamwork. Despite this simple paradigm, leadership is one of the most elusive concepts in management. J. M. Burns (1978) states that "leadership is one of the most observed and least understood phenomena on earth." It is difficult to delineate the characteristics of a "good" leader in a way that will differentiate such a leader from others. Perhaps a more salient question for the balance of this chapter would be whether an "effective" leader in this age of capitation must embrace the concepts and principles of epidemiology to be effective.

We are interested in leadership in the setting of the formal organization, particularly in the healthcare field: hospitals, nursing homes, ambulatory care centers, and managed care organizations. Consequently, theories of leadership must be linked to the organizational context in which they occur. Rakish and colleagues (1992) define leadership as the "process of influencing people to achieve particular goals." This is usually achieved by employing the motivational techniques discussed in the previous section.

For many years leadership has been considered synonymous with managerial behavior. Researchers have held the view that leadership is a critical role of any effective manager (Mintzberg 1973). However, some researchers have drawn more specific distinctions in the nuances of leadership and its role in management. One early work distinguishes leadership in terms of "an organizational function" versus "a set of personal abilities" (Bavelas 1942). The organizational function refers to the distribution of decision-making powers throughout the organization while organizational leadership consists of making choices to reduce uncertainty. Choices of this type are made using rational calculations, with maintaining organizational efficiency the chief aim in the organization. Personal leadership, on the

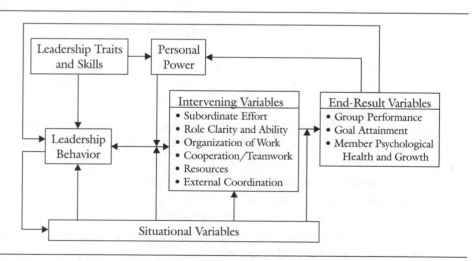

FIGURE 8.2
Integrative Conceptual Model of Leadership

Source: Rakich, J. S., B. B. Longest, and K. Darr. 1992. *Managing Health Services Organizations*. Baltimore, MD: Health Professions Press. Adapted from Yuki, Gary A. *Leadership Organizations, 2nd ed*. Copyright © 1998. Reprinted by permission of Prentice-Hall, Inc., Upper Saddle River, NJ.

other hand, involves the ability to innovate and take risks. However, a manager's propensity toward innovative thinking and risk-taking is more likely to decline as the organization moves along the business cycle from birth to maturity. This distinction between organizational and personal leadership is a corollary to the difference between management and entrepreneurship. Finally, Bavelas suggests a dual typology for leadership styles. The dyads are organizational leadership–middle management functioning and personal leadership–top administrative functioning. This typology creates a hierarchial structure of leadership segregating duties within levels of management responsibility.

Other researchers have made similar distinctions regarding managership versus leadership in the organizational setting. Zaleznik (1977) argues that organizational systems, with their bureaucratic structure, are innately conservative. Furthermore, only extremely conservative managers will be successful within such systems. The managerial culture in these systems are characterized by tradition, inertia, collective decision making, risk avoidance, and maintenance of the status quo. Zaleznik also contrasts this managerial culture with leadership in three respects:

1. The adoption of personal and active attitudes with respect to goal-setting, idea generation, and planning objectives.
2. The development of new and creative approaches to long-term organizational problems.
3. Empathetic communication toward subordinates and a strong focus on decision making and the reasons and potential outcomes of those decisions.

Sheldon and Barrett (1977) also present these same distinctions in the healthcare literature. They describe the leadership types that will create a convergence of healthcare organizations, which is much needed since many organizations compete for the same diminishing resources. Managership is contrasted with leadership as being a creation of efficient solutions rather than problem identification. Simply stated, leaders are more problem-centered at the organizational level rather than solution-based at the personnel level. Thus, leaders must implement a positive strategy toward both internal and external organizational problems. This is because long-range planning and resource development is essential for an organization's success and posterity. Within this organizational framework, managers have been defined as keepers of the status quo (Hutchens 1979), while leaders have been given the mantle of action and progressive change.

In summary, we characterize the organizational divide between managers and leaders in terms of (1) substance and (2) action: in other words, what decisions are taken and the methods for implementing those decisions. Managers get people to perform specific job requirements while leaders motivate performance in people that is above and beyond any job description.

Both managers and leaders would benefit from the integration of epidemiologic principles into the managerial "practice style." Managers need to motivate people at all levels of the organization to engage their skills and talents toward meeting the organizational objectives of providing cost-effective patient care. This may involve providing epidemiologic insight into the roles and responsibilities of the job, as discussed earlier in the section on motivation. Leaders, on the other hand, need to be proactive and visionary. They are regularly challenged by problems seeking creative solutions, the recognition, definition, and solution of which should be epidemiologically informed, if not derived.

Leader Traits and Skills

The search for the unique set of traits associated with leadership began with biographical studies of prominent political leaders. Such studies were soon complemented by more formal searches for traits that distinguished leaders from followers, effective from ineffective leaders, and higher-level from lower-level leaders. Bass (1982) lists 17 personality traits that have been correlated positively with leadership; these include dominance and self-confidence (the most frequently associated traits), and emotional control, independence, and creativity (the next most frequent traits). Social skills, such as sociability and administrative ability have also been associated with leadership. Some research evidence suggests that such traits have a limited ability to explain differences in leadership effectiveness. Finally, as Gibb (1947) discusses them: "Traits of leadership are any or all of those personality traits which, in any particular situation, enable an individual to (i) contribute significantly to group locomotion in the direction of a recognized goal, and (ii) be perceived as doing so by fellow group members." In effect, Gibb concludes that the traits associated with leadership are contingent on the nature of the task, the goal pursued, and the characteristics of group members.

In their recognition of the difficulties in documenting universal traits of leaders, many researchers have turned to other strategies. The new lines of inquiry are behaviorally oriented. The basic research question changes from "Which trait is associated with leadership?" to "What behaviors are associated with leadership?" and "What functions do leaders perform in effective groups?"

Gibb suggests that leadership traits depend on the nature of the task and on the goal(s) pursued. In the healthcare field the nature of the task is either directly or indirectly related to the practice of medicine, and the goal pursued is often patient care. Moreover, whether these leaders are senior-level executives, mid-level managers, or members of the governing board, healthcare leaders must regularly interact with physicians, nurses, and other medical professionals in group settings in order to be effective leaders. In group settings with clinicians, leaders are more likely to exhibit positive leadership traits, such as self-confidence, if they have a fundamental understanding of epidemiologic principles. They are more likely to be articulate in voicing administrative concerns if these issues are couched in a thorough understanding of risk, disease burden, and other epidemiologic concepts. In short, epidemiology can become a source of power for the healthcare leader.

Personal Power

Leadership ability is also closely related to the concepts of both power and influence. These terms differ in that power is a component of influence. By this we mean that power is defined as the "potential to exert influence" (Rakich, Longest, and Darr 1992), whereas the ability to influence people is the measurement standard of leadership in modern society.

There are five types of leadership power: legitimate, reward, coercive, expert, and referent (Rakich, Longest, and Darr 1992). Even though epidemiologic principles may not be completely applicable within the behavioral structure of all power types, there are epidemiologic applications for each type. **Legitimate power** is power based on authority. The fundamental tenet of this type of power is the right to tell subordinates what to do; it is similar to a contract labor relationship where subordinates relinquish all decision-making authority to the hiring agent. **Reward power** is defined as the ability to distribute a reward to subordinates for performing desired tasks. This type of power lies in the assumption that the people involved want the reward. The most undesirable type of power is coercive power. **Coercive power** is the opposite of reward power because it substitutes—for the ability to reward people for positive activity—punishment of people for engaging in undesirable behavior or performing undesirable tasks. **Referent power** is the power most closely identified with the personal characteristics—such as charisma—of the actual leader: this type of power uses the subordinate's desire to be in the company of a charismatic individual. Finally, **expert power** is based on the experience and expertise of the leader. Subordinates know that the leader is the expert in their field or industry and defer to this expertise.

The question here is whether a knowledge of epidemiology can be a source of power for the healthcare leader. Clearly, some people within the organization are able to claim legitimate power in this regard, perhaps the chief of infectious disease or the director of infection control. In addition, perhaps others may derive this power on the basis of recognized epidemiological expertise. Leaders who develop competencies in the area of epidemiology may be recognized by virtue of their power as experts and thus may be sought after for advice in addition to, or instead of, the more legitimate sources of advice. Thus, expert power becomes a source of "credibility."

Consider the ways in which power and leadership are exercised in the following encounter between the CEO of Bluegrass East, a 1,000-bed teaching hospital, and the hospital's chief of cardiology regarding balloon angioplasty:

Mr. Bottomline: I am on my way to a board meeting, Dr. Heart; now what was it you wanted to talk to me about?

Dr. Heart: We spoke briefly a month ago about opening up a balloon angioplasty lab on the third floor of the east wing. University Hospital across town has been doing these procedures for years now, and I'm afraid we are beginning to see a decrease in cardiology patients.

Mr. Bottomline: Oh really? Have you worked out the financials? How long do you think it will take to break even on this venture?

Dr. Heart: I'll talk to Mr. Noredline [the CFO] and get back to you by next week, but I'm convinced that we really need to move ahead before we lose market share.

Now consider a similar meeting between the COO, Mr. Epiwise, and Dr. Heart:

Mr. Epiwise: So nice to see you, Dr. Heart, and how is [your wife] Emily?

Dr. Heart: She just got promoted recently at Eastside, but what I really wanted to talk to you about was the proposed balloon angioplasty lab on the third floor of the east wing that we talked about last month.

Mr. Epiwise: I have given it some consideration. Have you seen any studies that have compared angioplasty to the more conventional alternatives in terms of outcomes? I would be particularly interested to see how the postsurgical mortality rates compare, and whether there are any other kinds of unwanted side effects. Are angioplasty patients at risk for other kinds of morbidity, for instance?

Dr. Heart: I will compare angioplasty to our alternatives and get you a report as soon as I can.

Mr. Epiwise: That's just great. A cost-effectiveness analysis would be wonderful. I am curious to see how the cost per symptom-free year of survival compares.

Epidemiology and Communication

The final section of this chapter presents a discussion of communication principles in healthcare organizations and the relationship between health communication and epidemiology. One basic definition of communication is the creation or exchange of understanding between sender(s) and receiver(s) (Rakich, Longest, and Darr 1992). From an applied clinical perspective, communication is the means by which information is obtained in order to make a diagnosis and prescribe treatment. It is also the way in which patients can obtain information in order to make informed decisions; understand their illnesses; participate in therapy; and share thoughts, ideas, and feelings. Since poor communication is the underlying cause of major managerial and patient conflict in healthcare, communication can be viewed as the crux of effective healthcare delivery.

Communication also has a major effect on healthcare satisfaction (for both patients and healthcare professionals), compliance, patient health outcomes, and medical malpractice litigation. In today's managed care environment, effective communication is critical to the changing roles of healthcare professionals and to the new, more active role of patients. Increased patient education is necessary, and the retraining of many healthcare professionals is mandatory. This new educational component of healthcare will provide a structured vehicle for introducing epidemiology concepts to the healthcare manager and subordinates.

Quality patient care demands enhanced history-taking, interviewing, and communication skills on the part of healthcare professionals. For example, a more thorough history on sexual behavior can identify those patients who are at risk for disease and injury. This process can also provide the opportunity to elaborate on the consequences of risk-taking behavior. These consequences can be expressed, of course, in epidemiologic terms, such as the number of times more likely a person is to develop AIDs if he or she engages in a high-risk behavior such as intravenous drug use. As an added benefit, effective communication plays a significant role in controlling healthcare costs and in improving access to healthcare services, and it will continue to do so in future healthcare reform. Reduced costs, ensured optimal outcomes, the delivery of quality patient care: these are the critical components in a managed care environment—and the one deciding element that drives these components is communication.

All managers in health services organizations depend on information within the context of intra-organizational relationships. Positive performance outcomes are directly linked to the degree of effective understanding that is transmitted and received through communication processes. Put another way, communication serves several functions within the realm of healthcare organization management: (1) an information function, (2) a motivation function, (3) a control function, and (4) an emotive function (Rakich, Longest, and Darr 1992). First, communication provides the basic information for healthcare managers in their decision making and for subordinates in the initiation of those decisions. Second, healthcare managers can create motivation in subordinates by informing them of the rewards that will result from their performance (positive reinforcement). Healthcare managers can manifest more effective leadership behavior by providing subordinates with the information that builds a commitment to the organizational objectives. Further, communication can be used to disseminate information that will fulfill an employee's personal needs and thus create positive motivation. Epidemiologic information can fulfill most of these functions. It certainly provides valuable information to managers for the strategic and tactical decisions they make, as discussed in Chapters 7 through 11. Moreover, it provides relevant information to clinicians for their patient treatment decisions, as discussed in Chapter 12. Finally, epidemiologic information can be motivational, in terms of performance evaluation and employee job satisfaction, as mentioned earlier in this chapter.

Environmental Barriers to Communication

Certain characteristics of an organization can block, filter, or distort communications between managers and subordinates. These are defined as environmental barriers (Rakich, Longest, and Darr 1992). Some examples of this type of barrier are competition for attention and time as well as personal bias issues. These barriers apply both to intra- and inter-organizational communication. Other environmental barriers that can filter, alter, or obstruct a message include the organization's managerial philosophy, multiple hierarchical levels, and power/status relationships between both senders and receivers. Multiple levels in an organization's hierarchy, and especially among organizations in a multi-organizational arrangement, tend to cause message distortion. Power/status relationships can also distort or inhibit the transmission of a message. The important question at this point is the extent to which epidemiology can break down some of these barriers. The issue is the distinction between clinical and managerial domains in terms of objectives, focus, and even language. If managers are encouraged to become proficient in epidemiologic concepts and thoughts, the communication between managers and medical professionals can be strengthened and the barriers between these two domains reduced.

Personal Barriers to Communication

Personal barriers (Rakich, Longest, and Darr 1992) arise from the nature of people and from their interaction with others of various cultural and personal backgrounds. These barriers manifest themselves constantly within what Rakish and colleagues refer to as an individual's "frame of reference." This can be defined as the act of encoding and sending messages, or decoding and receiving them through the filter of an individual's cultural background and past experiences. Frames of reference shape the ways in which messages are encoded and decoded through the process of "selective perception." The concept of frame of reference is exemplified in thoughts such as: "The manager is always right because he is the boss," or "Women are less competent than men for managerial positions," or "He doesn't understand medicine because he is only an administrator." Frame of reference, as a topic, is associated with the concepts of beliefs, values, and pre-judices that all individuals carry forward from their upbringing. All personal barriers create differences in the evaluating processes that form communications, and thus they make communication within healthcare organizations more difficult. Moreover, personal barriers can interfere with patient care—and with effective management, for that matter. An important question at this juncture is the degree to which managers and clinicians bring different frames of reference to their interactions, making it difficult to communicate. The point here is that epidemiologic insight can change a manager's frame of reference, and this will affect the way that messages are sent to and received by others, particularly clinicians. The frame of reference of clinicians may likewise change, based on experience with these managers, and the result will be enhanced communication between managers and clinicians.

Conclusions

This chapter has described the directing function of the healthcare manager, particularly in terms of motivating, leading, and communicating with the health-care workplace. In each case we have articulated the theory behind each role: the difference behind theories X, Y, and Z of management, for instance. An epidemiological approach to management would be motivational to the extent that employees—professionals and nonprofessionals alike—would more fully grasp the rationale behind their individual jobs and responsibilities. This type of practice style should favorably affect leadership, because epidemiology can become a source of power and credibility to the healthcare manager who must regularly interact with respected, powerful, and persuasive clinicians. Finally, epidemiology can improve communications, at least in part as a result of the usefulness of such information in making critical decisions. Perhaps more important would be the use of epidemiology to collapse, or at least lessen, the environmental and personal barriers to communication by circumscribing managers and clinicians by a common set of principles and vocabulary.

The point of this chapter, finally, has been to argue that managers can embrace a "practice style" of management that includes an appreciation for epidemiologic concepts, principles, and measures, and that brings forth their use, to the betterment of the organization and the patients it serves. Epidemiology, of course, is only one tool that managers can adopt as part of their practice style. It will not solve all of the problems that managers and clinicians face as they try to work together in today's complicated and ever-changing venue, but it should be a step in the right direction.

Case Study 8.1

Highgrounds Nursing Home is a 200-bed skilled nursing facility in a metropolitan area of the northeast. The administrator, Ms. Principal, has recently decided to reevaluate the performance appraisal system, partly as a result of the very high turnover of both nurses aides and staff nurses. Principal is also concerned with the high prevalence of decubitus ulcers (bedsores) and respiratory infections within Highgrounds. She would like to reward behavior on the basis of outcomes of care, motivate nurses and aides to provide high-quality care, and provide both extrinsic and intrinsic incentives. How can epidemiology be an important component of Ms. Principal's action plan?

Case Study 8.2

Saint Luke's is a 450-bed hospital in a suburban area of the deep South. The CEO, Mr. Burns, and the COO, Ms. Adams, come from different schools of management. Although each would admit to a managerial practice style based on Theory Y, Mr. Burns is borderline Theory X, with a somewhat abrasive and autocratic style of management. Although each executive regularly interacts with physician leaders, the clinicians consider Adams more approachable and less hostile then Burns. The chiefs of surgery and medicine routinely squabble with Burns over issues of resource allocation. The recent decision by Burns to postpone indefinitely a decision regarding establishment of a bone marrow transplant unit has infuriated the oncologists. Adams and Burns discuss how they can develop more favorable relations with the medical staff. How can epidemiology become part of this rebuilding process? How might epidemiology change the "frames of reference" for Burns, Adams, and the medical staff?

References

Bass, B. M. 1982. *Handbook of Leadership.* New York: Free Press.

Bavelas, A. 1942. "Morale and the Training of Leaders." In *Civilian Morale*, edited by G. Watson. Boston: Houghton-Mifflin.

Burns, J. M. 1978. *Leadership.* New York: Harper & Row.

Gibb, C. 1947. "The Principles and Traits of Leadership." *Journal of Abnormal Psychology* 42 (1): 267–84.

Hersey, R. E., and T. Blanchard. 1977. *Management of Organizational Behavior: Utilizing Human Resources.* Englewood Cliffs, NJ: Prentice Hall.

Hutchens, T. 1979. "Change: The Cornerstone of Leadership." *The Pathologist* 33 (3): 345–49.

Mintzberg, H. 1973. *Power In and Around Organizations.* Englewood Cliffs, NJ: Prentice-Hall.

Ouchi, W. G. 1981. *Theory Z: How American Business Can Meet the Japanese Challenge.* Reading, MA: Addison-Wesley.

Pearce, N. 1996. "Traditional Epidemiology, Modern Epidemiology, and Public Health." *American Journal of Public Health* 66 (5): 678–83.

Rakich, J. S., B. B. Longest, and K. Darr. 1992. *Managing Health Services Organizations.* Baltimore, MD: Health Professions Press.

Sheldon, A., and D. Barrett. 1977. "The Janus Principle." *Healthcare Management Review* 2 (2): 77–87.

Shortell, S. H. 1982. "Theory Z: Implications and Relevance for Health Care Management." *Health Care Management Review* 7 (Fall): 8.

Skinner, B. F. 1953. *Science and Human Behavior.* New York: Free Press.

Vroom, V. H. 1964. *Work and Motivation.* New York: Wiley.

Vroom, V. H., and P. W. Yetton. 1973. *Leadership and Decision Making.* Pittsburgh, PA: University of Pittsburgh Press.

Zaleznik, A. 1977. "Managers and Leaders: Are They Different?" *Harvard Business Review* May–June: 67–78.

Epidemiology and the Controlling Function

Steven T. Fleming

> *Mr. Practice drops a report (Massachusetts Rate Setting Commission 1995) on the CEO's desk that compares preventable hospitalization rates, by county, across the state of Massachusetts, and summarizes the hospital charges associated with these episodes of care. He indicates that Group Health East has a problem in this area, particularly with pediatric asthma cases among Medicaid enrollees. How can epidemiologic measures inform the CEO?*

The control function of a healthcare manager is perhaps one of the most critical components of health services management. It involves both assessment and intervention activities. Control activities link planning with operation; without planning, there is no direction, and without the control function, there is no assurance that what is planned will ever be accomplished. Most control activities for which the manager claims at least some responsibility can be classified as relating to either quality assessment/improvement or financial management. The former includes quality assessment and improvement, risk management, utilization review, and credentialing, whereas the latter consists of budgeting, case-mix accounting, and ratio or volume analysis, among others (Rakich, Longest, and Darr 1992). This chapter focuses on the integration of epidemiological thinking into the managerial control function with regard to quality of care. The purpose is not to train managers to replace or become hospital epidemiologists, but rather to cultivate a way of thinking that facilitates thoughtful discussion with clinicians and other experts, and thus enriches operational and strategic decisions. The concepts and principles of epidemiology for financial management are discussed thoroughly in Chapter 11.

A generic control system is illustrated in Figure 9.1 (Rakich, Longest, and Darr 1992). Inputs are converted through various processes into outputs with information generated at each stage. As the information is interpreted (assessment), intervention or change can occur at either the input stage or the process stage. Inputs and processes can be replaced, refined, or reconfigured. The control function is data driven; thus the need exists for information systems to collect and disseminate critical information to key decision makers. The concept of control involves monitoring, assessment, feedback, and regulation, and it implies the presence of standards, ideals, or objectives to which the organization is compared. If the standards are not met, then intervention through a corrective adjustment is required.

FIGURE 9.1
Generic Control
System

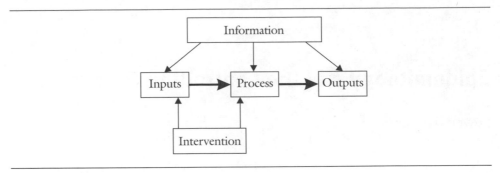

Source: Rakich, J. S., B. B. Longest, and K. Darr. 1992. *Managing Health Services Organizations.* Baltimore, MD: Health Professions Press.

Control should be simple, timely, flexible, directed at critical elements, and based on accurate and relevant information (Duncan, Ginter, and Swayne 1997).

The standards on which the organization is compared can be derived from and focused on inputs, processes, or outputs. Input standards refer to the characteristics and configuration of human and physician resources, a concept similar to what Donabedian refers to as "structure" (1980). The credentials of physicians and nurses are a simple example. Their defined relationships and turf are a more complicated one. Process standards are based on the machinations of healthcare delivery—the complex web of processes through which inputs are converted to outputs. Clinical guidelines, which describe ideal physician behavior, have been arduously developed and disseminated to the medical community. Critical pathways describe standardized care patterns. Although developed primarily for the hospital setting, these pathways have been expanded to include pre- and post-hospital care. The widespread adoption of a continuous quality improvement (CQI) philosophy signals a sincere interest on the part of healthcare providers in examining the processes of care and in setting standards or "benchmarks" to which healthcare organizations can compare themselves. Output standards refer to the characteristics of the product(s) of healthcare delivery, the most significant of which is the extent to which patients enjoy an improvement in health status or amelioration of symptoms. The outcomes research movement (Epstein 1998) should spawn clinical recommendations and expectations, outcome standards, and "best practices." It should be obvious to the reader that the structure-process-outcome paradigm of quality assessment so eloquently espoused by Donabedian captures the essence of the feedback control system illustrated in Figure 9.1, where the information useful for assessment can be generated from each of the three components of the model.

Duncan and colleagues distinguish between operational control, which focuses on individual performance or specific processes (e.g., operations and budgeting), from strategic control, which involves determining if an organization's strategy will result in progress toward meeting objectives (1997). The concept of input, process, and output standards for operational control has just been described. For strategic control, the standards are typically more financial and market oriented, such as market standing, innovative performance, productivity, liquidity and cash flow, and profitability (Drucker 1986). Perhaps in the future, quality will be more widely recognized as a performance standard to which organizations are compared both operationally and strategically. For this to happen, managers should develop at least some familiarity with the collection and interpretation of clinical data and an understanding of the basic concepts and principles of epidemiology.

The purpose of this chapter is to argue that the methods and tools of epidemiology are a critical means of converting the data gathered through the assessment of inputs, process, or outputs into useful information for the purpose of deciding whether or not intervention is necessary. Furthermore, a practical understanding of epidemiological principles will assist the manager with strategic control to the extent that performance standards are defined in clinical terms. Epidemiology and quality are defined and compared in section one. Rates and surveillance are discussed in section two. Complication rates are the focus of section three. Mortality rates and risk adjustment are described in section four. Managed care and avoidable hospitalization is the topic of section five. The integration of epidemiology and quality improvement is discussed in section six.

Epidemiology and Quality

According to most scholars, epidemiology is the study of the distribution and determinants of disease in human populations (see Chapter 2). Quality, at its fundamental level is derived from the judgments that clinicians make about balancing benefit and harm to achieve desirable patient objectives (Donabedian 1980). A more inclusive definition of quality would include such dimensions as access to care and patient satisfaction. Donabedian argues that quality of care also has an "epidemiology" in the sense that one can study the determinants of quality and its distribution among two different populations: providers and clients. Further, one can study quality against the framework of the traditional epidemiological triad: time, place, and person (Donabedian 1985). The manager should be familiar with the measurement and trend of quality over time, a topic to be discussed later in the chapter. Studies of this sort are particularly useful for strategic control where intervention and change of strategy(s) may result in more praiseworthy quality outcomes. Quality also has a distribution across settings and localities. Within the traditional epidemiology context, disease is investigated in different settings to identify particular agents, vectors, or risk factors that may be associated with disease. A study of quality within and across different settings (such as hospitals or nursing homes) and viewed through the epidemiology prism would be concerned with the determinants of quality in those settings. Within organizations, one should be concerned with the distribution of quality across units or clinics and the characteristics of those divisions that are associated with the higher levels of quality. In fact, a healthcare organization may be designed specifically to evaluate alternative interventions and outcomes of care in distinct units (see the discussion of hospital firms in Chapter 6). Finally, quality is distributed among the groups of people—providers and clients:

> Knowledge of the distribution of quality among providers of health services . . . is the product of the more usual studies of quality that throw light on the relation between structure, on the one hand, and either process or outcome on the other. . . . [Whereas] the distribution of specified levels of quality among various groupings of the consumers of care is, of course, the ultimate measure of the success or failure in achieving the social objectives of a health care system (Donabedian 1985).

The epidemiologist is concerned with identifying causal relationships between agents or risk factors and disease. At least to some extent, the incidence, severity, and progression of disease depends on the characteristics of the agent (e.g., virulence) or risk factor (e.g., strength) and the characteristics of the host or population (e.g., immunity or susceptibility). Quality is antithetical to disease in the sense that the former is desirable and beneficial. Therefore, the emphasis should be on identifying and measuring those provider characteristics, such as training, experience, specialization, and age (Donabedian 1985) that engender favorable outcomes of care. As difficult, perhaps, is the embarrassing task of identifying characteristics (such as race or socioeconomic status) that render patients susceptible to poor quality or inadequate care. For example, the recent study by Bindman et al. (1995), which examines access to care for preventable hospitalizations, suggests that uninsured persons—even if they are very ill—face a barrier to inpatient care.

Donabedian's thesis that quality has an epidemiology is appealing, partly because it validates our argument that the concepts and principles of epidemiology are relevant to the control function of the manager. Moreover, an extension of this thinking provides a useful metaphor through which to understand what quality is and how it can be controlled. Disease and quality are not quite two sides of a coin. Both have a distribution across time, place, and people that can be measured and analyzed. Both are derivative, in the sense that they can be causally related to an exposure—an agent, a risk factor, a provider, a setting, or a process of care. And both can be controlled through intervention such as elimination or modification of the exposure. This is where continuous quality improvement or risk management come into play.

Beyond the argument that quality of care has an epidemiology is the thesis that quality assessment or measurement has benefited greatly from the integration of epidemiological principles and methods into theory and practice. Donabedian suggests that epidemiology has contributed to QA in at least four different areas: (1) the specification of the standards and criteria of good practice; (2) the specification of those characteristics and configurations of providers and settings that are associated with good quality; (3) the development of measurement tools; and (4) the design and conduct of monitoring systems (1990). The first area relates primarily to the field of clinical epidemiology, which is discussed more thoroughly in Chapter 12: epidemiological studies can inform the clinical decision-making process with regard to choice of diagnostics or therapeutic strategies. The second area falls into the realm of health services research, inasmuch as the concern is with system design (refer to the discussion of "firms" in Chapter 6, for instance). In health services research, investigations are conducted to determine which attributes or characteristics of individual providers or systems of care are associated with better quality. Clearly, epidemiology can make significant contributions to the design and development of new measurement instruments, such as risk-adjusted outcomes, discussed later in this chapter. Donabedian's fourth area refers to monitoring and surveillance systems such as infection control programs, the topic of the next section.

Rates and Surveillance

A rate quantifies the number of healthcare events, such as disease or mortality, with reference to a defined population (e.g., 1,000 people) for purposes of comparison across intervals of time, geographic regions or settings, or different population groups. The epidemiologist is familiar with rates that express the mortality or morbidity experience of a population at risk, such as elderly females in the state of Kentucky. For the healthcare organization, the appropriate referent population at risk would be defined in terms of inpatient episodes (e.g., admissions); units of time (patient days); or, in the case of managed care organizations, enrolled members. Suppose, for example, that a growing managed care organization is interested in comparing preventable hospitalizations over time to determine if a new case manager program is effective. A crude count of these events over time would be misleading because enrollment has been rapidly increasing. The correct measure would be a rate that expressed the number of preventable hospital episodes per 1,000 enrolled members. A significant decrease in this rate over time would be a signal that the case manager program has been successful.

Most healthcare organizations have in place surveillance programs charged with the responsibility to monitor key indicators, such as infection rates. The focus should be on targeting infections that are frequent and preventable, and that generate high treatment cost or serious effects on either morbidity or mortality (Pottinger, Herwaldt, and Peri 1997). The "building blocks" of surveillance include a systematic collection of relevant data over a specific period of time; the management, organization, analysis, and interpretation of these data; and the communication of results to decision makers, at least some of whom will be healthcare managers (Pottinger, Herwaldt, and Peri 1997). Since the purpose of surveillance is to identify problems and intervene if necessary, it becomes the operational vehicle through which the manager delegates at least part of the control function to physicians, nurses, or other members of the epidemiology staff involved in these activities.

Historically, the "bread and butter" of surveillance has been nosocomial infections, which, by definition, originate from within the hospital setting. The difference between hospital-acquired illness and comorbidities is a difficult but critical distinction to make if quality of care judgments are in view. A comorbidity is a pre-existing illness that has existed before, or arises after, but is nonetheless unrelated to the hospital stay. Nosocomial infections, on the other hand, are hospital-derived and can become a reasonable measure of quality (if properly adjusted for risk). The timing of these events is crucial, which is why some have suggested labeling an infection as nosocomial only if it occurs at least two to three days after admission, within ten days after discharge, or with special exceptions for very short (e.g., the gastrointestinal Norwalk virus) or very long (e.g., hepatitus A) incubation periods (Pottinger, Herwaldt, and Peri 1997). Larson and colleagues report that approximately one-third of nosocomial infections are preventable and are therefore a reflection of quality of care. The remaining two-thirds are "much less amenable to intervention" because of intrinsic patient risk factors, such as age, gender, and chronic comorbidities, or differences in the "recognition" of these events by, for instance, the infection control staff (1988). A strong argument can be made for the surveillance of noninfectious outcomes of care as well, such as high-volume procedures, outcomes that are important to patients, or outcomes that reflect processes of care that are manageable. These could include accidents or adverse events related to procedures, equipment, or medications (Massanari, Wilkerson, and Swartzendruber 1995).

Fundamentally, surveillance involves the collection of data over time, to establish thresholds or baseline endemic rates, and the determination of whether the rates are stable or not and if they are higher than they should be. A significantly higher rate would trigger investigation, and even a statistically insignificant, but clinically "significant" increase might be worthy of inquiry (Pottinger, Herwaldt, and Peri 1997). In order for rates to be compared over time or to a threshold, they must be intrinsically comparable. Numerators should be based on precise definitions, reflecting the incidence or prevalence of adverse events, such as infection. Denominators should include only the population at risk, or the period of time during which the population is at risk, which means that these rates should also adjust for both intrinsic and extrinsic patient risk factors. Intrinsic risk would include the presence of comorbidities—immunodeficiency, for instance—that are patient-specific. Extrinsic risks are related to the hospital environment or exposures to medical interventions such as ventilators (Gayes 1997). For instance, duration of time in a hospital is a risk that can be adjusted by using patient days rather than admissions in the denominator (Pottinger, Herwaldt, and Peri 1997). The risk of infection associated with surgery or medical interventions such as ventilators can be adjusted by using total surgical procedures, or total patient hours of contact in the OR (or contact with an intervention), in the denominator. For these examples, one is measuring the incidence density rather than the cumulative incidence of these adverse events over time (Massanari, Wilkerson, and Swartzendruber 1995). The burden of controlling for intrinsic patient risk factors is discussed later in the section on risk adjustment.

Pottinger and colleagues (1997) discuss five distinct surveillance methods. **Hospital-wide** or **traditional surveillance** involves a prospective and continuous survey of all medical care areas so that the total incidence of nosocomial infections can be identified using microbiology reports and medical records as a source of information. **Periodic surveillance** is conducted routinely, but periodically; for example, the entire hospital may be surveyed one month each quarter, or a different unit may be surveyed each month. A **prevalence survey**, on the other hand, tabulates the total number of infections that are present and active within a specific time period. **Targeted surveillance** focuses on specific settings (e.g., critical care units); services, such as cardiovascular; or groups of high-risk patients. With **outbreak threshold surveillance**, the baseline endemic infection rates are used as triggers below which no surveillance activity would occur.

Complication Rates

The intrinsic and extrinsic risk mentioned earlier suggests that the occurrence of adverse events in healthcare settings is largely driven by factors related to patients, the environment in which they are treated, or the kind of treatment they receive. Fleming classifies adverse events along three dimensions: (1) whether procedures were good or deficient, (2) whether the disease process(es) was normal or abnormal, and (3) whether clinician skills were good or deficient (1996). These dimensions represent extrinsic (1, 3) and intrinsic (2) factors that may lead to poor outcomes. Clearly, an adverse event, such as infection, may result from a deficient procedure or practice, an abnormal disease process (i.e., unexpected disease course or complication), poor clinical skills, or from more than one factor. The surveillance system discussed earlier is typically unable to completely disentangle these factors, and it is difficult to make valid judgments about quality of care without knowing the cause of the adverse event.

Nonetheless, the literature offers some evidence that complication rates may be a useful measure of quality because they are more sensitive and directly related to the process of patient care than other, cruder measures of outcome such as mortality rates (Brailer et al. 1996). DesHarnais and colleagues, for instance, developed risk-adjusted indexes of mortality, readmission, and complications based on a sample of 776 short-term hospitals in 1983 (1990). The measures were shown to be stable over time and unbiased with respect to hospital size, ownership, and teaching status. The measures accounted for much of the variation across hospitals in the incidence of these adverse events. The complication measure, in particular, was adjusted for the risk associated with age and comorbidities.

More recently, Brailer et al. (1996) describe a comorbidity-adjusted complication measure which, like that of DesHarnais, is based on diagnoses reported on hospital claims. The Brailer measure, however, attempts to address at least two problems with some of the earlier measures: (1) the difficulty in distinguishing between a post-admission complication and a comorbidity occurring before or during hospitalization, and (2) the impact of multiple complications. This measure assigns a complication risk to each patient based on the secondary diagnoses recorded on claims data and the probability that each diagnosis is a complication for a specific admitting diagnosis. For example, if a patient is admitted with simple pneumonia, the probability that congestive heart failure, respiratory failure, and urinary tract infection are complications rather than comorbidities is 20 percent, 50 percent, and 90 percent, respectively. The authors discuss how this measure is highly correlated with other "gold standards," such as those based on chart review.

Iezzoni and colleagues identified 27 complications that "raise concern about the quality of care" (1994). The list includes such conditions as wound infections and decubitus ulcers. Each complication is assigned to a "risk pool" that represents the patients at risk for those complications. For example, only patients who endure major or minor surgery would be at risk for "postoperative complications." Observed-to-expected complication rates were compared across hospitals with the conclusion that larger and major teaching facilities, and those with open heart surgery, had higher relative complication rates. The Iezzoni study is especially relevant in this chapter for at least two reasons. The assignment of each quality indicator, in this case specific complications, to risk pools recognizes the importance of denominators in calculating rates. The incidence of adverse events, such as complications (the numerator), is derived from and must be compared only to the population "at risk" of the event (the denominator). Table 9.1 lists five complications and the associated risk group. Notice that some complications, such as aspiration pneumonia, should be associated only with a surgical risk group. Others, such as post-operative pneumonia, may arise from a somewhat larger risk group, which also contains patients subject to endoscopy and invasive cardiac procedures. Patients at risk of wound infections, on the other hand, comprise the largest group of medical and surgical patients, including those who endure endoscopic or invasive cardiac procedures.

The second reason why the Iezzoni study is relevant to the discussions of this chapter is the finding that complications were not significantly related to hospital mortality rates as calculated by the Health Care Financing Administration (HCFA). One explanation is that the latter measure is either too crude, poorly designed, or not particularly robust as an indicator of quality. Critics of this measure

TABLE 9.1
Complications and Associated "At-Risk" Categories

Aspiration pneumonia	Major, minor, or miscellaneous surgery
Postoperative acute myocardial infarction	Major, minor, miscellaneous surgery, endoscopy
Postoperative pneumonia	Major, minor, miscellaneous surgery, endoscopy, invasive cardiac procedures (e.g., catheterization)
Pulmonary embolism	Major, minor, miscellaneous surgery, endoscopy, invasive cardiac procedures (e.g., catheterization), medical patients
Wound infection	Major, minor, miscellaneous surgery, endoscopy, invasive cardiac procedures (e.g., catheterization), medical patients, complications pertaining to all patients

Source: Adapted from Iezzoni, L. I., J. Daley, T. Hereen, S. M. Foley, J. S. Hughes, E. S. Fisher, C. C. Duncan, and G. A. Coffman. 1994. "Using Administrative Data to Screen Hospitals for High Complication Rates." *Inquiry* 31 (1): 40–55.

are not shy with their disapproval. The larger question is whether mortality should even be correlated with complications, or whether each measures reflects a different dimension of quality of care.

Silber and colleagues evaluated the complication rate as a measure of quality of care and focused on coronary artery bypass surgery (1995). They compared actual death, complications, and failure to rescue (after complications develop) with expected rates, using variables that had previously been identified as predictive of these outcomes, such as severity of illness. Fifty-seven hospitals were rank-ordered with each of these three measures. The complications that were chosen were those that "increased the risk of dying and those that added complexity to the management of the patient." The complication measure correlated poorly with both failure to rescue and mortality, each of which was more often associated with hospital characteristics related to higher quality, such as the presence of an MRI facility or an approved residency program. The authors suggest that complications may not be a good indicator of quality because it may be measuring something different from either mortality or failure to rescue.

Several of these studies have raised cautionary flags with regard to the utility or validity of complications as a measure of quality given their poor correlation with other more acceptable measures, such as mortality. What remains unclear is if complications and these other quality measures should be associated—that is, whether indeed they move in the same direction at least—or if it may be misleading to applaud organizations with low complication rates, and vice-versa.

How would an epidemiologic frame of mind enable the health services manager to interpret these puzzling results and glean critical truths to apply in the practice of the management controlling function? An adverse event such as a nosocomial infection or a complication is clearly undesirable because it represents cost and suffering (Fleming 1996). These events should be monitored over time as rates, with the denominator of each rate representative of the patient population at risk of the event (Iezzoni et al. 1994). A more sophisticated surveillance program might include predicted rates, which include patient risk factors, such as age, that are unrelated to quality of care. The lack of association between complications and mortality does not exonerate complications as a cause for concern; rather, it suggests that confounding factors may be present that make it difficult to accept complications as an indicator of quality, particularly when comparing across organizations. It may be more useful to compare complication rates among providers or services within an organization, particularly if one can control for patient risk factors.

Mortality Rates and Risk Adjustment

Epidemiologists have long been interested in the study of mortality rates inasmuch as death is usually an easily defined event that is well-documented across cultures, and its incidence is routinely collected as part of the vital statistics collected by health departments. The cause of death can be studied with insurance claims data or with death certificates. Epidemiologists typically adjust mortality rates either directly or indirectly by age to compare trends across time, settings, or people (see Chapter 2). The concept of "risk adjustment" adds multiple dimensions to this process by recognizing that many factors, in addition to age, affect the likelihood of mortality.

The theory and methods of risk adjustment have been elaborated by Iezzoni and others (1997a, 1997b). Conceptually, risk adjustment is an extension of age-adjustment techniques that have graced epidemiologic tradition for years, in the sense that they are trying to "level the playing field" for the purposes of comparison. The process of adjusting for age, either directly or indirectly, facilitates a comparison of mortality rates across time, settings, or people, by accounting for differences in age mix that would otherwise confound the comparisons. Adjusting for risk extends this theory to include multiple risk factors, each of which potentially affects mortality rates. According to Iezzoni, risk adjustment can be used to "calculate the so-called algebra of effectiveness" in the sense that patient outcomes, such as mortality, are a function of clinical attributes (i.e., risk factors), random factors, quality, and effectiveness. The epidemiologist compares age-adjusted rates across time to detect any significant temporal differences unrelated to age. Clinicians and health services researchers use risk-adjusted rates to detect any significant differences across providers, settings, or patient groups that are unrelated to patient risk factors (i.e., presumably they are related to quality or effectiveness).

Iezzoni documents and explains the important risk-factors that affect patient outcomes as follows (1997a, 1997b). Age affects mortality rates to the extent that older people have lower "physiological reserve" and may be treated less aggressively. Gender affects mortality in that life expectancy and response to treatment may vary with anatomic, physiological, and hormonal differences. Moreover, some suggest a "gender bias" that affects the kinds of treatments made available to one or the other gender. Clinical attributes would include acute clinical stability, principal diagnosis, disease-specific severity, comorbidities, and functional status. Acute clinical stability refers to physiological functioning, as indicated by vital signs and serum electrolytes, for instance. Principal diagnosis represents a hypothesis of illness, a focal point of treatment, and the cause for making contact with the healthcare system, and as such it relates to the probability of survival. Disease-specific severity is a risk factor for mortality because it represents the intensity or seriousness of illness within a distinct category of disease. Comorbidities increase the risk of mortality in that they represent an additional disease burden that may complicate treatment, recovery, or prognosis. A permanent or temporary limitation in the ability to function—called functional status—influences mortality to the extent that everyday behavior affects one's sense of well-being and quality of life. Cultural, racial, ethnic, and socioeconomic factors may influence mortality through barriers to access (e.g., lack of insurance coverage), care-seeking behaviors, diet, and compliance, among others. Mortality is probably affected by other risk factors that are as difficult to measure as those just described, for instance, psychological, cognitive, and psychosocial functioning, health status, quality of life, and patient attitudes and preferences.

Iezzoni describes the "ideal" risk-adjustment process that would probably include most of the factors likely to affect mortality. Remember that the purpose of all of this is to gain the ability to compare outcomes across time, settings, and people. So far as the control function of the manager is concerned, the interest would be in comparing mortality rates among or within organizations and across providers of care, such as physicians or surgeons. Blumberg describes a generic Risk Adjustment Monitoring of Outcome (RAMO) system where one would compare expected-to-actual outcomes of care by hospital, physician, surgeon, payment method, or whatever (Blumberg 1986). The purpose of such a system would be to measure trends over time or to investigate unexpected clusters of adverse events: the nuts and bolts of epidemiologic inquiry. This system would need a methodology to adjust for the risk of death, such as one of the numerous severity-of-illness measures that are on the market today. These measures could be categorized into those based on claims and those derived from clinical data. Because the competing methods are not well correlated when they are used to rank hospitals on the basis of risk-adjusted mortality, each risk-adjustment method, it is suggested, may lead to a different judgment about a hospital's overall performance (Iezzoni 1997a, 1997b).

HCFA published annual risk-adjusted mortality statistics by hospital from 1986 until 1993, when the practice was discontinued. The statistics were the subject of intense criticism and controversy over the years, and the focus of contention was the Achilles' heel of most risk-adjusted measures, severity of illness. The measure had evolved considerably over the years: the final version was an elegant hazard function based on both short- and long-term risk, and patients were classified into 23 analytical categories (Fleming, Hicks, and Bailey 1995). It was argued, nonetheless, that this measure, which was based entirely on claims data, did not adequately adjust for severity of illness. Clearly, one cannot refute the limitations of claims-based data that are designed primarily for insurance purposes and not clinical decisions. However, there is some evidence that the measure could have been a useful screening tool to flag potential problem areas and prompt further investigation (Fleming, Hicks, and Bailey 1995).

More recently both New York and Pennsylvania have published "report cards" for cardiovascular surgery. Since 1992, the Pennsylvania Health Care Cost Containment Council has published risk-adjusted in-hospital mortality rates for for coronary artery bypass graft surgery (CABG). The rates compare in-hospital mortality to a range of expected rates by individual surgeon and hospital. The risk-adjustment methodology includes both severity of illness and comorbidities. The state of New York has also published risk-adjusted mortality rates for CABG since 1990, with a methodology that includes clinical risk factors, such as body mass index (BMI) and ejection fraction, as well as comorbid illness.

Both programs are intended to improve quality of care, in light of the choices that consumers and physicians can make regarding treatment or referrals based on these outcome scores. These programs have generated a fair amount of controversy. In fact, the New York State Department of Health had to be forced to release surgeon-specific risk-adjusted mortality rates through litigation, despite physician protests and the well-worn argument that the measures do not adequately adjust for severity of illness. The concern is not whether physicians like these measures—or even should like them, for that matter—but whether they find them credible and useful tools in decision making. A related issue is the extent to which managers would consider these measures informative and empowering in dealing with the medical staff. A final thought here involves consumers and the extent to which they should be involved in choosing a surgeon based on a report card score, the methods of which neither the patient nor the surgeon probably understands.

In terms of clinical utility, Schneider and Epstein (1996) surveyed a 50 percent randomized sample of Pennsylvania cardiologists and cardiac surgeons to assess the clinical impact of the Pennsylvania program. The mortality rates were "very important" in assessing surgical skills to only 10 percent of the sample, with 87 percent of cardiologists reporting that the "guide" had little or minimal influence on referral decisions. The majority of respondents questioned the inadequate risk adjustment, the absence of other quality indicators, and the lack of data reliability. The more compelling concern shared by 59 percent of the cardiologists was an increased difficulty in finding surgeons willing to perform CABG surgery on severely ill patients. Sixty-three percent of the cardiac surgeons agreed that, because of the Pennsylvania report cards, they would be less willing to operate on these patients.

The reluctance of surgeons to treat high-risk patients is a concern of the New York program as well (Green and Wintfeld 1995). The issue is whether reports cards such as these can adversely affect access to care for the severely ill. This effect on access should occur only if cardiac surgeons are not convinced that the measures accurately reflect the risk of surgery for these patients. Remember that the calculus of report cards depends on both actual and expected deaths. These scores can be improved in two ways: positive changes in quality (i.e., fewer actual deaths) or higher expected deaths (i.e., a sicker case mix). If surgeons eschew the sickest of patients with a view toward bettering their score, they are gambling that actual deaths will decrease more than the expected deaths associated with a healthier case mix. On the other hand, a more extensive coding of severity-related conditions would improve report card scores without the risk of mortality. If this occurs, we should see an increase in prevalence over time of conditions associated with higher severity of illness, for example, unstable angina. Anecdotal evidence would suggest that this has occurred (Green and Wintfeld 1995).

It appears that the New York program has had a clinical impact in terms of mortality rates, as reported by Hannan and associates (1994). Cardiovascular surgeons were categorized into high, middle, and low groups based on mortality ranking. Over a four-year period, each group showed improvement in risk-adjustment mortality, with the largest improvement being attributed to the group with the poorest outcome scores. The authors are willing to acknowledge a nation-wide reduction in CABG mortality as partial explanation. A more encouraging argument would suggest that hospitals used the information to make strategic changes in process and personnel that reduced preventable deaths (Chassin, Hannan, and DeBuono 1996). In another study, Hannan and colleagues describe shifts in surgical utilization among New York cardiovascular surgeons (1995). These include a decrease in low-volume cardiac surgeons and in the percentage of operations performed by low-volume cardiac surgeons, and increases in both high-volume cardiac surgeons and the operations they performed. This apparent shift from low- to high-volume surgeons is applauded given the lower risk-adjusted mortality rates among high-volume surgeons.

Other report cards are sure to appear in different settings and for physicians other than cardiac surgeons. Clearly the impact of these programs, in terms of "real" changes in quality, depends on the credibility of the risk-adjustment methodology, the ability of providers to "game" the system, and the willingness of managers and clinicians to implement the hard choices regarding the "practice" of medicine.

Managed Care

Clearly, managed care organizations (MCOs) require even greater accountability so far as quality of care is concerned because of the perverse incentives in this form of healthcare delivery. These responsibilities rest heavy on the shoulders of healthcare managers in their exercise of the control function of quality assurance and improvement. Report cards and physician profiling are becoming commonplace in managed care. Perhaps the most notable instrument in this context is the Health Plan Employer Data and Information Set (HEDIS) developed by the National Committee on Quality Assurance (NCQA). The initial version of HEDIS (1.0) was released in 1991, followed by a revised 2.0 version in October 1993 and the 3.0 version in early 1997. The most recent version contains 75 performance measures in eight different areas: effectiveness of care, access/availability of care, satisfaction, health plan stability, use of services, cost of care, informed healthcare choices, and health plan descriptives (Harris, Caldwell, and Cahill 1998). Only 14 of the performance measures are clinical quality indicators that more directly reflect the treatment of acute or chronic disease than did the earlier versions (Epstein 1998). Over 330 health plans voluntarily submitted these data for publication by NCQA. The purpose of HEDIS is to give employers an objective set of performance measures with which to judge the strengths and weaknesses of various managed care organizations. Physician profiles, on the other hand, are derived from administrative databases and are intended to provide feedback to physicians on costs, immunizations, screening, practice patterns, and appropriateness of care (Spoeri and Ullman 1997). Obviously, these profiles are intended to encourage physicians to practice medicine within the boundaries and norms established by their colleagues. Managerial control can be exercised directly through financial incentives, or with the requirement that physicians justify deviations from these norms. MCOs are particularly interested in specialist referrals and inpatient admissions.

Many hospital episodes may be potentially avoidable, particularly those related to ambulatory care–sensitive conditions (ASC) where treatment, monitoring, and follow-up outside the hospital may prevent these episodes from occurring in the first place. To go further, one can categorize ASCs into those conditions that are completely preventable (e.g., an immunizable disease such as measles), those in which earlier primary care would have prevented hospitalization (e.g., cellulitus), and those that require careful monitoring and treatment (e.g., asthma). All of these conditions are especially relevant under capitation, where the managed care organization is responsible for an enrolled population for whom it is at risk of bearing the financial burden of healthcare services. Given the incentive to underutilize under managed care, surveillance of ASCs would seem particularly appropriate. A reduction in unnecessary hospitalization affects quality, access, and cost. If patients can avoid hospitalization, they evade iatrogenic (Brennan et al. 1991) and other risks (Creditor 1993) associated with inpatient care. In short, quality of care is better if hospitalization can be legitimately avoided. This implies that patients have access to ambulatory care services. To the extent that these services prevent, replace, or reduce the duration of a hospital episode, then overall costs to the plan will be lower. A number of studies support these premises. Bigby and associates reports that 9 percent of 686 emergency hospital admissions were potentially preventable, and of these, two-thirds were caused by iatrogenic misadventures (1987). Solberg, Peterson, and Ellis (1990) studied 673 potentially avoidable hospital episodes for patients in 15 clinical conditions with rates ranging from one percent of asthma cases to 21 percent of hospital episodes for diabetes ketoacidosis. Another study compared uninsured to privately insured patients in terms of hospital admission for one of 12 potentially avoidable hospital conditions. Uninsured patients were 71 percent more likely to be admitted in Massachusetts and 49 percent more likely to be admitted in Maryland (Weissman et al. 1992). Bindman and colleagues showed that access to care across 250 zip code areas in urban California, as measured by insurance coverage and having a regular source of care, is more strongly related to preventable hospitalization than patient care–seeking behavior or physician practice style (1995). In Maryland, poor children with asthma had 40 percent fewer physician visits, but nearly twice the hospitalization rate and over three times the bed days (Halfon and Newacheck 1993). In another study using Maryland hospital claims data, the hospitalization rate for asthma among black children was nearly three times the rate for white children (Wissow et al. 1988). Clearly, the size of the preventable hospitalization problem is significant, and the cause(s), although still unclear, are coming into focus: they relate to issues of medical competence and to accessibility, particularly financial accessibility—and perhaps physical accessibility as well.

The studies just mentioned imply that quality assurance in a managed care organization should include the surveillance of ambulatory-sensitive conditions as well as preventable hospital episodes that can be traced back to deficient care in the ambulatory setting. Some ambulatory care–sensitive conditions include asthma, cervical cancer, hypertension, perforated/bleeding ulcer, diabetes, and ruptured appendix, to mention a few. The epidemiological insight in view here is the need to monitor changes in both the at-risk population (those with the ASC: the denominator) and the adverse outcome (the potentially avoidable hospitalization: the numerator) to calculate cause-specific avoidable hospitalization rates. For example, we need to know the prevalence of enrolled members with diabetes (the at-risk population) as well as the number of avoidable hospital episodes (for coma or ketoacidosis) during that same time. Changes in these cause-specific rates would inform managers of barriers to access of care for specific clinical conditions. A less useful approach would be to monitor changes in the rate of avoidable hospitalization expressed as the number of these hospital episodes per 1,000 enrolled members. Cause-specific rates would more accurately and specifically measure the ability of an MCO to control the burden of disease with the potential for exacerbation.

Total Quality Management

Many healthcare organizations today have adopted a philosophy of management referred to as total quality management (TQM) or continuous quality improvement (CQI). These programs have spread across the medical landscape with a kind of religious zeal (Fleming et al. 1993) in response to a number of factors, such as the escalation of healthcare costs and the variation in clinical practice. A number of key individuals were responsible for transplanting the TQM theories and concepts of earlier visionaries (Juran and Gryna 1988; Deming 1982) from industrial settings to the healthcare sector (Laffel and Blumenthal 1989; Berwick, Godfrey, and Roessner 1990). The premise underlying these theories is that quality can be improved by eliminating unwanted and nonrandom variation in the processes of healthcare. These techniques of statistical process control from industrial engineering fit nicely with the concepts of epidemiology, as we will see later.

Berwick discusses the basic principles of TQM (Berwick, Godfrey, and Roessner 1990), which include a focus on the processes of healthcare, with each employee playing the triple role of customer (receiving work from others), processor (adding value), and supplier (giving work to others). The main source of quality problems is the process, not the people performing it. To point the finger at a process rather than a "bad apple" (i.e., a hapless and probably innocent employee) was a major development in quality assurance (Berwick 1989). TQM should focus on the most vital healthcare processes, with a scientific and statistical mindset that encourages total employee involvement. In short, the TQM philosophy fosters employee empowerment with a corporate culture that rewards inquiry.

Organizations that have embraced TQM continuously engage in quality improvement project(s) through a number of different techniques, such as the Plan, Do, Study, Act (PDSA) cycle. In the "Plan phase," the project team diagrams a particular healthcare process with a flowchart, identifies sources of variation, and suggests potential changes. Changes are implemented on a small scale in the "Do phase" and observed during the "Study phase." Final changes are instituted across the organization in the "Act phase" (Sinioris and Najafi 1995). A related approach would be to (1) define the process, (2) collect data, (3) redesign the process, (4) implement changes, (5) measure results, and (6) hold the gains. Alternatively, some distinguish between the "diagnostic" and "remedial" journeys involved with quality improvement. TQM projects employing any of these three paradigms can be summarized as "storyboards" that detail the quality improvement process and lessons learned from each experience.

Quality improvement consists of a toolbox of descriptive and analytical techniques that are heavily grounded in statistics and either directly or indirectly related to epidemiological concepts. The flowchart used in CQI illustrates each step in a particular healthcare process. It displays the complexities of the process, identifies the decision points, and accentuates the critical junctures where timing is critical. The cause-effect or fishbone diagram classifies the potential causes of a problem by category, such as the Four M's (method, manpower, material, or machinery), the Four P's (policies, procedures, people, or plant), or other alternatives (e.g., people, methods, information, materials, or facilities) (Marszalek-Gaucher and Coffey 1993). A similar (albeit less fishy) approach would be to summarize a brainstorming session with an "affinity diagram" in which potential causes are fit into a classification scheme. Control charts and run charts depict trends over time, with or without confidence intervals, respectively. Histograms are simply bar graphs that illustrate frequency by category, and Pareto charts are histograms that have been sorted by frequency. Scatter diagrams portray the relationship between two variables. Each of these illustrative tools provides insight into the diagnostic or remedial process of quality improvement, and each has epidemiological relevance.

Figure 9.2 is adapted from Benneyan (1998) and depicts, by month, the trend of catheter-associated infections over a three-year period. Notice the mean of 4.22 infections per month and the upper confidence limit (UCL) of three standard deviations from the mean of 10.08. The purpose of TQM is to eliminate non-random variation from the process and thereby to improve quality. The control chart isolates specific points of non-random variation when the trend exceeds the upper (or lower) confidence interval, as is the case during months 28 and 29. Further inquiry into the matter would attempt to identify possible causes and suggest remedial action. The control chart illustrates the essence of what is called statistical process control (SPC) and is rich with epidemiological meaning. The purpose of SPC is to monitor a process over time (epidemiologists might call this surveillance) and distinguish between natural and unnatural variation in that process. With infections, for instance, the interest is in distinguishing between the endemic or underlying rate of disease and any abnormal (or epidemic) increase in that rate over time, perhaps during months 28 and 29. The threshold (UCL) represents an action limit that would trigger further investigation.

One can also use control charts to illustrate non-disease-related trends over time, such as daily emergency room admissions, average waiting time in minutes, or average time until referral in days. In each case, the purpose is to monitor the

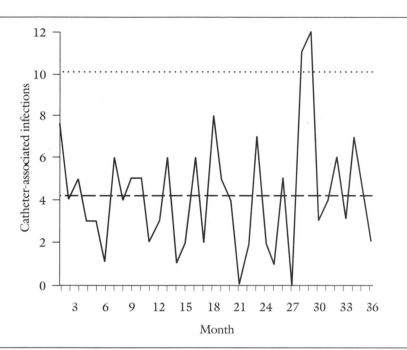

FIGURE 9.2
Control Chart of Catheter-Associated Infections

Source: Benneyan, J. C. 1998. "Statistical Quality Control Methods in Infection Control and Hospital Epidemiology. Part I: Introduction and Basis Theory." *Infection Control and Hospital Epidemiology* 19 (3): 194–214.

trend and identify the out-of-control points, which the epidemiologist would call "sentinel events." The circumstances that surround these events provide useful insights into potential causes of the problem.

Cause-effect or fishbone diagrams categorize the potential causes of process problems. Figure 9.3, for instance, illustrates a hypothetical cause-effect diagram for patient falls with four categories: weak mobility status, mental confusion, sedation, and environment. Note that the chart does not quantify the degree to which each factor contributes to the breakdown in process but merely illustrates the aggregation of factors into categories and subcategories. Epidemiologists search for the cause(s) of disease, disability, and other human suffering. Although these causes typically are not summarized in a cause-effect diagram, some have elaborated webs of causation for chronic disease. Refer to Timmreck (1998) for webs of causation for coronary heart disease, myocardial infarction, and heart disease. A "web of causation" would advance the cause-effect diagram one step further because it depicts the intricacy of causal relationships among various factors, not simply the categories to which they belong. For example, in Figure 9.3, sedation could also cause mental confusion. Clearly, it would be more efficient to eliminate the root rather than the derivative causes of process problems.

A Pareto chart is simply a sorted bar graph which is used to prioritize. Figure 9.4 illustrates a contrived Pareto chart associated with the cause-effect diagram of Figure 9.3. Notice that the top three reasons for falls comprise 85 percent of the risk of this process failure. The Pareto chart assumes that each instance of process

FIGURE 9.3
Cause-Effect
Diagram for Falls

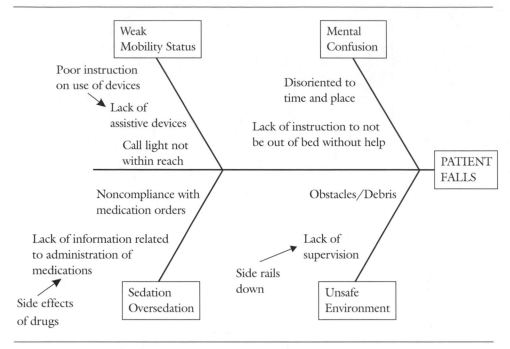

Source: Adapted from Al-Assaf, A. F., and J. A. Schmele. 1993. *The Textbook of Total Quality Management in Healthcare*. Boca Raton, FL: St. Lucie Press.

FIGURE 9.4
Pareto Chart:
Patient Falls

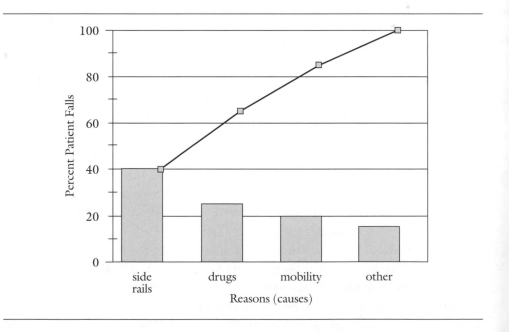

failure (e.g., patient fall) can be attributed to one distinct cause (e.g., side rails). In fact, these charts are derived by identifying which cause is responsible for each process failure. This is akin to the epidemiologist recognizing one specific agent at a time responsible for disease.

The multi-cause model of chronic disease consists of numerous interrelated risk factors, each of which acts both individually and severally to increase the probability of developing disease. Thus, the attributable fraction (see Chapter 4) is calculated as a measure of the extent to which a particular risk factor is responsible for disease in the population, given the relative risk and prevalence of the risk factor in the population. Although this is typically not done, TQM teams could design studies to determine the relative risk (or odds ratio) of each specific cause that is associated with a process failure—for example, of those patients who are sedated, the proportion who fall out of the bed. A simple case control or cohort study should be adequate here. Ideally the study should control for all proposed causes (i.e., it probably needs to be a multivariate analysis). Once the relative risk of each specific cause is determined along with the prevalence of the cause in the population, the attributable fraction of each cause can be calculated. A Pareto chart derived from these results would identify the most important causes of process failure, assuming that each cause does not cause process failure all of the time and that more than one cause may cause process failure some of the time.

The statistical tools discussed in this section and others are used by TQM teams to determine the cause(s) and remedies for process failures, with an eye to improving quality. Clearly, epidemiology should play a pivotal role in the design and implementation of these studies. The concepts of causal relationships, risk, rates, and surveillance are fundamental to total quality management.

Conclusions

An epidemiological frame of mind is particularly relevant to the health services manager in terms of the control function. The focus has been on measuring and managing quality of care using the fundamental principles of epidemiology: (1) the distribution of disease in human populations across time, place, and people; (2) the measurement and study of risk factors that increase the probability of adverse outcomes such as morbidity and death; and (3) the surveillance, monitoring, and identification of atypical clusters of disease or death. The concepts of rates and at-risk populations, and the definition and measurement of such quality indicators as complications, mortality, and avoidable hospitalizations, have been discussed. Further, we have described how the traditional epidemiological concepts of age adjustment can be extended further to include a multifactorial model of risk adjustment. Finally, the basic principles and tools of quality improvement have been described with an epidemiological interpretation.

Eighty years ago or so, Ernest Amory Codman was engaged in a struggle for the recognition and reputation of an idea that brings us back to the future. Codman passionately advocated the idea that physicians be held accountable for the care that they provide. The symptoms, main diagnosis, treatment plan, complications, and one-year follow-ups for each patient would be summarized on an "end-results card." Codman's passion foresaw what we call "the outcomes movement" and provider report cards. His ideas anticipate clinical quality improvement and clinical practice guidelines because the end results system would reveal to each doctor:

> an undistorted picture of both his successes and failures . . . [from which] he could then learn which cases he could treat better, which cases he should refer to others, and which subjects are deserving of further research . . . the first inklings of a discovery would appear in the end results attained by individual physicians as they introduced their particular innovations. It would be the responsibility of the hospital, then, to take note of the events, and to subject those innovations that seemed promising to a more thorough test, always guided by end results. The innovations that survived would be referred to the committee of the college [American College of Surgeons] which, in turn, would select the more worthy ones for further testing at other collaborating hospitals (Donabedian 1989).

Let us remember the foresight of Codman as we close this chapter on the relevance of epidemiology to quality measurement and control. Codman knew that accountability was the key to quality improvement and the advancement of clinical science, and that surveillance of entire patient populations was the essence of innovation.

Case Study 9.1

Totalhealth is a 50,000-member group model HMO in a northeastern SMSA of about two million people. It holds affiliations with two major teaching hospitals. Totalhealth has a sophisticated surveillance program that monitors the incidence of nosocomial infections in each of the two hospitals by month. This HMO also tracks hospital case mix by DRG as well as the case mix of ambulatory care episodes. The surveillance program indicates an upward shift in the incidence of pneumonia beyond the trigger threshold and persisting for the most recent three months. The analysis of ambulatory care episodes also indicates an upward shift in the incidence of pneumonia that has persisted for the last four or five months:

1. Assuming that the HMO has a prospective and continuous surveillance system in place, what kinds of other surveys might you want to initiate given these results?
2. How would the HMO distinguish between nosocomial pneumonia and pneumonia as a comorbidity?
3. Could the characteristics of your membership have changed (e.g., age, comorbidities), and if so, how would this affect the results?

Case Study 9.2

Boondocks Hospital is a 50-bed hospital located in a small Midwestern town of 10,000 people. Although the hospital has struggled financially over the last ten years or so, it has been able to maintain a 70 percent occupancy. The hospital boasts two operating rooms, an active general surgery service, and an obstetrical service that has recently partnered with a teaching hospital 25 miles away. The hospital has decided to monitor quality of care with several different measures, including a risk-adjusted measure of complications (Iezzoni et al. 1994). The developers of the measure report observed-to-expected rates of complications as follows:

	Major Surgery	Minor Surgery	Medical
Large hospitals	1.15	1.14	1.33
Small hospitals	0.82	0.89	0.94
Teaching hospitals	1.00	1.00	1.10
Nonteaching hospitals	0.89	0.95	0.94

Boondocks Hospital calculates an index of of 1.2 for minor surgery and 1.1 for medical patients:

1. Why might you expect the complications measure to be higher for the large and/or teaching hospital?
2. Describe some plausible explanations for Boondocks Hospital.
3. What kinds of action should Boondocks take?

Case Study 9.3

Mountain Medical Center is a 329-bed hospital located in New York state that boasts a full range of cardiovascular services including cardiac catheterization, open heart surgery, cardiac intensive care, and angioplasty. According to the recent report (http://www.health.state.ny.us/nysdoh/consumer/heart/cabg935.pdf) summarizing coronary artery bypass surgery (CABS) from 1993 through 1995, Mountain had a significantly higher mortality rate than expected given the risks associated with the case mix of patients. Mountain treated 1,130 CABS patients, 34 of whom died, for an observed mortality rate (OMR) of 3.01 percent. The expected mortality rate (EMR) was 1.66 percent (or 18.7 patients), which was calculated based on the individual patient's risks. In other words, older and female patients are more likely to die, as are those with an unstable hemodynamic state, shock, severe atherosclerosis, a previous heart attack, malignant ventricular arrhythmia, congestive heart failure, renal failure, or previous open heart operations. If Mountain had the same patient mix as the entire state of New York, the risk-adjusted mortality rate (RAMR), would be 4.66 percent with a high and low confidence limit of 3.23 and 6.51, respectively. The lower confidence limit is higher than the statewide mortality rate of 2.52 percent, meaning that Mountain is a high outlier. The hospital should evaluate quality of care with regard to CABS. Table 9.2 identifies the number of cases, deaths, OMR, EMR, RAMR, and confidence interval for the cardiovascular surgeons with privileges at Mountain:

1. What kinds of quality assessment activities should be pursued at this point?
2. Do you need to collect more epidemiological data?
3. Should doctors A, B, and C be reviewed?
4. Do any other cardiovascular surgeons need to be evaluated?
5. Offer another explanation for these results.

TABLE 9.2
Mortality Rates for Cardiovascular Surgeons at Mountain Medical Center

	Cases	Deaths	OMR[†]	EMR[‡]	RAMR	95% C[§] for RAMR
Doctor A	326	5	1.53	1.74	2.26	(0.73, 5.27)
Doctor B	286	11	3.85	1.71	5.79[*]	(2.89, 10.36)
Doctor C	206	7	3.40	1.44	6.06	(2.43, 12.49)
All others	312	11	3.53	1.67	5.43[*]	(2.71, 9.72)
Total	1,130	34	3.01	1.66	4.66[*]	(3.23, 6.51)

[*]significantly higher than the statewide rate.
[§]Confidence interval.
[†]Observed mortality rate.
[‡]Expected mortality rate.

Case Study 9.4

Valley Medical Center is a 300-bed hospital in the southeastern United States that is concerned about the relatively high rate of return of asthmatic patients to the emergency room department. Asthma is an ambulatory-sensitive condition that may exacerbate and require hospitalization if it is not adequately monitored. Valley is the sole acute care provider for SunHealth, a 50,000-member IPA. Valley contacted the IPA and expressed concern for the asthma hospitalizations. SunHealth had also noticed a significant increase in asthma hospitalizations over the last year or so. They agreed to jointly participate in a total quality management study to reduce the number of these preventable hospitalizations:

1. Define the problem that needs to be solved by this study.
2. Who should be included in this multidisciplinary TQM team?
3. What kinds of epidemiological data need to be collected?
4. What might be some of the problems and how can they be corrected?

References

Al-Assaf, A. F., and J. A. Schmele. 1993. *The Textbook of Total Quality Management in Healthcare.* Boca Raton, FL: St. Lucie Press.

Benneyan, J. C. 1998. "Statistical Quality Control Methods in Infection Control and Hospital Epidemiology. Part I: Introduction and Basis Theory." *Infection Control and Hospital Epidemiology* 19 (3): 194–214.

Berwick, D.M. 1989. "Continuous Improvement as an Ideal in Health Care." *The New England Journal of Medicine* 320 (1): 53–56.

Berwick, D. M., A. B. Godfrey, and J. Roessner. 1990. *Curing Health Care: New Strategies for Quality Improvement.* San Francisco: Jossey-Bass.

Bigby, J., J. Dunn, L. Goldman, J. B. Adams, P. Jen, C. S. Landefeld, and A. L. Komaroff. 1987. "Assessing the Preventability of Emergency Hospital Admissions: A Method for Evaluating the Quality of Medical Care in a Primary Care Facility." *American Journal of Medicine* 83 (6): 1031–36.

Bindman, A. B., K. Grumbach, D. Osmond, M. Komaromy, K. Vranizan, N. Lurie, J. Billings, and A. Stewart. 1995. "Preventable Hospitalization and Access to Care." *Journal of the American Medical Association* 274 (4): 305–11.

Blumberg, M. S. 1986. "Risk-Adjusting Health Care Outcomes: A Methodological Review." *Medical Care Review* 43: 351–93.

Brailer, D. J., E. Kroch, M. V. Pauly, and J. Huang. 1996. "Comorbidity-Adjusted Complication Risk: A New Outcome Quality Measure." *Medical Care* 34 (5): 490–505.

Brennan, T. A., L. L. Leape, N. M. Laird, L. Hebert, A. R. Localio, A. G. Lawthers, J. P. Newhouse, P. C. Weiler, and H. H. Hiatt. 1991. "Incidence of Adverse Events and Negligence in Hospitalized Patients: Results of the Harvard Medical Practice Study." *The New England Journal of Medicine* 324 (6): 370–76.

Chassin, M. R., E. L. Hannan, and B. A. DeBuono. 1996. "Benefits and Hazards of Reporting Medical Outcomes Publicly." *New England Journal of Medicine* 334 (6): 394–98.

Creditor, M. C. 1993. "Hazards of Hospitalization of the Elderly." *Annals of Internal Medicine* 118 (3): 220–23.

Deming, W. E. 1982. *Quality, Productivity, and Competitive Position.* Cambridge: Massachusetts Institute of Technology, Center for Advanced Engineering Study.

DesHarnais, S. I., L. F. J. McMahon, Jr., R. T. Wroblewski, and A. J. Hogan. 1990. "Measuring Hospital Performance: The Development and Validation of Risk-Adjusted Indices of Mortality, Readmission, and Complications." *Medical Care* 28 (12): 1127–41.

Donabedian, A. 1990. "Contributions of Epidemiology to Quality Assessment and Monitoring." *Infection Control and Hospital Epidemiology* 11 (3): 117–21.

———. 1989. "The End Results of Health Care: Ernest Codman's Contribution to Quality Assessment and Beyond." *Milbank Quarterly* 67 (2): 233–67.

———. 1985. "The Epidemiology of Quality." *Inquiry* 22 (Fall 1985): 282–92.

———. 1980. *The Definition of Quality and Approaches to Its Assessment.* Chicago: Health Administration Press.

Duncan, W. J., P. M. Gunter, and L. E. Swayne. 1997. *Strategic Management of Health Care Organizations.* Malden, MA: Blackwell Publishers.

Drucker, P. F. "If Earnings Aren't the Dial to Read." *The Wall Street Journal.* (30 October 1986): 32.

Epstein, A. M. 1998. "Rolling Down the Runway: The Challenges Ahead for Quality Report Cards." *Journal of the American Medical Association* 279 (21): 1691–96.

Fleming, S. T. 1996. "Complications, Adverse Events, and Iatrogenesis: Classifications and Quality of Care Measurement Issues." *Clinical Performance and Quality Health Care* 4 (3): 137–47.

Fleming, S. T., K. D. Bopp, and K. G. Anderson. 1993. "Spreading the 'Good News' of Total Quality Management: Faith, Conversion, and Commitment." *Health Care Management Review* 18 (4): 29–33.

Fleming, S. T., L. L. Hicks, and R. C. Bailey. 1995. "Interpreting the Health Care Financing Administration's Mortality Statistics." *Medical Care* 33 (2): 186–201.

Gayes, R. P. 1997. "Surveillance of Nosocomial Infections: A Fundamental Ingredient for Quality." *Infection Control and Hospital Epidemiology* 18 (7): 475–78.

Green, J., and N. Wintfeld. 1995. "Report Cards on Cardiac Surgeons: Assessing New York State's Approach." *The New England Journal of Medicine* 332 (18): 1229–32.

Halfon, N.,and P. W. Newacheck. 1993. "Childhood Asthma and Poverty: Differential Impacts and Utilization of Health Care Services." *Pediatrics* 91 (1): 56–61.

Hannan, E. L., D. Kumar, M. Racz, A. L. Siu, and M. R. Chassin. 1994. "New York State's Cardiac Surgery Reporting System: Four Years Later." *Annals of Thoracic Surgery* 58 (6): 1852–57.

Hannan, E. L., A. L. Siu, D. Kumar, H. Kilburn Jr., and M. R. Chassin. 1995. "The Decline in Coronary Artery Bypass Graft Surgery Mortality in New York State: The Role of Surgeon Volume." *Journal of the American Medical Association* 273 (3): 209–13.

Harris, J. R., B. Caldwell, and K. Cahill. 1998. "Measuring the Public's Health in an Era of Accountability." *American Journal of Preventive Medicine* 14 (3, Supplement): 9–13.

Iezzoni, L. I. 1997a. *Risk Adjustment for Measuring Healthcare Outcomes.* Chicago: Health Adminstration Press.

Iezzoni, L. I. 1997b. "The Risks of Risk Adjustment." *Journal of the American Medical Association* 278 (19): 1600–07.

Iezzoni, L. I., J. Daley, T. Heeren, S. M. Foley, J. S. Hughes, E. S. Fisher, C. C. Duncan, and G. A. Coffman. 1994. "Using Administrative Data to Screen Hospitals for High Complication Rates." *Inquiry* 31 (1): 40–55.

Juran, J. M., and F. M. J. Gryna, eds. 1988. *Juran's Quality Control Handbook, 4th ed..* New York: McGraw-Hill.

Laffel, G., and D. Blumenthal. 1989. "The Case for Using Industrial Quality Management Science in Healthcare Organizations." *Journal of the American Medical Association* 266 (20): 2869–73.

Larson, E., L. F. Oram, and E. Hedrick. 1988. "Nosocomial Infection Rates as an Indicator of Quality." *Medical Care* 26 (7): 676–84.

Marszalek-Gaucher, E. J., and R. J. Coffey. 1993. *Total Quality in Healthcare: From Theory to Practice.* San Francisco: Jossey-Bass.

Massachusetts Rate Setting Commission. 1995. *Improving Primary Care Using Preventable Hospitalization as an Approach.* A Report of the Massachusetts Rate Setting Commission. Springfield, MA: MRSC.

Massanari, R. M., K. Wilkerson, and S. Swartzendruber. 1995. "Designing Surveillance for Noninfectious Outcomes of Medical Care." *Infection Control and Hospital Epidemiology* 16 (7): 419–26.

Pottinger, J. M., L. A. Herwaldt, and T. M. Peri. 1997. "Basics of Surveillance: An Overview." *Infection Control and Hospital Epidemiology* 18 (7): 513–27.

Rakich, J. S., B. B. Longest, and K. Darr. 1992. *Managing Health Services Organizations.* Baltimore, MD: Health Professions Press.

Schneider, E. C., and A. M. Epstein. 1996. "Influence of Cardiac Surgery Performance Reports on Referral Practices and Access to Care." *The New England Journal of Medicine* 335 (4): 251–56.

Silber, J. H., P. R. Rosenbaum, J. S. Schwartz, R. N. Ross, and S. V. Williams. 1995.

"Evaluation of the Complication Rate as a Measure of Quality of Care in Coronary Artery Bypass Graft Surgery." *Journal of the American Medical Association* 274 (4): 317–23.

Sinioris, M. E., and K. L. Najafi. 1995. "Epidemiology and Health Care Quality Management." In *Epidemiology and the Delivery of Health Care Services: Methods and Applications*, edited by D. M. Oleske. New York: Plenum Press.

Solberg, L. I., K. E. Peterson, and R. W. Ellis. 1990. "The Minnesota Project: A Focused Approach to Ambulatory Quality Assessment." *Inquiry* 27 (4): 359–67.

Spoeri, R. K., and R. Ullman. 1997. "Measuring and Reporting Managed Care Performance: Lessons Learned and New Initiatives." *Annals of Internal Medicine* 127 (8): 726–32.

Timmreck, T. C. 1998. *An Introduction to Epidemiology.* Boston: Jones and Barlett Publishers.

Weissman, J. S., C. Gatsonis, and A. M. Epstein. 1992. "Rates of Avoidable Hospitalization by Insurance Status in Massachusetts and Maryland." *Journal of the American Medical Association* 268 (17): 2388–94.

Wissow, L. S., A. M. Gittelsohn, M. Szklo, B. Starfield, and M. Mussman. 1988. "Poverty, Race, and Hospitalization for Childhood Asthma." *American Journal of Public Health* 78 (7): 777–82.

Epidemiology and the Organizing and Staffing Functions

Lyle Snider and Steven T. Fleming

Mr. Jones, the CEO of Group Health East, has been approached by Dr. Wheez, a prominent and influential member of the board of directors, to consider asthma as a specific product line. What kinds of epidemiologic data and/or studies does Mr. Jones need to evaluate?

I n the coming years, the performance of medical care organizations and health-care systems will increasingly be assessed by health status and outcomes measures derived, at least in part, from the methods of epidemiology (Kindig 1997; MCH Model Standards Working Group 1997). Because these outcomes can have a substantial influence on the design of healthcare organizations and their delivery systems, a valid and precise measurement of these variables is critical. Moreover, changes in the environment—in technology, demography, and reimbursement, and in the healthcare industry as a whole—may require organizational redesign, for instance, a move to product line management or "centers of excellence" (Shortell, Gillies, and Devers 1995). Epidemiology can provide critical input in this decision-making process.

The staffing function is an important component of organizational design. Successful medical care organizations (MCOs) evaluate staffing continuously to ensure the optimal array of healthcare workers and the optimal staffing level for each type of worker (Ruzek et al. 1999). For example, the advent of minimally invasive surgery using fiber optics in the ambulatory care setting has increased the rate of same-day surgeries and has reduced the number of overnight hospital stays. This development has reduced the demand for hospital beds and the staff for those beds, but it has increased the demand for health workers in home health (Buerhaus, Staiger, and Douglas 1996). A change in health worker staffing may also be caused by new diseases. The AIDS epidemic caused a dramatic increase in the demand for health educators for unique target audiences: gay men and IV drug users (Guenther-Grey et al. 1992). Epidemiology is used to assess health outcomes and predict future staffing needs as the organization adapts to a rapidly changing healthcare environment.

This chapter discusses the ways in which the concepts and methods of epidemiology can inform the organization and staffing functions of the healthcare manager. We discuss the organization design process as a continuous activity over time, in which epidemiologic measurement can inform the manager by assessing organizational performance and characterizing the needs of the population served. We then discuss three major building blocks of organizational design (division of work, span of control, and coordination) and three major types of organizational design (functional, divisional, and matrix). In each case, epidemiology provides critical information to the manager as these building blocks are chiseled into different configurations or design structures. We then discuss the development of product lines and the role of epidemiology in providing crucial information to that process. Finally, we consider the staffing function of a manager and develop a simple model to predict human resources by describing the needs of the population served with epidemiologic measures.

Epidemiology and Continuous Organizing

Successful MCOs must continuously evaluate their organizational design and staffing and make the necessary changes as a routine component of the organization's management. Some modifications in organizational design are required as routine evaluation of the organization's performance reveals problems. A more important cause of organizational redesign is the increasingly rapid change throughout the healthcare system. The list of health system components that can change quickly includes technology, reimbursement systems, the incidence and prevalence of disease, and ownership.

One event that may inspire a change in organizational design is an unacceptably low level of performance (Avery 1999). The organization may not facilitate collaboration in critical areas, or it may not create the required incentives among departments and workers. For example, managers may apply epidemiologic concepts (e.g., routine surveillance) to discover that the level of nosocomial infections in a hospital is higher than that of competitors because of inadequate infection control by the housekeepers as they move from room to room to clean and empty the trash. To remedy this problem, for instance, a change in organizational design would place the housekeeping department under the supervision of the director of nursing. This example illustrates both the routine use of epidemiology by managers to assess the management process and the need to assess and change organizational design to achieve optimal performance.

A major cause of transformation in organizational design is a change in the "environment" (Shortell, Gillies, and Devers 1995). An organization's environment includes competitors, clients, reimbursement systems, available healthcare technology, and characteristics of the local community (population demographics, schools, social welfare agencies, law enforcement, transportation, communications, and so on). Unfavorable changes in the environment often result in financial losses. New healthcare technology presents both opportunities and risks for the organization, particularly during the technology's early years of implementation. If the organization adapts to changes in the environment by changing types of services ("product lines"), or by changing leadership, these developments usually require a change in organizational design (Leatt, Shortell, and Kimberly 1994). Managers can use measures of morbidity (such as case mix in the hospital setting and incidence/prevalence of disease in the ambulatory setting) to evaluate ways in which the organization should respond to environmental change in terms of new product lines. Moreover, as managers implement organizational redesign, epidemiology becomes an essential managerial tool to assess the effect of the organizational changes on healthcare outcomes.

Financial losses are a strong motivator for organizational change, not only in healthcare but also in other organizations and agencies (Norton and Lipson 1998). In healthcare, the losses are frequently concentrated in a specific area of the healthcare organization, such as obstetrics. Common environmental changes for obstetrics are changes in reimbursement and the emergence of competitors. A reorganization of obstetrics or the discontinuance of obstetrical services is often sufficient to reverse the financial losses. Epidemiologic measures can be used to forecast the need for obstetrical services in the community. The epidemiologic forecast would provide an understanding of the relative risk of neonatal intensive care and other special obstetrical services given the kinds of risk factors (or exposures) in the hospital service area, such as smoking, substance abuse, AIDS, and lack of prenatal services use. Managers can also use epidemiology to identify the most important determinants of optimal obstetric outcomes as they develop a new organizational design for obstetric services that includes the proper mix of prevention, technology, and workforce (Sachs et al. 1999). For example, the organization may want to evaluate epidemiologic studies that compare outcomes for obstetricians, nurse practitioners, and midwives, or consider the studies that examine the routine use of ultrasound for normal pregnancies (Ewigman et al. 1993). Occasionally, a healthcare organization faces losses in most areas of its service that require a complete overhaul of the entire enterprise's organizational design or dissolution of the organization.

New technology is another force that may prompt a change in the nature of healthcare work; such deep-seated change will require a modification of organizational design. The new technology may involve pharmaceuticals, surgical techniques, information technology, behavior modification programs, or types of health providers. For example, older men must make a decision on whether or not to be screened for prostate cancer. A positive test result means more decisions about diagnostic follow-up and treatment alternatives should prostate cancer be confirmed. Men are becoming better informed about these issues from a variety of sources. One important source of information is the Internet, which gives men access to prostate cancer information at many different levels of complexity. As a result, men are better informed, although some may be misinformed by a "cyberspace" that is not subject to the normal peer review of most respectable journals (Lindberg and Humphreys 1998). As technology enables more health information to be stored in a digital format, men with prostate cancer who move to a new region when they retire will find that their new healthcare providers have comprehensive records that even include the latest images of the prostate showing the progression of the disease. These developments will foster a greater coordination of healthcare among providers and with the client. The cost of this technological adventure will be a change in the nature of the provider-client relationship. The character of the work performed by physicians, radiation technicians, and record and billing clerks will be markedly changed. New organizational designs may be necessary to function effectively within this data-driven and information-charged kind of environment. The increased availability of epidemiologic information can be a blessing to physicians, however, despite the changes in organizational designs that may be necessary as a tradition-based style of practice is replaced with evidence-based medicine (see Chapter 12 for a discussion of this transition).

Another important characteristic of an organization's environment is the preferences, needs, and health status of the client population. Many factors affect a client population, including natural birth, death, and aging, migration into (or out of) the service area, and the emergence of new diseases. Over the past two decades, the proportion of the population over 65 has increased dramatically in several areas of the country because of the in-migration of retirees. This regional aging of the population has markedly changed the demand for certain kinds of healthcare services, such as arthritis treatment, artificial knees and hips, cancer diagnosis and treatment, and heart disease, while less emphasis has been placed on obstetrics, pediatrics, family planning, and sports medicine. Epidemiologic measures can identify market opportunities that may result from a changing client population. For example, a high level of late-stage breast cancer diagnoses in a retirement destination area may indicate a market opportunity for better patient education and access to mammography screening. Referring to Table 10.1, which ADD offers the best mammography screening market opportunity for radiologists and surgeons in the area on the basis of these breast cancer incidence rates? A change in organizational design (the focus of the next two sections) may facilitate the creation of a breast cancer screening program.

TABLE 10.1
1997–1998 Two-Year Age-adjusted Breast Cancer Incidence Rates in Kentucky by Selected Area Development Districts

ADD District	All Stages		Early Stage		Late Stage	
	Cases	Rate	Cases	Rate	Cases	Rate
Cumberland, Valley	259	88.5	144	49.1	88	30.9
Gateway	109	132.2	63	75.0	42	52.5
Purchase	393	136.0	268	92.6	109	39.1
Kentucky total	5,993	119.6	3,889	78.0	1,828	36.6

The incidence rates for breast cancer by stage at diagnosis for the entire state of Kentucky and for selected Area Development Districts (ADDs) are displayed.
Source: Adapted from Kentucky Cancer Registry. "Cancer Incident Reports (1991–1998)." University of Kentucky. [Online]. http://www.kcr.uky.edu. April 26, 2000.

Epidemiology and Organizational Designs

The major building block of organizational design is "division of work." Each organization is characterized by the degree of worker specialization and expertise. In healthcare some aspects of the work have become highly specialized, and the work of many workers is defined by licensure and regulation. For example, the only workers allowed to perform brain surgery are those who are licensed physicians and have completed a neurological surgery residency. Similarly, the administration of intramuscular injections is limited to nurses and physicians in most settings. Many health workers must receive specific training that leads to licensure. However, even unlicensed workers may be specialized. The housekeeping staff are not licensed, but they have more knowledge of cleaning solutions, buffers, and other cleaning equipment than other workers. The healthcare organization that divides work to promote the efficient completion of tasks should reasonably be expected to be effective. Epidemiology is one set of tools used to assess the outcomes that result from the current division of work. Because outcomes are such an important indicator of health system performance, it will be necessary for every healthcare worker to have a basic understanding of epidemiology. Each employee should understand the critical bearing that the performance of their work has on outcomes and the job performance factors that lead to most optimal outcomes (see Chapter 8 for a discussion of this concept).

Consider the "division of work" within a typical soccer team, the objective of which is to place the ball past the opponent's goal line and within the net boundary. Soccer players as young as 12 years know that they can be more effective in accomplishing this objective by "dividing" the work, or specializing. The task of the goalie is the most specialized: the goalie generally stays close to the goal, wears a distinctively colored uniform, and is the only player allowed to use arms and hands to accomplish the task of keeping the ball from crossing "into the net." This task is also highly specialized because it requires a unique set of skills. The remaining players also specialize (defense, midfield, or attack), but less so than the goalie since they share more skills and attributes (ball handling skills, kicking power, and speed). Another indication of the lack of specialization of the remaining players is their ability to switch positions and roles during the course of the game. Practice involves the rehearsal of plays or "procedures" that involve the division and coordination of the "work" of everyone on the team. When soccer teams review the opponent's previous games, they search for patterns of play that lead to the opponent's success or failure, such as a player's favorite position for shooting on goal.

Healthcare organizations can be compared to soccer teams inasmuch as the work is divided among multiple specialists, each of whom contributes to the "goal" of quality care. There may be some position switching, as in nurses assigned to different wings but (to switch metaphor), a division of work "fabric" is defined by licensure and certification constraints—call it starch if you will. The role of epidemiology so far as this fabric is concerned is to evaluate and measure the degree to which the current division of work results in optimal outcomes. Epidemiology can also be used to predict whether changes in the division of work adversely affect patient care. An example of this would be the move to allowing allied health professionals with multi-disciplinary training more freedom in performing tasks outside their principal area of expertise.

Large organizations with many employees must allocate workers into groups of a manageable size, because a single manager is unable to successfully manage more than 10–15 individual workers. For the first 50–60 years of the 1900s, these similar kinds of workers were aggregated into units called departments, for example, nursing, housekeeping, and laboratory. More recently, employees have been grouped on the basis of involvement in specific projects. Project organization, as it is called, places employees from a variety of departments in close proximity to work on a task that requires coordination and collaboration from a variety of workers with different skills and experience. Project organization has been particularly effective for innovative initiatives such as the development of the first atomic bomb, landing a man on the moon, and the development of early computers and their programs. Product line organization is another form of project organization that brings together workers from a variety of disciplines to provide a set of services. For example, prostate patients who visit a prostate cancer center can obtain a variety of services that may include laboratory tests, x-rays, and physician examination and evaluation by staying in one location rather than by having to walk from one end of the hospital to the other to visit several departments.

Span of control is an important organizational design concept that refers to the number of workers or lower-level managers who should report to a higher-level manager (see Figure 10.1). One example of a broad span of control is the direction given to pharmacists in a hospital pharmacy organization. Because a pharmacist's work is highly standardized, one manager is able to direct a large number of pharmacists successfully in this setting. On the other hand, the management of an operating room for highly specialized surgery may require a narrow span of control. The nurse manager is unable to manage a large group of workers in this setting because the work is not standardized and will change as new

FIGURE 10.1
Broad and Narrow
Spans of Control

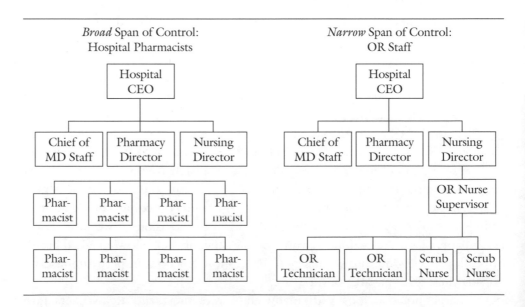

procedures and techniques are developed. A common strategy to reduce costs is the reduction or eliminatation of middle managers so that the span of control for remaining managers is increased. As employers and consumers demand better-quality healthcare, epidemiology will be used to determine if the reduction of the middle managers has been successful both in lowering costs and in maintaining or improving outcomes.

Coordination of the work within an organization was involved in many of the examples cited here, although it was not explicitly described. The *Oxford American Dictionary* defines "coordinate" as "to work or cause to work together efficiently" (Ehrlich et al. 1980). Coordination is achieved through communication among different units of the organization and by workers within each unit. One important form of coordination for most organizations is a regular meeting of program and department heads, and these meetings often occur on Monday mornings. These meetings define the organization's short-term goals for the week as well as the plan to achieve the goals in a manner that will facilitate the efforts of all workers to efficiently complement each other. Some workers are frustrated at "long" coordination meetings that distract them from their urgent work. Successful managers conduct brief coordination meetings that concisely define the issues and outline the required collaboration and that discourage long explications not required to conduct the week's work.

Another important form of coordination is voluntary or informal coordination (Rakich, Longest, and Darr 1992) that occurs either through worker or group communication, or both, conducted in the course of work performance. Rakich notes that this type of voluntary, informal coordination makes an important contribution to organizational efficiency and effectiveness. An important requirement for voluntary coordination is workers who are empowered to take this level of initiative. Managers with a basic understanding of epidemiology are more likely to coordinate work in a manner that furthers the primary goal of the medical care organization: quality patient care. Coordination should be facilitated as managers (1) develop credibility among medical professionals; (2) reduce communication barriers that separate managers from medical professionals; and (3) communicate to employees, in epidemiologic terms, the effect of their jobs on outcomes and the importance of their work to patients (Chapter 8).

Epidemiology tools can also be used to design product lines, describe the market population, and evaluate the outcomes of changes in organizational design outcomes. This use of epidemiology has been used extensively by the public health sector to prevent the transmission of diseases. For example, HIV infection control efforts have used epidemiology to identify the people who are at greatest risk of contracting HIV as well as the behaviors that place them at risk. These programs have identified shared needles and unprotected sexual intercourse as common causes of HIV transmission. Epidemiology was used to locate the highest-risk population geographically so that the most effective behavior modification interventions could be concentrated on those with the highest risk.

Organizational Designs

Three common organizational designs for healthcare entities are the functional, divisional, and matrix structures (Leatt, Shortell, and Kimberly 1994). The **functional design** allocates workers into departments based on function or on discipline. Typical departments in an organization with a functional design are administration, dietary, housekeeping, nursing, and physical therapy. The major advantage of this design is that managers in each department are usually from the same professional discipline as their workers and have a good understanding of the tasks performed by each worker. The advantage of placing discipline-specific managers in high-level positions is illustrated by the director of hospital physical therapy who combines substantial administrative power and influence with clinical physical therapy experience. Physical therapists who face administrative obstacles to high-quality physical therapy care have a powerful advocate for action to remove the obstacles. The major disadvantage is that the design encourages discipline-oriented thinking that may limit the range of potential solutions considered by workers and managers. In addition, this design's concentration of decision making at the top level of management inhibits spontaneous collaboration among disciplines in the clinics and wards where healthcare is delivered. As a result of this process, the organization is unable to initiate those collaborations and adaptations to changing conditions that emanate from the lower-level healthcare workers.

One example of the functional design is a nursing home in the 1980s in which many different workers—including the head cook, the housekeeping maintenance supervisor, and the nursing director—report directly to the nursing home director. As nursing home care has become more complex in the 1990s with the addition of social workers, physical therapists, and occupational therapists, as well as with more process measures of quality, nursing homes have adopted a more flexible organizational design that facilitates greater levels of collaboration among disciplines and faster adaptation to changing conditions.

The **divisional design** allocates workers by departments and disciplines. In the 1980s and early 1990s, many academic medical centers and other large hospitals used this design with departments based on medical specialties (such as medicine, surgery, and pediatrics) and discipline-specific management structures within each division. The advantage of this design is a congruence with physician training and specialties. The major disadvantage is that patients have healthcare needs that draw on skills from a wide variety of health professions. The divisional design often hinders collaboration across specialties and disciplines. Another disadvantage is that divisional management structures sometimes come into conflict with departmental management structures. For example, the nursing and medicine division policies for the roles of nurses and physicians may interfere with an efficient use of personnel in certain specialized wards that require unique functions for both nurses and physicians.

An example of a divisional design is the radiology department of a large hospital that performs both diagnostic and treatment procedures. The radiology equipment and personnel are located in one area of the hospital, and patients from throughout the facility as well as ambulatory patients go to that area for radiology services. Because all of the personnel are in close proximity, the divisional design facilitates management of the radiology services by the chief of radiology to achieve the optimum quality of services. On the other hand, the design makes it difficult for the nursing vice president to coordinate an efficient utilization of nurses and to co-ordinate their continuing education. Another problem with this divisional design is that patients who require other services at the hospital (e.g., physical therapy, lab, specialty physicians, and so on) must travel to the far reaches of a large hospital and must make appointments and wait in line in many different departments.

The **matrix structure** became much more popular in the 1990s as health-care organizations developed product lines (family-centered obstetrics, heart attack rehabilitation, women's health, and so on) to improve marketing and performance. Many institutions call their specialized service sites "centers of excellence." The matrix structure retains the discipline-specific departments of the functional design and adds the horizontal lines of authority for programs or product lines (see Figure 10.2). The advantage of the matrix structure is that it facilitates effective collaboration among workers from a variety of disciplines to deliver care to select groups of patients. "This seems particularly appropriate given that many of the major diseases of the 1990s—AIDS, Alzheimer's, cancer, trauma, and behavioral problems—are not diseases that single departments can handle but, rather, illnesses that require an entire system of care" (Shortell, Gillies, and Devers 1995). Product

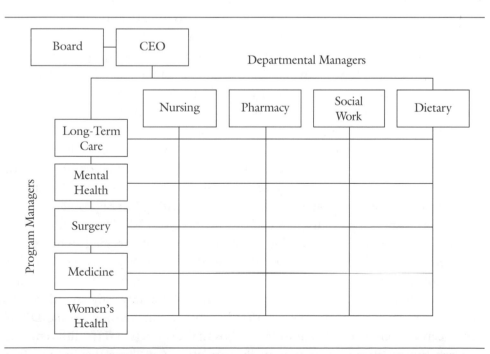

FIGURE 10.2
Matrix Organizational Design

Source: Baker, G. R., L. Narine, and P. Leatt. 1994. "Organizational Designs for Health Care." In *The AUPHA Manual of Health Services Management*, edited by R. J. Taylor and S. B. Taylor. Gaithersburg, MD: Aspen Publishers, Inc.

line patients receive one-stop shopping for all of their required services. Another advantage is that it allows managers to focus cost-control efforts on specific kinds of diseases, selected on the basis of cost, frequency, preventability, or other critical factors. One disadvantage of the matrix design is the conflicting lines of authority that appear among disciplinary departments and product line organizations. One example of the conflicting values between departments and product lines is the desire of laboratory technicians to perform all lab work in the centralized hospital lab to promote efficiency and quality control, while "centers of excellence' clinics want to perform lab tests in the clinic to facilitate prompt results. In addition, not all patients require services that comprise a product line, and they may have to obtain services from sectors of the hospital that do not receive the resources and management attention received by the centers. For example, few hospitals have "lupus centers." Lupus erythematosus patients, who face the same problems outlined under the divisional design, must travel all over the hospital to obtain services from a wide variety of departments.

Product Lines

Suppose that an organization were interested in moving away from a functional or divisional structure to a matrix model. The challenge would be to identify and to develop relevant product lines or programs. At least initially this would involve a **needs assessment** both in terms of an internal assessment of capacity (i.e., current products, and current physical and human resources) and an external assessment of the environment (markets, competitors, needs of the population, and so forth). The latter, of course, is characterized by epidemiological measures such as the incidence/prevalence of acute and chronic disease. Within the hospital, one could examine case-mix patterns over a period of years, say ten. Diagnosis-related groups represent specific hospital products for the Medicare population, whose data have been available since 1983. It would be useful to examine changes in DRG mix over time, and across competitors in the hospital service area, to describe the need for specific "hospital" products in the service area. If the organization is a managed care organization, then one may also want to get measures of ambulatory care need, if available, such as a breakdown of visits to physicians by diagnosis. It would also be worthwhile to collect data on the enrolled population, in terms of various risk factors that lead to disease, such as obesity, smoking, and hazardous workplaces. This information would be key to forecasting future product lines.

Consider Group Health East (GHE), the fictitious 100,000-member managed care organization introduced in Chapter 1, which has decided to move to a matrix model of organization with specific product lines or programs. The enrolled population is characterized on three dimensions: acute care, ambulatory care, and risk factors. For acute care, the prevalence of disease/disability is measured by case mix and described over a five-year period by DRGs. Furthermore, some DRGs have been clustered together into larger hospital products. GHE differentiates between those DRGs that are potentially avoidable from those that are not (see Chapter 9). In terms of ambulatory visits, members are grouped into classes based on diagnosis. For risk factors, members are assessed based on smoking, obesity, substance abuse, and employment in a hazardous workplace. The three dimensions are then integrated into potential product lines or programs. For example, the acute care DRG profile reported 250 hospitalizations for asthma in 1999, at least some of which were avoidable, for a rate of 2.5 per 1,000 population. Although the incidence of asthma in the United States and throughout the world has increased dramatically over the past several decades (Pearce 1998; Chadwick and Cardew 1997), the GSE rate was considerably higher than the statewide average. The ambulatory visit profile showed 3,500 physician visits for asthma for a rate of 4 per 100 enrolled members, somewhat lower than the state average. In terms of risk factors, 35 percent of the enrolled population were considered regular smokers, a suspected risk factor for pediatric asthma. Based on these data, and on discussions with the medical staffs from both affiliated group practices, GHE decides to consider developing the prevention and treatment of asthma into a distinct program. The purpose of this structural change would be to improve the management of asthma in the ambulatory setting and reduce that incidence of avoidable hospitalization.

Group Health East is aware that childhood asthma has received substantial attention from health services managers as one of the most common causes of preventable hospitalizations. The reduction of preventable hospitalizations is a high priority for organizations such as GHE as they strive to lower costs and improve outcomes. In addition, childhood asthma illustrates the important potential contributions of people and organizations outside of the traditional healthcare process. The causes of preventable hospitalizations from childhood asthma include poor access to ambulatory care, lack of utilization of the most effective drug protocols by the healthcare provider, school and after-school teachers' lack of knowledge about the disease process, school policies that prevent the administration of inhalers and other pharmaceuticals at school, and tobacco smoke in the home (Second Expert Panel on the Management of Asthma 1997). Although traditional healthcare services are an important component of a healthcare system to reduce morbidity and hospitalizations, there are other components that are equally important. These components would include 18- to 24-hour access to ambulatory care; adoption of the most effective treatment protocols by healthcare providers; 24-hour access to inhaler treatments; and education of the patients, parents, and teachers on the most effective procedure to administer inhalants. GHE believes that the structural change to a distinct asthma program will allow more careful monitoring of members with asthma, a reduction in avoidable hospitalizations associated with this disease, and the development of innovative outreach programs to embrace others, outside of the traditional healthcare system, who also have an effect on outcomes of care.

Epidemiology and Information Systems

The focus on outcomes will transform the information systems of organizations that provide medical care as well as other policymaking and collaborating agencies

(Rivers and Bae 1999; Roos et al. 1996). Traditional information systems were designed primarily to collect cost information and expedite patient billing. The information specialists for these systems often had a background in business or accounting. Although some software systems exist that monitor outcomes and risk factors, most organizations collect data on outcomes and risk factors for a very limited number of health conditions. In the future, medical care organizations and integrated systems may compete on the basis of comprehensive programs to track and monitor outcomes. To do so will require the employment of specialists in outcome measurement and biostatistics, and the collection of additional data on both outcomes and risk factors. These data must be accurately and efficiently compiled and fashioned into valid measures of organizational effectiveness for the purpose of comparison with other competitors.

Outcomes specialists will improve the accuracy and validity of the outcomes assessments. To manage these specialists effectively, managers will need an understanding of epidemiology. This understanding will enable administrators not only to evaluate the performance of the specialists, but also to describe and disseminate the outcome assessments more effectively. For example, to accurately evaluate the success of a program to reduce cardiovascular disease morbidity and mortality, the administrator needs to review heart disease mortality rates and compare them to regional and national benchmarks. The validity of this comparison will depend on a variety of epidemiological issues, including sample size and adjustment for income, age, gender, race, and other cardiovascular risk factors (Alter, Naylor, and Tu 1999).

Epidemiology and Staffing

One critical function for successful managed care organizations is the achievement of optimal health professions and health worker staffing because employee benefits comprise a substantial portion of hospital expenses. Two major components to optimal staffing must be considered: (1) the selection of the optimal types and mix of healthcare workers, and (2) obtaining the minimum number of worker hours required to provide the services. To select the optimal types of workers, workers with the lowest levels of training and the lowest salary levels necessary to perform the required tasks are employed. As organizations strive to achieve optimal staffing, they must employ epidemiology to ensure that changes in staffing patterns do not have a negative effect on health status and health outcomes. Since nurses are the most numerous healthcare professionals, healthcare organizations for many years have devoted substantial resources to the development of optimal nurse staffing levels. Nurses and their employers have used epidemiology to document outcomes in their ongoing debates on the adequacy of the number and skill mix of nurses. One factor that forces constant reassessment of staffing patterns is the rapid rate of healthcare technology development and change. The second factor that influences optimal staffing is changes in reimbursement for specific professions.

The implementation of managed care causes enormous changes in health-care worker staffing patterns for many types of healthcare workers. For example, managed care strives to promote the utilization of primary care physicians, nurse practitioners, and physician assistants as case managers and the initial entry point into the healthcare system. Also, these organizations seek to reduce utilization of highly paid specialists and their relatively expensive procedures and operations. The research is somewhat mixed with regard to this new model of healthcare delivery, which focuses on primary care and away from expensive specialists and hospitalization. It is unclear whether managed care has an adverse effect on patient outcomes and, if so, what the primary reasons are (Barber 1997; Clement et al. 1994; Krieger, Connell, and LoGerfo 1992; Miller, Weissert, and Chernew 1998). Any of a number of factors may affect outcomes (either favorably or unfavorably), such as the mix of primary care versus specialists and use of lower-cost physician extenders.

Rakish, Longest, and Darr (1992) describe human resources planning as a five-step process: profiling, estimating, inventorying, forecasting, and planning. Profiling involves estimating the quantity and mix of employees who are needed to staff the organization. With the estimating step, industry standards, such as staffing ratios, are used to project the number of employees necessary. The skills of current employees are assessed in the inventory step. Forecasting involves estimating workforce changes such as deaths, retirements, and transfers. In the planning stage, the organization articulates a plan based on the assumptions of the previous four steps to meet the anticipated needs of the organization. Epidemiology should play a significant role, particularly in the profiling stage of human resource planning, inasmuch as the organization must estimate the need for human resources based on the expected demand for services.

Some of the theory and techniques that have been developed to estimate the need for physician workforce in the aggregate (i.e., across the United States) could be adapted for organization-wide workforce profiling. This would not be as relevant in a nonintegrated, fee-for-service environment, in which each level of care (ambulatory, acute, and long-term care) provide separate, and not necessarily coordinated, services. In a managed care environment, however, it seems reasonable to estimate the need for workforce by describing the kinds of present and future morbidity that can be expected among enrolled members.

A simplified version of the Donabedian (1973) model is illustrated in Figure 10.3, in which "need" can be associated with service equivalents, which can then be associated with resource equivalents. This paradigm was anticipated by Lee and Jones (1933), who were probably the first to estimate the need for physician workforce in their classic study. They estimated the number of people in a population who should receive different kinds of services based on the prevalence of disease, and they estimated the amount of time and number of services that would be required for each disease: this latter relates to the "strategy" of care. Finally, they predicted the number of services that could be provided by each professional, obviously a measure of physician productivity. Thus, in this model,

The Relationship
Among Need,
Services, and
Resources

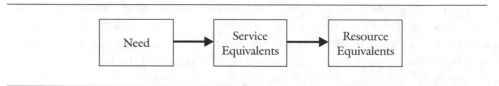

Source: Based on Donabedian, A. 1973. *Aspects of Medical Care Administration*. Cambridge, MA: Harvard University Press.

need (as measured by the prevalence of disease) could be translated into services (using strategies, "guidelines," standards, or whatever), which could then be translated into workforce based on productivity. Clearly, productivity depends on type of practitioner, setting, organization, and even gender.

The major shortcoming of the "needs-based" methods of Lee and Jones and Donabedian, in terms of forecasting workforce, is that it is based entirely on a "normative" rather than an "actual" measure of the services required by each type of morbidity. In other words, with Lee and Jones, a panel of physicians would prescribe the kinds of services that "ought" to be provided for each kind of disease. The modern-day approach would be to use a practice guideline, "clinical trajectory," or critical pathway to predict a mix of services. Regardless of time frame, the point is that normative prescriptions for service delivery may not directly translate into utilization because of access barriers, financial or otherwise. Lack of insurance may prevent a patient from securing medical care regardless of the practice guideline's specifications. Because of this dilemma, some of the more recent models to predict physician workforce, such as the approach by the Graduate Medical Education Advisory Committee, or GMENAC (McNutt 1981), have attempted to factor market behavior into the projections. Thus the requirements for workforce are based at least in part on a predicted demand for services.

Even the rather simple needs-based model (need → services → workforce) is encumbered with complexity and cannot be fully understood or developed without epidemiologic concepts and insight. Clearly, the model is only as good as the measures to assess "need." The measurement of need is doubtless an epidemiologic concept, expressed formally as the incidence and prevalence rates discussed in Chapter 2. The accuracy of the model also depends on the set of "standards" that are used to translate need into service equivalents. For instance, the organization that is trying to predict workforce needs may choose standards that are less than "best practice," in which case workforce needs may be overestimated. Services are translated into workforce through productivity norms that may vary, of course, by type of setting or organization: physician office, hospital, clinic, and so on.

Suppose you are the CEO of a large managed care organization—Mr. Jones with Group Health East, for instance. You are trying to anticipate the future need for staffing, particularly with regard to physicians and nurses, and others in the allied health workforce, such as physical therapists. The simplest approach would be to describe your present need based on the prevalence of cardiovascular morbidity in the enrolled population, as illustrated in Figure 10.4. You could predict the number of physician visits (generalist and specialist), nursing services, surgical procedures, laboratory tests, and so on, that would be associated with each cardiovascular diagnosis. The number of professional and support personnel that would be required to deliver and support those services could be extrapolated from these data using productivity norms.

A more "upstream" approach to predicting staffing requirements is illustrated in Figure 10.5, where risk factors of disease (such as smoking) are expected to increase the incidence of various kinds of morbidity (such as lung cancer, heart disease, and emphysema). For example, smoking makes one twice as likely to get heart disease and ten times as likely to get lung cancer (refer to Chapter 12). Future incidence of these diseases can be predicted for those with and without a particular risk factor using one or more of the observational and experimental studies described in Chapters 4, 5, and 6. The incidence of these diseases can then be associated with services and workforce resources, as was the case earlier, in Figure 10.4.

Clearly, the issue is the extent to which medical care organizations even care about predicting future staffing based on risk factors in a population, or whether staffing requirements can be developed solely on the basis of current morbidity. For hospitals and group practices that are not affiliated with managed care organizations, staffing can be determined on the basis of current patient

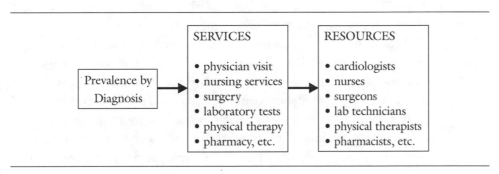

FIGURE 10.4
Need, Services, and Resources for Cardiovascular Disease

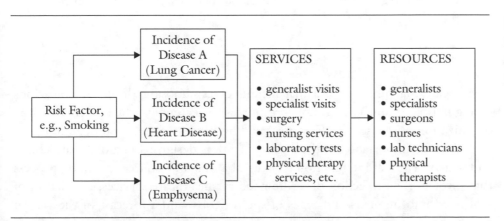

FIGURE 10.5
Risk Factors, Need, Services, and Resources

load as measured by case mix—for example, DRGs for hospitals, CPT codes for physicians. This information would have to be projected into the future, taking into consideration any expected changes in the demand for services or the market share. If managed care organizations recognize the promotion of health as a priority, then they should care about risk factors and the ultimate translation of risk into future incidence of disease—at the cost of more resources. It is clear that society has an interest in reducing risk factors. Few managed care organizations have that same interest because consumers (not always willingly) tend to change health plans regularly. The poignant question is whether these organizations will operate within a short time horizon rather than a long one, in the expectation that future morbidity will be somebody else's problem.

Performance Appraisal

Epidemiology can play a key role in performance appraisal—particularly the performance of medical professionals—by using outcomes as a measure of performance. We discussed in Chapter 8 the use of outcomes (such as bed sores) as a measure of performance for nurses aides in a nursing home. In Chapter 9, we described report card systems in New York and Pennsylvania, in which cardiovascular surgeons are evaluated based on expected and actual mortality subsequent to cardiovascular surgery. To integrate epidemiology into the performance appraisal process, one must identify those key outcomes that are particularly relevant for each employee, if any, and devise a surveillance system for these outcomes. Moreover, it is important to identify and measure the risk factors that make patients more likely to suffer these adverse events (see the discussion on risk adjustment in Chapter 9). For example, paralyzed patients are more at risk for bed sores, and employees should not be penalized for taking care of these patients, in terms of performance appraisal. Likewise, the systems in New York and Pennsylvania adjust mortality rates to give cardiovascular surgeons "credit" for operating on the more severely ill patients who are at increased risk of death. In epidemiologic terms, employees whose performance is being assessed based on patient outcomes must be given credit for patient "exposures" (such as comorbidities and clinical instability) that put them at increased risk of death.

Summary

The organizing function of a manager involves choosing the most efficacious configuration of human and capital resources to accomplish the objectives of the organization. We describe the major building blocks of organizational design as well as three important healthcare organization designs: functional, divisional, and matrix. The staffing function consists of a human resources planning process that involves the projection of future need for healthcare services, translation of that need into numbers and types of specific jobs, and a forecast of the way in which the organization will meet that need in the future. The purpose of this chapter is to convince the reader that epidemiologic measures can inform the healthcare manager in terms of the requirements for employee organization and staffing. Measures of morbidity, such as hospital case mix, characterize the need of the population to be served in a way that will assist the manager in identifying "centers of excellence," product lines, or specific kinds of programs that should be organizationally distinct. Epidemiologic measures are also necessary to project staffing patterns for the future based on an assessment of current morbidity and risk factors. Future managers will be making decisions in a healthcare landscape that is continually changing, not just in terms of patterns of morbidity, but also of reimbursement, insurance, technology, and healthcare delivery systems. Epidemiology measures must be in use to trace this changing "topography of risk." Advances in information systems, such as electronic patient records, should be available to allow managers to assemble immediate profiles of patient need—by diagnosis or risk factor, for instance. Thus, their ability to reorganize or change staffing patterns on the basis of morbidity burden will be better informed.

Case Study 10.1

Pediatric Asthma

A traditional managed care organization finds that the prevalence and hospital utilization for pediatric asthma are much higher in one tertiary care region than in the others in its service area. The hospital utilization and prevalence rates are presented in Table 10.2 and Figure 10.6. Managers are puzzled about this pattern because the tertiary care hospital has a national reputation for the quality of its pediatric intensive care unit. Further investigation reveals that this particular service area is characterized by the following indicators related to pediatric asthma: high levels of poverty, substandard housing, unemployment, and low levels of education. Although effective interventions for pediatric asthma require close collaboration among hospitals, ambulatory medical care providers, schools, health departments, social service agencies, and parent groups, the region's hospitals and ambulatory care providers have little experience in working with schools or parent groups.

| | Tertiary Service Areas | | | |
	All areas	1	2	3
Number of Asthma-Related Hospital Admissions per 1,000 Children	7.1	7.2	5.8	12.9
Number of Asthma-Related ER Visits per 1,000 Children	8.7	12.3	4.6	4.9
Percentage of Children with a Primary Diagnosis of Asthma	6.5	5.3	5	9.9

TABLE 10.2
Prevalence of Asthma and Utilization of Services

Source: Adapted from Snider, L. B., and L. Piecoro. (13 November 1998). "Rates of Pediatric Asthma Prevalence, ER Utilization, and Hospitalization Among Kentucky Medicaid Recipients in 1996." Presentation to the Reducing Childhood Asthma Morbidity and Mortality Conference Series. University of Kentucky Center for Health Services Management and Research, Lexington, KY.

FIGURE 10.6

Asthma: Prevalence
and Utilization of
Services

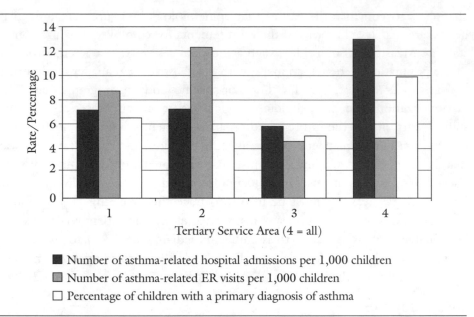

■ Number of asthma-related hospital admissions per 1,000 children
■ Number of asthma-related ER visits per 1,000 children
□ Percentage of children with a primary diagnosis of asthma

Source: Adapted from Snider, L. B., and L. Piecoro. 1998. "Rates of Pediatric Asthma Prevalence, ER Utilization, and Hospitalization Among Kentucky Medicaid Recipients in 1996." Presentation to the Reducing Childhood Asthma Morbidity and Mortality Conference Series. University of Kentucky Center for Health Services Management and Research, Lexington, KY.

Can we conclude from the foregoing data that asthma outcomes are worse in the tertiary care region? What are the threats to the validity of the conclusion? What type of organizational design will facilitate this collaboration within the next five years? Will a different design be required 5–15 years from now?

Case Study 10.2

Care of Heart Attack Patients

The service areas for three regional referral hospitals share common boundaries with substantial population and market share in the boundary areas. In all three of the service areas, the referral hospitals hold a variety of relationships with the primary and secondary hospitals in the service area. The relationships range from full ownership and management of the local hospital by the referral hospital to a referral hospital that has no organizational relationship and little influence over operations in the local hospital. Within the past two years, HMOs serving the boundary areas have contracted with only one of the hospitals (Hospital A) to the exclusion of the other referral hospitals (Hospitals B and C) for the treatment of heart attack victims. The HMOs state that they have selected Hospital A because it has demonstrated better outcomes for acute myocardial infarction (AMI), related to increased utilization rates of the most effective AMI treatments, than the other two hospitals. If this pattern of health plan selection continues for another two or three years, Hospitals B and C will lose an important part of their service areas to Hospital A. The HMO's assessment of heart attack outcomes is based on the following data presented in Table 10.3.

Quality Indicator	Mean % Following Guidelines			
	Region Average	Hospitals		
		A	B	C
Aspirin prescribed during the hospitalization	88	95	70	75
Aspirin prescribed at hospital discharge	76	90	50	60
[beta]-blocking agents prescribed at hospital discharge	50	85	40	0
One year post-AMI survival	60	70	35	42

TABLE 10.3
Adherence to Quality Indicators and Outcomes for Heart Attack Victims by Hospital Service Areas

Source: O'Connor, G. T., H. B. Quinten, N. D. Traven, L. D. Ramunno, T. A. Dodds, T. A. Marciniak, and J. E. Wennberg. 1999. "Geographic Variation in the Treatment of Acute Myocardial Infarction: The Cooperative Cardiovascular Project," *Journal of the American Medical Association* 281 (7): 627.
Copyright © 1999, American Medical Association.

Is the behavior of the HMOs based on a valid interpretation of the data presented in the table? Identify three potential threats to the validity of the interpretation. What organizational designs are recommended for Hospitals B and C to increase utilization of the most effective treatments in their own hospitals *and* in the local hospitals in their referral areas?

Case Study 10.3
Uninsured Migrant Workers

An HMO serving a rural area finds that a rising population of transient migrant farm workers is having an adverse effect on its balance sheet. This adverse effect is the result of four factors: (1) many of the migrants are uninsured and are reluctant to seek Medicaid because they fear possible deportation; (2) the migrants suffer from markedly higher rates of infectious diseases, and many of the infections are resistant to standard U.S. treatment regimens and antibiotics; (3) the migrants' morbidity and need for healthcare is markedly increased by high rates of occupational accidents and exposures to agricultural chemicals; and (4) language barriers between the migrants and healthcare workers impede effective implementation of treatment plans. Table 10.4 displays the prevalence of tuberculosis among migrant workers and permanent residents, and the drug resistance status of the infections to INH, the drug used most frequently for treatment and prophylaxis.

Is it possible for the HMO to formulate a remedy to the drug resistant TB problem in the region based on the data from Table 10.4? If not, what additional information is needed? Outline an organizational design to gather the necessary information, and address the HMO's problems in caring for migrant workers and their families. Integrate many of the following organizational entities into the design: farm owners, public health, social services, migrant advocates, the U.S. Immigration and Naturalization Service, infectious disease specialists, Spanish-speaking lay health outreach workers, and farm worker injury specialists.

TABLE 10.4
Tuberculosis
Prevalence and
INH Resistance

	Prevalence per 100,000	Percent INH Resistant
Permanent Residents	7.0	6.0%
Migrant Workers	31.3	9.5%

Source: Dye, C., S. Scheele, P. Dolin, V. Pathania, and M. C. Raviglione. 1999. "Consensus Statement. Global Burden of Tuberculosis: Estimated Incidence, Prevalence, and Mortality by Country. WHO Global Surveillance and Monitoring Project." *Journal of the American Medical Association* 82 (7): 677–86.
Copyright © 1999 American Medical Association.
Centers for Disease Control and Prevention. 1998. *Recommendations for Prevention and Control of Tuberculosis Among Foreign-Born Persons: Report of the Working Group on Tuberculosis Among Foreign-Born Persons.* MMWR: 47 (No. RR-16).

Case Study 10.4

Information Systems

A 100-bed independent rural hospital had an information system (IS) that met its needs for billing, personnel management, and financial management through the early 1990s. The first sign of IS inadequacy was its inability to produce a report of its HCFA 94 forms for the state hospital database. However, with great difficulty, the hospital was able to upgrade the information system to produce the required report for the state. When the hospital signed a contract with an MCO to care for a cohort of patients and to document the outcomes of its care, no amount of upgrading enabled the IS to produce the required outcomes reports that were adjusted for age, gender, and comorbidity.

1. Does the need to produce outcomes reports require a new organizational design?
2. List the types of workers whose job descriptions will change in the production of the outcomes reports, and describe how the job description will change for each type of worker.
3. Will the hospital need to hire new types of workers? If so, what new types of workers will need to be hired? Briefly outline the job description of any new workers required.

References

"AIDS Community Demonstration Projects: Implementation of Volunteer Networks for HIV-Prevention Programs: Selected Sites, 1991–1992." 1992. *Morbidity and Mortality Weekly Report* (41): 868–72.

Alter, D. A., C. D. Naylor, and J. V. Tu. 1999. "Effects of Socioeconomic Status on Access to Invasive Cardiac Procedures and on Mortality After Acute Myocardial Infarction." *The New England Journal of Medicine* 341 (18): 1359–67.

Avery, S. 1999. "A Limited-Service Rural Hospital Model: The Freestanding Emergency Department." *The Journal of Rural Health* 15 (2): 170–79.

Baker, G. R., L. Narine, and P. Leatt. 1994. "Organizational Designs for Health Care." In *The AUPHA Manual of Health Services Management*, edited by R. J. Taylor and S. B. Taylor. Gaithersburg, MD: Aspen Publishers, Inc.

Barber, M. J. 1997. "Outcomes for Patients with Stroke in Managed Care vs. Fee-for-Service." [letter; comment]. *Journal of the American Medical Association* 278 (16): 1315; discussion 1316.

Buerhaus, P. I., and D. O. Staiger. Managed Care and the Nurse Workforce. *Journal of the American Medical Association* 276 (18): 1487–94.

Centers for Disease Control and Prevention. 1998. *Recommendations for Prevention and Control of Tuberculosis Among Foreign-Born Persons: Report of the Working Group on Tuberculosis Among Foreign-Born Persons.* MMWR: 47 (No. RR-16).

Chadwick, D., and G. Cardew. 1997. *The Rising Trends in Asthma.* New York : Wiley.

Clement, D. G., S. M. Retchin, R. S. Brown, and M. H. Stegall. 1994. "Access and Outcomes of Elderly Patients Enrolled in Managed Care." *Journal of the American Medical Association* 271 (19): 1487–92. [published erratum appears in *Journal of the American Medical Association* 272 (4): 276].

Donabedian, A. 1973. *Aspects of Medical Care Administration.* Cambridge, MA: Harvard University Press.

Dye, C., S. Scheele, P. Dolin, V. Pathania, and M. C. Raviglione. 1999. "Consensus Statement. Global Burden of Tuberculosis: Estimated Incidence, Prevalence, and Mortality by Country. WHO Global Surveillance and Monitoring Project." *Journal of the American Medical Association* 82 (7): 677–86

Ehrlich, E., S. B. Flexner, G. Carruth, and J. M. Hawkins, eds. 1980. "Coordinate" [entry]. *Oxford American Dictionary.* New York: Avon Books.

Ewigman, B. G., J. P. Crane, F. D. Frigoletto, M. L. LeFevre, R. P. Bain, and D. McNellis. 1993. "Effect of Prenatal Ultrasound Screening on Perinatal Outcome: RADIUS Study Group." *The New England Journal of Medicine* 329 (12): 821–27.

Guenter-Grey, C., S. Tross, A. McAlister, A. Freeman, D. Cohn, N. Corby, R. Wood, and M. Fishbein. 1992. "AIDS Community Demonstration Projects: Implementation of Volunteer Networks for HIV-Prevention Programs, Selected Sites, 1991–1992." *Morbidity and Mortality Weekly Report* 41 (46): 1.

Kentucky Cancer Registry. "Cancer Incident Reports (1991–1998)." University of Kentucky. [On-line]. http://www.kcr.uky.edu. April 26, 2000.

Kindig, D. A. 1997. *Purchasing Population Health: Paying for Results.* Ann Arbor, MI: The University of Michigan Press.

Krieger, J. W., F. A. Connell, and J. P. LoGerfo. 1992. "Medicaid Prenatal Care: A Comparison of Use and Outcomes in Fee-for-Service and Managed Care." *American Journal of Public Health* 82 (2): 185–90.

Lee, R. I., and L. W. Jones. 1933. *The Fundamentals of Good Medical Care.* Publication of the Committee on the Costs of Medical Care, No. 22, pp. 302. Chicago: The University of Chicago Press.

Leatt, P., S. M. Shortell, and J. R. Kimberl. 1994. "Organizational Design." In *Health Care Management: Organization, Design, and Behavior*, edited by S. M. Shortell and A. D. Kaluzney. Albany, NY: Delmar Publishers, Inc.

Lindberg, D. A. B., and B. L. Humphreys. 1998. "Medicine and Health on the Internet: The Good, the Bad, and the Ugly." *Journal of the American Medical Association*, 280 (15): 1303–304.

MCH Model Standards Working Group. 1997. Maternal and Child Health Model Indicators: Executive Summary. (Contract Number 240-94-0047). Washington, D.C.: Maternal and Child Health Bureau, HRSA, December.

McNutt, D. R. 1981. "GMENAC: Its Manpower Forecasting Framework." *American Journal of Public Health* 71 (10): 1116–24.

Miller, E. A., W. G. Weissert, and M. Chernew. 1998. "Managed Care for Elderly People: A Compendium of Findings." *American Journal of Medical Quality* 13 (3): 127–40.

Norton, S. A., and D. J. Lipson. 1998. "Public Policy, Market Forces, and the Viability of Safety Net Providers." Assessing the New Federalism Occasional Paper No. 13. Washington, DC: The Urban Institute.

O'Connor, G. T., H. B. Quinten, N. D. Traven, L. D. Ramunno, T. A. Dodds, T. A. Marciniak, and J. E. Wennberg. 1999. "Geographic Variation in the Treatment of Acute Myocardial Infarction: The Cooperative Cardiovascular Project," *Journal of the American Medical Association* 281 (7): 627

Pearce, N. 1998. *Asthma Epidemiology: Principles and Methods.* New York: Oxford University Press.

Rakich, J. S., B. B. Longest, and K. Darr. 1992. *Managing Health Services Organizations.* Baltimore, MD: Health Professions Press, Inc.

Rivers, A. P., and S. Bae. 1999. "Aligning Information Systems for Effective Total Quality Management Implementation in Health Care Organizations." *Total Quality Management* 10 (3): 281–89.

Roos, N. P., C. Black, N. Frohlich, and C. DeCoster. 1996. "Population Health and Health Care Use: An Information System for Policy Makers." *The Milbank Quarterly,* 74 (Spring): 3–32.

Ruzek, J. Y., L. E. Bloor, J. L. Anderson, and M. Ngo. 1999. *The Hidden Health Care Workforce: Recognizing, Understanding and Improving the Allied and Auxiliary Workforce.* San Francisco, CA: UCSF Center for Health Professions, July.

Sachs, B. P., C. Kobelin, M. A. Castro, and F. Frigoletto. 1999. "The Risks of Lowering the Caesarian-Delivery Rate." *The New England Journal of Medicine* 340 (1): 54–57.

Second Expert Panel on the Management of Asthma. 1997. *Guidelines for the Diagnosis and Management of Asthma.* (NIH Pub. No. 97-4051). Washington, DC: National Institutes of Health, July.

Shortell, S. M., R. R. Gillies, and K. J. Devers. 1995. "Reinventing the American Hospital." *The Milbank Quarterly* 73 (1): 131–60.

Snider, L. B., and L. Piecoro. 1998. "Rates of Pediatric Asthma Prevalence, ER Utilization, and Hospitalization Among Kentucky Medicaid Recipients in 1996." Presentation to the Reducing Childhood Asthma Morbidity and Mortality Conference Series. University of Kentucky Center for Health Services Management and Research, Lexington, KY.

Epidemiology and Financial Management

Keith E. Boles and Steven T. Fleming

> *At a recent executive staff meeting, the medical director of Group Health East, Dr. Practice, reports that a number of physicians have been lamenting over the amount of time that is spent counseling patients to give up smoking. They are amazed that so many enrolled members smoke, especially since smoking has been linked to a number of different illnesses, such as lung cancer and heart disease. Can Group Health East afford to ignore risk factors, such as smoking, in setting capitation rates?*

The healthcare landscape is ever changing, particularly now, making it necessary to view the finance function through a wide-angle lens. Managed care, specifically, has broadened the horizon of financial managers, and the landscape is not without faults and crevices. This new panoramic view is driven by the additional risks to be considered if managed care is to succeed and if the health of the population is to improve.

The new healthcare landscape has several features that stand out. The first is **risk**: most of this chapter will discuss the implications of the changing risk "topography" for the financial manager. The second feature is the need for **information**. The identification, measurement, and management of risk requires a great deal of information. More information supplied on a timely basis can lead to a greater reduction in risk—or a greater degree of planning activity. We will not discuss the validity of information per se; for our purposes we will assume that information is accurate and timely. The science of decision making has always been based on the premise that more information is better than less and that decisions are better made when the information is more accurate and timely. This premise is becoming ever more critical in the health industry.

Healthcare Delivery: Reactive or Proactive?

Healthcare costs are driven by the healthcare needs of the population. Historically, these needs have been determined by the occurrence of disease. This disease-based approach to medical care has been the cornerstone philosophy of medical schools, in which physicians are trained to diagnose and treat disease. Thus, the primary focus of educating health providers, regardless of type, is "reactive." The healthcare provider reacts to the healthcare needs presented in the office—when the patient has specific signs and symptoms, what is the disease? The patient is the one who has historically decided when it is time to make a visit to the physician and who that physician should be.

Within the historical context of the health system, the individual man, woman, or child has been referred to as a patient. This has seemed appropriate, since an individual entered the health system only when the need for health services arose, that is, when specific signs and symptoms signaled that the individual should take action. After the disease was successfully treated, the patient left the healthcare system until another event occurred. Individuals entered the healthcare system, became patients, and left the system, hopefully as healthy people. These behaviors, both on the part of the healthcare provider and the individual consumer of health services, determined the growth and development of the healthcare industry through most of the century. These modes of behavior within the healthcare system have changed with the advent of managed care.

The primary objective of the illness or sickness system, misnamed the healthcare system, is to heal the sick and injured. This system is meant to be reactive in form and is designed that way given the objective. This objective is taught in the medical schools, and most systems have been constructed to engage in a battle with disease after it develops. But the primary objective of a health system should be to place the emphasis on individual health and, in so doing, to maximize the health of the population. This statement recognizes the interaction and interdependencies among people. The health status of one individual may have an impact on the health status of others.

Costs in the health system are driven by a variety of factors. The most obvious ones are those associated with the direct delivery of health services. These costs are usually associated with a physical structure, with state-of-the-art equipment and supplies, and with plenty of labor to provide the services. The list includes drugs, primary care physicians, specialty physicians, nurses, therapists, pharmacists, dentists, behavioral health specialists, magnetic resonance imagers, lithotripters, and so on.

Under managed care, coordinated care, or whatever it is called, the primary emphasis has shifted from battling disease to maximizing the health of a population. This redirected emphasis changes the focus of the system described earlier, and it requires a different way of looking at the world—through that wider-angle lens. This new approach is "proactive," one where all parties (consumers and providers) are involved in the production function for health. This means that the individual previously described as a patient is now a client or a consumer of health, and must become a co-producer in the health production function.

This approach also requires a much broader view of what is inclusive and exclusive to the health system. Earlier we described costs as being driven by physical structures and by medical training designed to react to sick individuals accessing the healthcare system. With managed care and the focus on the health status of a population, the view of the world has changed. This new vista includes a variety of other risks, those risks believed to play a much greater role in the determination of health system costs than the physical equipment and personnel factors previously addressed.

Healthcare Risks

Cost drivers and associated risks can be separated into three categories: (1) genetic risks, (2) behavioral risks, and (3) environmental risks. Remember the discussion in Chapter 2, where "exposure" was defined as anything that increased or decreased the probability of disease or injury. All of these risk categories are types of exposure. Furthermore, the three risk categories straddle the **agent**, **host**, and **environment** triad also discussed in that chapter. Genetic and behavioral risks are associated with the host, whereas environmental risks are clearly associated with the environment.

Genetic risks are congenital and often are passed down from generation to generation. The Human Genome Project is engaged in the research necessary to identify the extent to which genes play a role in the human body: physical shape, metabolism, susceptibility to disease, and immunological defensive posture. Genetic risks are defined to be the risks linking what is commonly referred to as genetic predisposition with certain acute or chronic diseases. It is known that diabetes, asthma, hypertension, cardiovascular disease, some forms of cancer, and Alzheimer's tend to be familial. This form of risk is believed to account for approximately 20 percent of total health system costs, although it is difficult to be precise here because genetic risks are, at least to a large extent, operationalized through behaviors.

Behavioral risks are believed to account for 50 percent of total health system costs and are assumed to be under the control of the individual. We will sidestep the debate surrounding the extent to which genes are responsible for certain behaviors. Some individuals engage in behaviors known to be risky because they have been linked to disease, such as smoking, eating and drinking to excess, unprotected and prolific sexual activities, illicit drug use, and a sedentary lifestyle.

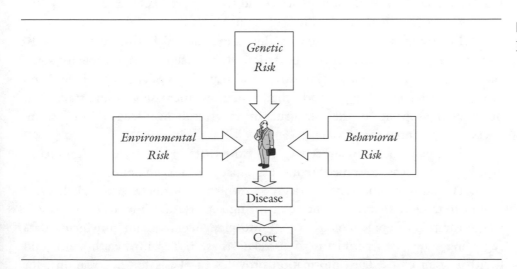

FIGURE 11.1
Healthcare Risks

Some behaviors are known to exacerbate conditions linked to genetic risk, such as eating a high-fat diet if one has a gene for hypercholesterolemia. Some behaviors delay or eliminate the onset of disease, exercise and heart disease, for instance. Other behavioral risks include those more likely to result in trauma should an accident occur, such as skydiving, flying an airplane, scuba diving, hang gliding, driving fast, drinking to excess, and so on. Since behavioral risks are most likely associated with conditions that must be dealt with by the health system, it is important to recognize that these risks have both internal and external components. The internal components are those that have an effect on physiological functions and pathology—blood pressure, cholesterol levels, and other bodily functions—while the external components create risks that are most likely to result in external causes of distress, such as broken bones.

The third form of risk is called **environmental risk**, which originates from a number of different sources. One form of environmental risk is associated with the commonly recognized forms of pollution: air, water, and even sound. These risks, derived from living in our modern industrialized world, include radiation (both solar and otherwise), ozone depletion, global warming, and any other form of pollution that is relatively universal and difficult to avoid. Many of these risks fall under the purview of the Environmental Protection Agency (EPA). Environmental risks also arise from a number of other venues, including the workplace, the home, the roads, and wherever recreation activity occurs. The workplace introduces risk through stress, poor ventilation, exposure to noxious or poisonous fumes, and unsafe work conditions. Many of these risks are regulated through the Occupational Safety and Health Administration (OSHA). Risks occurring in the home are not regulated to any great extent, except in cases where children or others are at risk of disease or injury. Home-involved risks include many of those associated with the workplace, in addition to others, such as physical and/or mental abuse. Although many of these environmental risks are often regulated to some extent, they still result in healthcare costs. These risks can be categorized as those primarily having internal implications (i.e., pathogenesis) and those more likely to result in bodily distress from the outside (e.g., injury or trauma).

Environmental risk is also introduced by external factors, such as roads, railways, and other routes for transportation. Road design is responsible for some accidents, while lack of railway infrastructure creates risks of eroding rail beds and of poorly maintained bridges and other structures. Increasing airline travel that outpaces the capacity of the infrastructure may result in increased congestion, stress, and potential for incidents.

It appears that few aspects of life exist that do not have an impact on health status, at least to some extent. This impact will also influence health system costs. The dilemma concerns the degree to which we formally acknowledge and assimilate these risks into healthcare financing activity, and how to do it. This is where the role of epidemiology comes into play. Accurate and convincing data regarding these risks permit us to correlate these risks with health status and health system costs. This information provides the basis for negotiations, for management controls, for cost estimation, and most important, for the development of proactive health management strategies to address as many of these forms of risk as possible.

The Role of Epidemiology in Finance

What is the role of epidemiology in this discussion? It should be obvious that the use of epidemiologic data and information can help the financial manager to forecast the costs associated with taking care of a defined population. More important, these data are capable of providing information that redirects the focus to activities of health promotion and to areas that may have the greatest potential for health improvement and cost reduction.

The financial manager should use this information judiciously to evaluate those areas with the greatest cost implications. It is important, at this juncture, to put on the wide-angle lenses discussed earlier and recognize the expanded role of the healthcare system. This expanded role means that, without exception, all aspects of life that have an impact on health must be considered in the health services equation. These include genes, individual behaviors, the physical and social environment, highways, intersections, roads without sidewalks, dangerous curves, speeding vehicles, and so on. The modern financial manager, who sees a much wider landscape of risk than his or her predecessors, must be able to forecast the costs associated with maximizing the health of a defined population and devise a reasonable pricing mechanism and structure to use in contract negotiations. This is no simple task.

It is extremely important for the financial manager and all key decision makers in the organization to have a clear objective in mind when negotiating contracts. If that objective is to maximize the health of the population, then two premises must be acknowledged. First, all components of the health system are co-producers in the production of health. The payers, the providers, and the clients all play integral roles in the production function. They are a team and must act as a team, in the production of health. And second, all parties to the transaction react to the incentives with which they are faced. This is rational, economic behavior. Therefore, it is important to ensure that any pricing and regulatory mechanism is evaluated with regard to appropriate incentives, so that incentives do not stand in the way of achieving the desired result.

Managed care has developed a long list of tools to be used in the attempt to manage care. This list includes utilization review, protocols and guidelines, preadmission certification, discharge planning, case management, capitation, and numerous other mechanisms. These mechanisms might appropriately be categorized as regulatory, legalistic, or financial. They create conditions wherein different parties to the interaction have incentives to act in specific ways. Most of them are designed to influence the behavior of the providers (guidelines, protocols, case management, formularies, capitation, fee schedules, and so on). Some are designed to influence the behavior of the client (co-payments, use of gatekeepers, emergency room use restrictions) or the behaviors of the health plan or third party payers.

One of the tools of managed care is capitation. This is the payment of a fixed amount on a per-member-per-month (PMPM) basis. Unfortunately, this tool has been used inappropriately to provide incentives that are sometimes at odds with the objectives of managed care. Capitation is designed to shift at least a portion of the financial risk associated with the health needs of a client onto the provider of health services. Capitation can be paid to a primary care physician or a specialist for a defined set of services, to a hospital, to a behavioral health organization, to a dentist, or to one or more of these in combination with one or more of the others. When the capitation is paid separately to the different providers, incentives are created that may be at odds with the team requirements of managed care.

Capitation: An Introduction

Clearly, the move to capitation has sent ripples through the healthcare delivery system, not only in terms of financing, but also in patterns of delivery, in access to care, and in quality of outcomes. These effects are driven by the change in provider incentives to perform healthcare services within a fixed PMPM budget constraint. The incentive, therefore, is to provide fewer resources (physician visits, diagnostic testing, hospital days) than are collected in PMPM revenues. This can be accomplished in a number of ways, including process-of-care efficiencies as well as selection of risks. Newhouse (1998) argues that price competition in managed care should be based on more efficient delivery rather than on a search for better risks.

The process of enrolling in a capitated healthcare plan involves two kinds of choices: (1) choice of one plan from among a limited menu of plans by the consumer, and (2) selection of members by capitated plans. Both kinds of choices can lead to selection bias to the extent that patients with more or less risk of incurring healthcare costs either choose, or are chosen by, a capitated healthcare plan. Newhouse and colleagues (1989) distinguish between active and passive selection by the capitated plan. Active selection occurs as the plan proactively chooses lower-risk patients through the process of "cream skimming" or selective disenrollment strategies. Passive selection occurs if the plan is organized or marketed in such a way as either to attract lower-risk patients or repel higher-risk patients. This process of actively or passively segmenting risks (Giacomini, Luft, and Robinson 1995) implies conscious effort and activity to "choose" more profitable (or less costly) patients.

Giacomini and colleagues (1995) suggest that plans can be attractive to lower-risk patients with higher copays and lower premiums, less comprehensive services, exclusions for pre-existing conditions, restricted networks rather than free choice of providers, and the location of facilities in healthier areas. To the extent that this occurs, there can be favorable risk selection. Adverse selection, on the other hand, occurs if capitated plans attract higher than average risks because of the types of services that are offered, the cost-sharing arrangements, and the delivery network, in terms of choice and location of physicians and facilities.

Adverse selection may also occur if high-risk patients selectively choose certain plans (perhaps because of their benefit and cost-sharing characteristics). Thus, passive risk selection and patient choice are two sides of the same coin. Both involve encouraging patients to choose certain capitated plans. Adverse selection is fueled by two concepts: moral hazard and information asymmetry. **Moral hazard** refers to the relationship between insurance and utilization. It poses a hazard to the insurance companies inasmuch as patients use more services if they have insurance. Whether this is amoral or immoral will be left up to the reader. Thus, the principle of moral hazard dictates that patients often choose insurance plans based on expected use (Luft 1995). A high-risk patient will probably choose a capitated plan with comprehensive benefits and low cost-sharing based on the anticipation of using services in the future. Adverse selection is also fueled by **information asymmetry**, which simply means that not all parties to the relationship or interaction have access to the same kind and quality of information. To the extent that the patient and the capitated plan have access to a different level and quality of information regarding past and present health status, adverse selection may occur. Patients may withhold information regarding pre-existing conditions, for instance, in order to secure enrollment in a healthcare plan at a premium that probably does not reflect their risk of using services.

The literature is unclear about whether capitation plans, such as health maintenance organizations, experience adverse or favorable selection. Certainly, healthier patients are less likely to have forged strong ties with their providers and are more likely to switch to an HMO plan with which their physician may not be affiliated (Lubitz 1987). But the comprehensive nature and low cost-sharing of many HMO benefits packages is definitely attractive to the higher risks. A literature review by Hellinger (1987) concludes that HMOs do not experience favorable selection. Furthermore, measurement issues may cloud the results. The better health status of individuals enrolled in HMOs vis-à-vis fee-for-service means either favorable selection or successful health improvement activities directed to current members (Lubitz 1987). The fear of adverse selection may also result in perverse effects on healthcare delivery. The chronically ill would benefit greatly from the coordinated care of many capitated plans. Unfortunately, these patients are viewed as high-risk patients whom the plan would prefer to avoid. Moreover, the temptation to compete on the basis of what Donabedian would refer to as "structure" quality (e.g., the new heart unit) is dampened by the harsh reality that patients may self-select into the plan with a view toward using these expensive services (Lubitz 1987).

The historical underpinnings of these selection issues are embodied in the "community" versus "experience" rating literature. Community rating was the basis on which the original Blue Cross plans were founded. Under this approach, a single premium is based on the experience of all policyholders within a group who are provided the same benefit package. The idea here is that low-risk groups or individuals cross-subsidize high-risk groups. The result is not only a sharing of risks across individuals, but a transfer of income from the low-risk groups to the high-risk groups. This is inefficient because the premium "price" to low-risk groups is greater than the marginal costs of services consumed. The smart and healthy consumer will avoid this type of insurance—he or she may find a better value elsewhere. Community rating may be equitable if income redistribution is a policy objective and if one assumes that the high-risk groups tend to be poorer than the low-risk groups—although this is not always the case (Cave, Schweitzer, and Lachenbruch 1989). Experience rating, on the other hand, purports to adjust premiums based on expected use, with the high-risk groups being charged higher rates than the low-risk groups. The debate here is one of "actuarial fairness," that is, whether premiums should reflect expected use (Luft 1995). However, even if all relevant risk factors could be identified and incorporated in premium differentials, it is obvious that random variation would still occur. After all, that is what insurance is all about. But actuarial fairness may come into conflict with our notions of equity, with what is fair and just and the right thing to do.

So how do these discussions of selection and risk segmentation affect the financial manager, who is responsible for negotiating capitated risk contracts? And how can an epidemiologic perspective be part of the solution? If actuarial fairness is the operating assumption, then experience rating is the prescription. Premiums should be adjusted on the basis of expected use. This can be done retrospectively, using historical patterns of utilization; concurrently, based on morbidity profiles of the enrolled population; or prospectively, using risk factors for disease, such as high blood pressure, inactivity, lipids, and cholesterol. These will be discussed further on in this chapter under the topic of risk adjustment. On the other hand, equity may be an important policy objective with the desire to subsidize those with a heavy burden of illness by reducing their healthcare premiums below the actuarially fair level. If this were only to occur within and not across healthcare plans, this community rating solution would place some healthcare plans (i.e., those that attract high-risk patients) at a serious disadvantage. Their rates would be too high and unattractive to healthier patients. If the burden was shared across healthcare plans, extra monies to healthcare plans, based on their share of high-risk patients, would be distributed from a high-risk pool by some fourth party. In this case, a much larger group would bear the burden of serious illness and the community-rated premiums would be more tolerable to the healthy. Under this approach it would be necessary for the healthcare plan to apply the tools of epidemiology to assess the morbidity and risk factors of its enrolled population with a view to capturing extra monies from the high-risk pool.

A number of policy or management tools might be useful in limiting the extent to which risk selection occurs across healthcare plans (Kronick, Zhou, and Dreyfus 1995). A third party agency may be necessary to manage enrollment while enforcing guaranteed issue and renewability provisions. This would provide the checks and balances among plans regarding enrollment and re-enrollment applications. The same agency could monitor disenrollment to prevent plans from dumping their sickest members. A standardized benefit package would prevent plans from designing benefits specifically to attract the healthier risks or to discourage high risks. Community rating of some sort would ensure that plans do not avoid the higher-risk population by charging exorbitant premiums. Oversight of marketing strategies would ensure that plans are not intentionally catering to the better risks while discouraging the sickest. Finally, the publication of consumer satisfaction and quality information would promote accountability.

Community and experience rating may involve social policy questions, in which case the issue will not be discussed further. However, the adjustment of capitation rates to reflect different population risk characteristics is pertinent. The following sections will discuss capitation and methods of risk adjustment.

Capitation Basics

The revenues generated by a capitated healthcare plan are derived from fixed monthly premiums (PMPM) collected from enrollees or their employers. Financial solvency, therefore, depends on keeping per capita costs at or below these levels. Per capita costs are driven by at least three factors: population risk, efficiency, and quality of services (Giacomini, Luft, and Robinson 1995). Thus, costs can be lowered by enrolling a healthier population (lower population risk), increasing efficiency, or modifying quality. Selective enrollment was discussed earlier; suffice to say that strong financial incentives exist to enroll the healthier patients. The value of information about the client cannot be overstated in this instance. More information about enrollees permits the organization to do a much better job of forecasting health status, and of establishing mechanisms for providing for health along with the associated costs. Efficiencies may involve providing more cost-effective services or eliminating marginally less-effective services. It may also involve substituting less costly but equally effective resources—nurse practitioners for physicians, for instance. Striving for efficiency is hazardous when the necessary and marginally effective services are eliminated, either intentionally or in ignorance. Therein lies the well-known dilemma: how to distinguish between essential and superfluous services. This issue also encompasses prevention activities. In the past, the refrain has always been, "No one pays for prevention." In a capitated environment, however, preventive programs such as smoking cessation and weight loss may be encouraged if it can be demonstrated that these programs result in lower costs to the managed care organization in the long run.

Per capita costs are also related to quality, although the relationship is far from simple (Fleming 1991; Fleming and Boles 1994). Improvements in quality may indeed be costly, particularly if they involve substituting new technologies. In addition, in this chapter we have been stressing the additional risks to be dealt with on a proactive basis: genetic risks, behavioral risks, and environmental risks. These risks pose the danger of additional costs, together with opportunities for cost reduction.

Because the focus of this chapter is on the use of epidemiology in healthcare finance, we will not describe in detail the concepts of efficiency, quality, and cost, although the excellent work of Donabedian and colleagues would be the place to start (1982). Population risk, however, should be explored in more detail, for it is a major purpose of epidemiology. Manton, Tolley, and Vertrees (1989) discuss financial risk within the context of health maintenance organizations, making the distinction between random and systemic variation. Random variation represents the totally unexplainable and unpredictable acts of God, for which the concept of insurance was originally designed. One cannot control or adjust for random variation, only expect and prepare for it. Stop-loss, risk-pooling, and reinsurance mechanisms are three ways in which the industry copes with this kind of uncertainty. Systemic variation, on the other hand, refers to the potentially explainable uncertainty that relates to beneficiary characteristics (e.g., age, sex, and comorbidities), as well as to differences in treatment strategies, provider costs, and location (Manton, Tolley, and Vertrees 1989). Differences in treatment strategies have been well studied by Wennberg (Wennberg and Gittelsohn 1973) and others resulting in specific methodologies for small area variation studies. Provider costs depend on the cost of resource inputs and on the efficiencies with which they are combined; for instance, location determines local wage level, among other things. Our concern, from an epidemiologic point of view, is with beneficiary characteristics and the extent to which these characteristics can predict resource use. A critical question is the proportion of total financial risk that is predictable. Newhouse has estimated that we can expect to explain only 20 percent (1982) or 14.5 percent (Newhouse et al. 1989) of healthcare expenditures unless they are outpatient expenditures, in which case the proportion is higher, up to 50 percent (Newhouse et al. 1989). We believe that a greater percentage can be predicted when we approach the management of the different risk forms proactively. At the present time, however, this is only a hypothesis to be tested. In the meantime, we present a capitation calculation model that can be used to determine this risk adjustment. The following section discusses the use of risk information to adjust capitation rates.

Risk Adjustment: The Basics

Giacomini, Luft, and Robinson (1995) describe "risk" as a population's innate need for, and propensity to use, healthcare services, whereas Hornbrook and Goodman (1991) describe risk in a more traditional economic sense as the "expected value of the distribution of per capita costs of efficiently produced preventive, diagnostic, and therapeutic health care services delivered to a defined group of enrollees for a specific future period." Earlier we described three kinds of risk: genetic, behavioral, and environmental. In any case, risk represents "burden" to the capitated system in terms of future expenditures. The question here is whether, and how, one can use population-based and epidemiologically-derived risk factors to "adjust" capitation payments to reflect the burden of present and future illness. The purpose of risk-adjusting capitation payments would be to "level the playing field" with regard to patients and force capitated plans to concentrate on efficiencies and quality of care rather than on the selection of healthier patients.

A population can be broken down into four basic groups (Robinson 1993), each with different epidemiologic features: (1) healthy people using few if any medical services, (2) relatively healthy people who are not hospitalized but use some ambulatory services, (3) people who are hospitalized for routine or nonrecurrent admissions, and (4) high-cost users of inpatient and outpatient services. Although each of these groups consists of a heterogeneous mix of clinical conditions, a similar epidemiology may exist within groups and different ways of capturing the burden of illness may occur across groups. Group 4, for instance, is likely to be composed of many people with chronic illness, for whom inpatient diagnoses may be important predictors of future expenditures. It is important, however, to attempt to identify the most likely future candidates for group 4 in order to take actions to delay or eliminate their entry into group 4. These diagnoses may be less important in predicting group 3 expenses, given the nonrecurrent or "acute" nature of the hospital episode. It may be very difficult to predict the expenses for group 1, whose illnesses would fall within the category of random rather than systemic variation, as discussed earlier. Clinical conditions within these four groups are those that have been categorized in the public health literature as preventable and non-preventable. Preventable exposures, such as those associated with food and waterborne illness and communicable diseases, can all be managed to some extent. Trauma cases might be reduced through a variety of actions, discussed previously. It is also important to recognize that the content of each of the four categories is not stable—that is, over time, individuals move from one category to the next. The lowest cost category is the first, the highest the last. It could very well be, however, that increased expenditures on individuals in the first category, may slow their progression into the higher-cost categories.

Manton and colleagues (1989) describe a number of distinct beneficiary characteristics that are probably related to utilization of services and that potentially could be used to risk-adjust capitation payments. These include health-related characteristics, demographic and social characteristics, prior use of health services, and mortality (as an index of severity). Health-related characteristics are those that pertain to the mix of diseases and disorders of an enrolled population—call them disease profiles. Certainly the case-mix measure used by the Medicare prospective payment system provides one example, where a resource-related weight is assigned to each hospitalized patient on the basis of diagnosis-related group, and the index (CMI) is simply the average of all of these weights. Conceivably, one could develop case-mix weights for a capitated population on the basis of the "burden of illness" as it relates to expected resource use. Ideally, this measure should go beyond the presence or absence of a set of diagnoses to include such things as severity of illness and response to treatment (Manton, Tolley, and Vertrees 1989). An elderly patient may have a physiological response to illness that is very different from that of a younger patient—the former reflected in higher resource use than the latter. Demographic characteristics would include such classic epidemiologic variables as age and sex, which are consistently predictive of both resource use and patterns of illness. Socio-economic status is a rich variable that reflects a complex set of environmental risks and behavioral risks, such as neighborhood environment, housing, and preferences for and access to healthcare. Prior use of healthcare is related to its future use as a proxy for chronicity of illness. The use of prior use as an adjuster to capitated rates, however, is not without its critics. Past inefficient patterns of healthcare delivery may be perpetuated if capitated plans are rewarded for such behaviors. Mortality can be used to adjust capitation rates as an index of illness severity and to recognize the high cost of end-of-life care.

Other beneficiary characteristics of interest should include health status factors, obtained perhaps through health status surveys and clinical risk factors, such as smoking and genetic screenings, that are precursors to illness (Giacomini, Luft, and Robinson 1995). Health status surveys are useful instruments to obtain information from the patient perspective. Hornbrook (1999) discusses surveys, but cautions that they may be subject to misrepresentation or gaming. Clearly, patients would have an incentive to overestimate their health status if they were facing the burden of a higher premium. Patients have been misrepresenting pre-existing conditions for years to avoid higher premiums. Alternatively, Hornbrook asserts, patients may be coached by providers to deflate health status scores if a third party payment to the provider (e.g., from Medicare) is higher. Thus, any attempt to incorporate self-reported health status scores may result in a kind of "health status creep," similar in concept to the "DRG creep" that occurred during the 1980s. Clinical risk factors may also be used to adjust capitated payments. However, only some of these may be available on existing databases or patient records. From an epidemiologic standpoint, risk factors represent an "upstream" rather than "midstream" kind of adjustment. According to Figure 11.2, risk factors lead to the onset of disease in a certain proportion of cases. This is captured by the epidemiologist's notion of relative risk— how many times more likely you are to have cardiovascular problems if you are a smoker. Cardiovascular disease as a morbidity in prevalence data is then associated with the risk of future inpatient and ambulatory care services. Presumably then, capitated payments can be adjusted upward to reflect both increased risk factor burden and increased disease burden.

Schauffler, Howland, and Cobb (1992) suggests that chronic disease risk factors, such as cigarette smoking (behavioral risk), systolic blood pressure (genetic risk, environmental risk), cholesterol level (genetic risk, behavioral risk), and blood glucose level (genetic risk, behavioral risk) may be used to adjust Medicare capitation. Using Framingham data on 1,162 persons, these authors explained 5–6.5 percent of the variance in Medicare Parts A and B payments with chronic risk factors alone. They suggest that these measures are strongly associated with chronic disease and are predictive of future expenses. They can be objectively measured and verified, although there may be a perverse incentive for managed

FIGURE 11.2
Risk Factors, Morbidity, and Cost

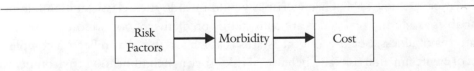

care organizations to reduce health promotion and prevention in the elderly if capitation is somehow tied to the prevalence of these chronic risk factors. The challenge is to develop a way to risk-adjust capitation by taking into consideration chronic risk factors (as indeed predictive of future expense) while, at the same time, rewarding those providers whose programs decrease the prevalence of these risk factors among enrollees.

Figure 11.2 also suggests that morbidity is an important beneficiary characteristic that is related to future costs and can be used to risk-adjust capitated payments. Morbidity is an epidemiologic concept and a direct measure of disease burden. One would expect chronic illness to be a better predictor of future expense than acute illness, unless, of course, the acute illness has been found to result in long-term complications or future morbidity (for example, strep throat and rheumatic fever). One can measure morbidity by inpatient and ambulatory diagnoses that are recorded on insurance claims. These data are a rich source of morbidity information that are routinely collected by third party payers such as Medicare. Since the data are a secondary source of information collected by others, primarily for the purpose of documenting financial information, they are subject to a number of biases related to the methods by which they are collected and to underlying incentives. In short, claims data are not without problems and limitations (Fleming and Kohrs 1998). In a literature review of risk factors, Giacomini, Luft, and Robinson (1995) reported that age and gender explain 1–4 percent of the variance in healthcare expenditures, 3–6 percent of self-reported health status, 5–11 percent of physiologic measures, and 4–21 percent of prior use. The prior use measures, which included inpatient diagnoses, explained a larger proportion of the variance. Using up to three years of hospital diagnoses would improve predictability even more, according to a recent study of the Netherland Sickness Fund by Lamers (1999). Hornbrook (1999) suggested that ambulatory diagnoses should be able to predict expenses even better than hospital diagnoses for the following reasons. The diagnoses represent a burden of disease that may be missed by inpatient claims only. Further, there is probably less variation in ambulatory expenses vis-à-vis inpatient expenses because ambulatory care is more frequent and typically less expensive. And, finally, many chronic diseases involve continuing care patterns, a large part of which occur in an ambulatory setting.

Newhouse (1998) describes a number of reasons why risk-adjustment is difficult to accomplish. The first relates to a reluctance to charge the higher premiums to bad risks. Although this is the crux of experience rating, our charitable nature goes against forcing those with chronic disease or pre-existing conditions to pay exorbitant premiums. Second, if we want the bad risks and good risks to pay the same premium, then some fourth party will be needed to redistribute monies from healthcare plans with proportionately fewer bad risks to those with proportionately more of them. Furthermore, it may be costly to get reliable data that predict spending, and, even if these adjusters can be obtained, they may distort provider behavior. For example, inpatient diagnoses may be more reliable than ambulatory ones, but we would not want to create incentives to hospitalize patients for the purpose of boosting capitation. Also, to the extent that risk-adjusters are derived from fee-for-service (FFS) claims databases, they may not reflect optimal patterns of care in non-FFS settings. Moreover, if physicians or healthcare plans have just slightly more information on enrollee health status than the risk-adjustment formula has, there remains considerable incentive to profit through cream skimming or dumping patients. Finally, with regard to geographic variation in treatment costs, it may be difficult to disentangle true health status differences in the population from differences in practice patterns.

Adjusting Capitation Rates

If we are to avoid some of the perverse incentives regarding risk-segmentation and selective enrollment, it may be necessary to risk-adjust capitation rates and design a methodology to charge community-rated premiums to enrollees by subsidizing higher-risk plans through some redistributive mechanism. If we assume that a community-rated premium is desirable, then the high-risk plans (i.e., those with sicker patients) will get more per member per month than the quoted premiums. In other words, they will have to be subsidized by the low-risk plans through some fund-distributing mechanism or fourth party. Thus, according to Giacomini, Luft, and Robinson (1995), risk-adjustment will raise the "effective price" of the low-risk plans as it lowers the "effective price" of the high-risk plans.

The previous section discussed risk-adjustment and described a number of potential risk-adjusters. If the goal is to charge enrollees a similar community-rate premium across healthcare plans, then it will be necessary to employ a risk-adjustment method to calculate the degree to which enrollee expected costs exceed or fall short of this premium. One method is to associate a marginal excess premium with each risk factor (e.g., smoking or a specific type of morbidity). The excess premium would represent the degree to which a high-risk enrollee is expected to incur costs in excess of the community-rated premium. These marginal excess premiums would be distributed to the high-risk plans from high-cost condition pools. Contributions to the high-cost condition pools would be derived from the "taxation" of low-risk plans, which would donate "marginal deficit premiums" to the pool. Alternatively, one could use general revenues, such as state or federal income taxes, to stock the high-cost pools with funds. The assumption with all of this, of course, is that social health insurance rather than actuarial fairness is the desirable objective (Giacomini, Luft, and Robinson 1995).

The question of whether or not capitation premiums should be risk-adjusted does not have a simple answer. Clearly, unadjusted capitation rates create incentives to attract low-risk enrollees and to disenroll the high-risk members. Adjustments to these rates would reduce the risk of enrolling an atypical population. This would be more attractive to providers of care (Manton, Tolley, and Vertrees 1989) and would perhaps prevent some health plans with higher-risk populations from leaving the market (Rogal and Gauthier 1998). On the other hand, capitation systems are supposed to create incentives different from those created by a fee-for-service system. If incentives are created only through risk, one might question the extent to which risk-adjustment would compromise managed care. As managed care markets mature, however, the relative profitability of improvements in efficiency may decrease. With no more "fat" left in the system, the relative profitability of risk selection would rise (Giacomini, Luft, and Robinson 1995). Risk-adjusted capitated rates would at least mitigate the process by which plans are forced to look for good risks in order to have a healthy bottom line.

Ellis and colleagues (1996) developed and tested a methodology using diagnosis and procedure information on claims data to risk-adjust the Medicare capitation payment known as the adjusted average per capita cost (AAPCC). Ellis et al. used total Medicare program expenditures for 1991 and 1992 on a 5 percent sample of Medicare beneficiaries. These expenses included hospital inpatient, outpatient, physician, home health, hospice, skilled nursing facility, laboratory, durable medical equipment, and other services. The basic approach used principal inpatient diagnoses from the preceding year as risk adjustors. One extension to this approach added secondary diagnoses from inpatient and outpatient claims, with the individual classified by the highest cost diagnosis. Another extension adjusted for the presence of multiple comorbidities by developing a hierarchy of coexisting conditions. A third extension included life-sustaining medical procedures. A final extension attempted to predict both concurrent (same year) and prospective (subsequent year) expenses. The hierarchy of coexisting conditions models (HCC) actually aggregate the marginal predicted cost payments for each coexisting condition to get a total payment. Ellis et al. found that the inpatient diagnosis model explained about 5.53 percent of the total variance in expenditures, whereas the most robust model with hierarchical coexisting conditions and inpatient diagnoses, procedures, age, and sex explained 9.01 percent of the variance.

The Ellis methodology is particularly interesting because it suggests an epidemiological approach to adjusting capitation payments based on the prevalence of multiple comorbid conditions. The approach could essentially derive a type of marginal excess premium, described earlier: that high-risk plans could be reimbursed from a high-cost illness pool of some sort. Table 11.1 illustrates the incremental payments derived by Ellis et al. for ten illustrative conditions.

Breakeven Analysis

Breakeven analysis is a common tool used by financial managers to demonstrate the volume of goods or services that must be sold in order for the organization to break even, that is, for revenues to equal expenses. Boles and Fleming demonstrate that the concept of breakeven analysis within a capitation environment is far from "pure and simple" and that the incentives with regard to utilization rate in fee-for-services and capitation are diametrically opposed (Boles and Fleming 1997). The authors believe that breakeven analysis in a fee-for-service environment is relatively stable and straightforward, with net income (revenues minus expenses) increasing as long as the number of patients or the utilization rate of existing patients increases. In

TABLE 11.1
Hierarchical
Coexisting
Conditions and
Incremental
Payment Weights

		Incremental Payment	
HCC	Example	Diagnoses	With Procedures
High-cost infectious diseases	AIDS	$4,116	$3,045
High-cost cancers	lung cancer	4,226	3,457
High-cost nervous system	MS	1,556	1,436
Cardiac arrest/Shock	—	1,759	1,271
Congestive hearth failure	—	3,063	2,873
Coronary artery disease	angina pectoris	1,049	995
Respiratory arrest	—	9,282	6,561
Chronic obstructive pulmonary disease	emphysema	1,555	1,448
Higher-cost pneumonia	pneumoccocal	2,943	2,673
Hip and vertebral fractures	—	1,109	998

Source: Adapted from Ellis, R. P., G. C. Pope, L. I. Iezzoni, J. Z. Ayanian, D. W. Bates, H. Burstin, and A. S. Ash. 1996. "Diagnosis-Based Risk Adjustment for Medicare Capitation Payments." *Health Care Financing Review* 17 (3): 101–28.

a managed care environment, breakeven analysis is more dynamic, "driven by the utilization rate of existing enrollees and the cost per unit of utilization" (Boles and Fleming 1997). With fee-for-service, breakeven analysis can be represented by a two-dimensional graph, with revenues/expenses on the y-axis and volume on the x-axis. Both revenues and expenses increase with volume, and the point at which the lines intersect represents the breakeven point. With capitation, breakeven is a three-dimensional concept, with revenues/expenses on one axis and number of enrollees and utilization on the other two. Total revenues increase as membership increases. Total costs increase with both membership and utilization rates. Thus, as utilization rates increase, the number of enrollees required for breakeven increases exponentially, rather than linearly. Furthermore, net income, or profit, increases with either increasing membership or decreasing utilization rate. The authors contend that it makes sense to view the three-dimensional breakeven analysis as a "trajectory over time" that relates profits to the future growth of the organization.

The breakeven formulations in either a fee-for-service or capitation environment make a number of assumptions regarding economics and epidemiology. With regard to economics, one must assume that the expenses incurred by the organization are determined by a production function, which describes the manner in which inputs are combined to produce outputs. Thus, the efficiency with which organizations and/or physicians choose, combine, and sequence resources, such as doctors, nurses, pharmaceutical, and imaging technology, determines the costs that are incurred. Insofar as epidemiology is concerned, the breakeven model makes no distinction among patients in terms of morbidity or disease severity. It may assume a nonlinear relationship between cost and volume of patients treated, so that it is proportionately more or less costly to increase volume. Presumably one could expand the three-dimensional breakeven model to include a fourth dimension, say, case mix. In this case, one could show that the breakeven point increases as case mix or disease severity increases. Another approach would be to weigh volume (i.e., membership) by some measure of case mix or resource use. Giacomini, for instance, suggests that one could associate a relative risk with each risk factor or risk-adjuster, such as those described earlier in this chapter (Giacomini, Luft, and Robinson 1995). In this case, the relative risk has a financial rather than epidemiologic meaning. A relative risk of 1.2 would mean that the risk factor is likely to be associated with costs exceeding the "average" by 20 percent. This would only be useful for enrollees with one or no risk factors, in which case the volume for breakeven analysis would be the aggregated sum of the relative risks. For patients with multiple risk factors, one would have to combine this risk-relative concept with the "hierarchical coexisting conditions" method discussed in the last section and to determine a way to assign a relative risk to each patient enrolled in the managed care organization. Breakeven analysis would simply aggregate these relative risks and represent the total as the volume of patients or membership.

Summary

We have described a changing, perhaps more colorful, and certainly expansive healthcare landscape, over which managed care has redirected the focus from sick patients to healthy populations. The fissures and faults of risk have been categorized as genetic, behavioral, and environmental, with the burden placed on financial managers to recognize and measure the seismic potential of these "exposures." We have described the basic principles of capitation, the problem of adverse selection, and the potential to incorporate risk into the process of setting capitation rates. The measurement of risk for the purpose of developing risk-adjusted capitation rates can include both upstream and midstream features. Upstream measures of risk include exposures of genetic, behavioral, or environmental risk that make the insured more or less likely to develop disease and incur costs to the healthcare system. Midstream measures would include measures of current morbidity burden. Even if we could develop these sophisticated systems to measure disease profiles, the more poignant question is, should we?

Case Study 11.1

Group Health East decides to incorporate several risk factors into the capitation rates that are charged to area employers. The risk factors include smoking, obesity (defined as a body-mass index of at least 30), and high cholesterol (more than 240 mg/dl). Each of these risk factors has been linked to coronary heart disease (CHD), and each of these factors can be substantially reduced in a population through behavioral and pharmaceutical intervention. Assume that the prevalence of smoking in GHE is 30 percent, 25 percent of the members are considered obese, and 30 percent have high cholesterol. Assume that the relative risks of CHD for smoking, obesity, and high cholesterol are 1.7, 2.0, and 3.0, respectively (Valanis 1999) and that the percentages of CHD attributed to smoking, obesity, and high cholesterol are 15.6, 21.0, and 21.0, respectively. The rate of discharges from short-stay hospitals for heart disease is 161 per 10,000 population (Graves and Owens 1998). Assume that the percentage of physician office visits for obesity in the 25–44 and 45–64 age groups is 8.7 percent and 14.7 percent, respectively (Valanis 1999) and that 2.7 percent of physician office visits were for heart disease. Assume that the average cost of a hospitalization for acute myocardial infarction (AMI) is $7,000 and that the average physician office visit is $100.

1. What interventions could GHE implement to reduce the three risk factors?
2. What are the costs that would be associated with these interventions?
3. Assume that the 100,000 GHE members have 500,000 office visits per year. How could one estimate the reduction in physician and hospital costs associated with reducing the prevalence of all three risk factors to 20 percent of GHE enrollees?
4. Could the information in the case be used to estimate what additional premiums should be charged to enrollees with smoking, obesity, or high cholesterol risk factors?
5. What additional information would be useful to calculate these premiums?
6. The relationship between risk factors and disease is probabilistic. Only some people with these risk factors will develop disease. The time lag between exposure and disease onset is uncertain. The onset of a cost-related event, such as acute myocardial infarction, may (or may not) occur at some near (or distant) time in the future. Would this capitation system based on the prevalence of risk factors be "actuarially fair?" In other words, is it "fair" for GHE to collect additional premiums from the employers of members with each of these three risk factors if someone else will have to bear the burden of disease?
7. What are the ethical issues associated with this case, in particular the dilemma of taxing people with a risk factor that may be genetically predetermined?

Case Study 11.2

Apparently it is possible to estimate the effects of malicious and protective exposures on survival by calculating a "real age," which takes into account the effects of various kinds of "exposures" on age (http://www.realage.com). Table 11.2 separates these exposures on the web site into seven different categories. For example, a person who sleeps, on average, 6.5–7.5 hours per night can subtract one year from his or her actual age. Those who sleep 7.5–8.5 hours can subtract 0.5 years from the actual age. Those who sleep fewer than 6.5 hours or more than 8.5 hours must add 0.5 and 1.5 years to the actual age, respectively (Roizen 2000). Presumably, these relationships are based on epidemiologic data that link various kinds of exposures with survival. Because many of these exposures are related to increased morbidity as well, managed care organizations may want to consider the extent to which capitation should be adjusted for members with some of these exposures. Suppose that the chief financial officer of a large health maintenance organization plans to incorporate health risks into its capitation rates:

TABLE 11.2

Exposures That
Affect "Real Age"
Calculation

General Health	Stress and Social Support	Physical Activities
Self-reported health status	Marital status	Aerobics, etc.
Educational level	Dog ownership	Group sports
Employment status	No. close friends	Individual sports
Amount of sleep	Attend church	Bicycling, etc.
Height	Stressful events	Outdoor activities
Weight	Unemployed, etc.	Hunting, etc.
	Group membership	Walking for exercise
	Parents divorced, separated?	

Nutrition	Medical History	Lifestyle and Safety
Breakfasts per week	Parents age when died	Wear seat belts
Breads, rice, pasta	Heart rate	Car airbag
Fiber	Blood pressure	Car phone
Fruits	Cholesterol	Size of car
Vegetables	HDL cholesterol	Miles per year
Dairy products	Ever have or treated for	Drive speed limit
Meats, smoked meats	Clogged arteries	Driver drinks
Fish	Asthma	Drive motorcycle
Oils	Heart attack	Smoking
Coffee, tea, wine, water	Stroke	Second hand smoke
Chocolates, sweets	Cirrhosis	Marijuana smoke
Juices, tomatoes/juice	Diabetes	**Medications**
Salt	Kidney disease	
Vitamins, aspirin daily	Periodontal disease	
		Aspirin daily
		No. prescriptions daily
		No. over-the-counter drugs daily

Source: Adapted from "The Real Age Quick Test." [On-line]. http://www.realage.com.

1. Can the various kinds of exposure listed in Table 11.2 be categorized as environmental, behavioral, or genetic?
2. Which of these exposures are linked to both morbidity and mortality?
3. For which of these exposures can the member be held liable in terms of increased premiums?
4. How can the managed care organization guarantee the accuracy of the reporting of these exposures?
5. How can the managed care organization know if a member has changed an exposure level in some area?

References

Boles K. E., and S. T. Fleming. 1997. "Why Traditional Breakeven Analysis Doesn't Work with Managed Care." *Health Care Systems Economics Report* 1 (9): 7–12.

Cave, D. G., S. O. Schweitzer, and P. A. Lachenbruch. 1989. "Adjusting Employer Group Capitation Premiums by Community Rating by Class Factors." *Medical Care* 27 (9): 887–99.

Donabedian, A., J. R. C. Wheeler, and L. Wyszewianski. 1982. "Quality, Cost, and Health: An Integrative Model." *Medical Care* 20 (10): 975–92.

Ellis, R. P., G. C. Pope, L. I. Iezzoni, J. Z. Ayanian, D. W. Bates, H. Burstin, and A. S. Ash. 1996. "Diagnosis-Based Risk Adjustment for Medicare Capitation Payments." *Health Care Financing Review* 17 (3): 101–28.

Epstein, A. M., and E. J. Cumella. 1988. "Capitation Payment: Using Predictors of Medical Utilization to Adjust Rates." *Health Care Financing Review* 10 (1): 51–69.

Fleming, S. T. 1991. "The Relationship Between Quality and Cost: Pure and Simple?" *Inquiry* 28 (1): 29–38.

Fleming, S. T., and F. P. Kohrs. 1998. "Linking Claims and Registry Data: Is It Worth the Effort?" *Clinical Performance and Quality Health Care* 6 (2): 88–96.

Fleming, S.T., and K. E. Boles. 1994. "Financial and Clinical Performance: Bridging the Gap." *Health Care Management Review* 19 (1): 11–17.

Giacomini, M., H. S. Luft, and J. C. Robinson. 1995. "Risk Adjusting Community-Rated Health Plan Premiums: A Survey of Risk Assessment Literature and Policy Applications." *Annual Review of Public Health* 16: 401–30.

Graves, E. J., and M. F. Owens. 1998. *1996 Summary: National Hospital Discharge Survey.* Advance Data from Vital and Health Statistics, no. 301. Hyattsville, MD: National Center for Health Statistics.

Hellinger, F. J. 1987. "Selection Bias in Health Maintenance Organizations: Analysis of the Evidence." *Health Care Financing Review* 9 (2): 55–63.

Hornbrook, M. C. 1999. "Commentary: Improving Risk-Adjustment Models for Capitation Payment and Global Budgeting." *Health Services Research* 33 (6): 1745–51.

Hornbrook, M. C., and M. J. Goodman. 1991. "Health Plan Case Mix: Definitions, Measurement, and Use." *Health Services Research* 26 (1): 111–148.

Kronick, R., Z. Zhou, and T. Dreyfus. 1995. "Making Risk Adjustment Work for Everyone." *Inquiry* 32 (1): 41–55.

Lamers, L. M. 1999. "Risk-Adjusted Capitation Based on the Diagnostic Cost Group Model: An Empirical Evaluation with Health Survey Information." *Health Services Research* 33 (6): 1727–44.

Lubitz, J. 1987. "Health Status Adjustments for Medicare Capitation." *Inquiry* 24 (4): 362–75.

Luft, H. S. 1995. "Potential Methods to Reduce Risk Selection and Its Effects." *Inquiry* 32 (1): 23–32.

Manton, K. G., H. D. Tolley, and J. C. Vertrees. 1989. "Controlling Risk in Capitation Payment: Multivariate Definitions of Risk Groups." *Medical Care* 27 (3): 259–71.

Newhouse, J. P. 1998. "Risk Adjustment: Where Are We Now?" *Inquiry* 35 (2): 122–31.

———. 1982. "Is Competition the Answer?" *Journal of Health Economics* 1 (1): 109–15.

Newhouse, J. P., W. G. Manning, E. B. Keller, and E. M. Sloss. 1989. "Adjusting Capitation Rates Using Objective Health Measures and Prior Utilization." *Health Care*

Financing Review 10 (3): 41–54.

"The Real Age Quick Test." [On-line]. http://www.realage.com.

Robinson, J. C. 1993. "A Payment Method for Health Insurance Purchasing Cooperatives." *Health Affairs* (Supplement): 66–75.

Rogal, D. L., and A. K. Gauthier. 1998. "Are Health-Based Payments a Feasible Tool for Addressing Risk Segmentation?" *Inquiry* 35 (2): 115–21.

Roizen, M. 2000. "What's Your Real Age?" *Reader's Digest* (January): 33–36.

Schauffler, H. H., J. Howland, and J. Cobb. 1992. "Using Chronic Disease Risk Factors to Adjust Medicare Capitation Payments." *Health Care Financing Review* 14 (1): 79–90.

Valanis, B. 1999. *Epidemiology in Health Care.* Stamford, CT: Appleton & Lange.

Wennberg, J. E., and A. M. Gittelsohn. 1973. "Small Area Variations in Health Care Delivery." *Science* 182 (117): 1102–108.

Clinical Epidemiology

Kevin A. Pearce and F. Douglas Scutchfield

Introduction

For the purposes of this chapter, **clinical epidemiology** refers to the use of evidence, derived from observational and experimental studies of human illness or risk factors for illness, in medical decision making. Rational and critical synthesis of the available information is a prerequisite. Clinical epidemiology differs from population epidemiology in that the denominator is usually a subpopulation of patients regarded in the context of healthcare. This chapter addresses the evolving applications of clinical epidemiology in routine medical practice and discusses some areas ripe for expansion of this type of thinking, all from the viewpoint of the practicing generalist physician. Consider these scenarios:

1. You have recently been given the responsibility of coordinating cardiovascular disease screening and prevention services for a small regional managed care organization. Two of the large local employers that currently offer your health plan to their employees are especially interested in cholesterol screening and treatment as criteria for continued participation. Your MCO contracts with 175 primary care physicians and 12 cardiologists. You decide to query these physicians for suggestions regarding covered services. Their responses range from "screening for high cholesterol is a waste of time, because people won't change their habits anyway, and the medicines do not work very well," to "every enrollee over the age of 30 should have their cholesterol levels checked regularly, and those with high levels should have lifelong medication as a covered benefit." Several respondents cite research findings to support their opinions.
2. You are the manager for a 20-physician family practice/internal medicine group that is shopping for an electronic medical records system. They want to be sure that the system will include prompts and evidence-based guidelines to help them optimize preventive services as well as the medical management of the four most common chronic diseases in their practice, and that they can update the system as new evidence emerges. Your task is to identify the top three vendors in terms of meeting the group's criteria.
3. As the CEO of an MCO, you are subjected to strenuous lobbying by several contracting employers and physicians. They want your MCO to offer a smoking cessation program as a covered benefit, citing the cost savings to be expected from the prevention of tobacco-related diseases.

In all of these scenarios, and in hundreds of similar ones played out each week, American healthcare managers must navigate through a morass of bias, opinions, and even ulterior motives, to arrive at the best solution. Assuming that the sought-after solution transcends political and fiscal expedience, *clinical evidence* will have to be understood and weighed in order for the manager to foster the best outcome. Implicit is the fact that clinical medicine is moving away from practices based on opinion and tradition toward those based on scientific evidence (Sackett et al. 1997). This paradigm shift represents a true revolution in healthcare. Although much of what most physicians do today lacks solid supporting evidence, the increasing pace of high-quality clinical research coupled with an information management revolution promises sweeping changes in physician decision making. Indeed, many practicing physicians are already using clinical epidemiology to guide more and more of their opinions and actions. An understanding of the uses, abuses, and pitfalls of clinical epidemiology will serve to strengthen the influence of healthcare managers, while it increases their value to physicians and healthcare organizations. That value will ultimately be manifest in improved health for the patients served.

Experience and Tradition in Medical Practice

Consider another scenario. In 1984 a 60-year-old man was admitted from the emergency department to the coronary care unit with a myocardial infarction (MI). His physician knew that the first 48 hours after an MI are a time of high risk for severe or fatally abnormal heartbeat rhythms (arrythmias). Following the advice of his past teachers and the custom of his colleagues, the physician ordered the drug lidocaine to prevent such arrythmias (the drug has been proven to suppress these arrythmias once they occur). He also ordered complete bedrest for three days, followed by a strictly graduated exercise program in the hospital over the next ten days. The man was released home on the 11th day. This physician, lacking reliable clinical evidence to prove or disprove his course of action, relied heavily on experience and tradition. In the light of scientific evidence available in 1999, we now know that the lidocaine he prescribed was more likely to cause serious problems in this type of case than to prevent them, and that for most patients there is no need for an expensive ten days of graduated activity in the hospital after an MI.

Although we often think of medicine as a science, clinical practice relies heavily on experience and tradition as handed down from teacher to student and shared among colleagues. Medical education is generally divided into the **basic sciences** (e.g., anatomy, physiology, biochemistry, and genetics) and the **clinical sciences** (e.g., physical diagnosis and the behavioral, medical, and surgical disciplines). The science of medicine is firmly rooted in knowledge derived from the basic sciences. But the complexity of the human body as a whole, multiplied by the intricacies of human experience and a person's interactions with his or her entire environment, makes clinical practice as much an art as a science.

Currently, there is simply a lack of scientifically derived information available to inform practitioners as they make many of their clinical decisions (Shaughnessy, Slawson, and Becker 1998). This is especially problematic in situations where lifelong treatment (e.g., oral medications for diabetes) is considered, because data on long-term outcomes are lacking. Thus, practitioners must often rely on their own experience, that of their teachers and colleagues, logic, intuition, and the traditions upheld by generations comprising a lore of unproven concepts so well-worn that they are assumed to be true. This reliance on nonscientific means has its advantages; if physicians insisted on rigid adherence to scientific proof for their treatments, most patients would get no treatment, whereas, instead, many do receive sensible (if unproven) treatments. Furthermore, experience and tradition humanize the application of science to medicine and encourage caution against the wholesale adoption of scientifically "proven" ideas that run counter to experience (Shaughnessy, Slawson, and Becker 1998). The fallibility of science applied to the human experience justifies such caution. Still, there are obvious dangers associated with medical practices guided by what is presumed to be "best," as opposed to reliance on best practices supported by rigorous scientific evaluation. More scientifically derived information is needed continuously to inform clinical practices.

The Evidence Base of Clinical Practice

In light of the current information explosion, the limitations of the evidence base applied in clinical practice are astonishing. As of early 1999, the National Library of Medicine's MEDLINE (www.nlm.nih.gov) database of medical journal articles contained about nine million references, and at least 400,000 new entries are added each year. Billions of dollars in public and private funds are spent on medical research each year. Why, then, is clinical practice not primarily evidence based? In our opinion, the main reasons are (1) the gap between the kinds of scientific medical evidence produced and the kinds needed to reliably inform best clinical practices, and (2) barriers that prevent practicing physicians from assimilating the rapid changes and expansions of pertinent scientific information. These barriers slow the transfer of new knowledge from the lab to the bedside.

Much of medical research is disease oriented—focused on the basic sciences. As such, it advances knowledge about the biophysical mechanisms of disease. This type of new knowledge forms the basis for many of the advances in the clinical sciences that follow. However, advances in the basic sciences rarely, if ever, address the length or quality of any patient's life and are usually not directly applicable to clinical decision making. An example of a basic science advance is the elucidation of hormonal mechanisms important to the development of high blood pressure (Ferrario 1990).

Clinical research may be disease oriented or patient oriented. The latter refers to new knowledge that directly addresses length or quality of life, and it is relatively rare. Only a small portion of all medical research published each year

produces patient-oriented evidence that can be relied on to improve clinical practices (Slawson, Shaughnessy, and Bennett 1994; Ebell et al. 1999). An example
of a disease-oriented advance in clinical science is the demonstration that a certain
class of drug (called "statins") lowers cholesterol without negative biochemical
side effects (Davignon et al. 1994; Nawrocki et al. 1995). This research has led
to patient-oriented studies that show this type of medication to actually prevent
heart attacks without serious negative side effects (Shepherd et al. 1995; Sacks et
al. 1996; Downs et al. 1998). These studies lasted for four to five years, but the
question remains about whether or not lifelong treatment with statins is good for
people at high risk of heart attack.

Rarely is clinical practice informed by *proof* from patient-oriented research.
Rather, evidence is compiled from multiple sources and weighed. Evidence that
most strongly influences clinical practice satisfies the criteria for causality (see
Table 12.1), first proposed by Koch for acute infectious diseases and since revised
to be applicable to chronic diseases as well (Evans 1978). Fulfillment of these
criteria can be applied to evidence about the causes of disease, disease prevention,
screening, diagnosis, or treatment of disease. In addition to addressing these
criteria, high-quality evidence must be based on valid measurements and must
be as free as possible from bias and error. Furthermore, to be applied confidently
by clinicians, the evidence must be generalizable from the group of people studied
to the patients whom the physician actually sees.

Clinical evidence is derived from observational and experimental studies.
It is generally held that well-controlled clinical experiments (i.e., randomized
controlled trials, or RCTs) provide a higher quality of evidence than do observational studies (i.e., case reports, cohort or case control studies). This is because
observational studies are more prone to bias than are well-controlled experiments.
In practice, experimental investigations usually follow observational studies as a

---

TABLE 12.1
Criteria for
Causality

Strength of association. Exposure is strongly associated with disease; treatment
strongly associated with improvement.

Consistency of association. The apparent relationship between exposure and disease
is consistent from study to study and/or population to population.

Temporality of relationship. Hypothesized cause precedes hypothesized effect (i.e.,
exposure precedes disease, or treatment precedes improvement).

Specificity of effect. Exposure always causes only one disease and is the sole cause
for that disease; treatment brings about specific improvement (this criterion often is
not applicable in multifactorial diseases).

Dose-response gradient. The duration and/or intensity of exposure are associated
with more severe or frequent disease; more treatment is associated with more
improvement (obvious toxicity limitations on the latter).

Biological plausibility. Basic science evidence supports a cause-effect relationship
between exposure and disease or treatment and improvement.

Experimental confirmation. Controlled experiments confirm the hypothesized
cause-effect relationship (preferably in real patients when ethically feasible).

---

way to confirm hypotheses generated by the observations. The results of these clinical experiments can be used to guide medical practices in a process called evidence-based clinical decision making.

As an example of applying these rules of evidence to a clinical problem, let us revisit the scenario in which you are the CEO of an MCO who is being pressured to offer a smoking cessation program as a covered benefit. Believing short-term political expedience to be insufficient for your decision, you ask the medical director of your MCO to help you look at the evidence that such programs can be expected to actually improve enrollees' health. The medical director convinces you to focus on the most common (heart disease) and most feared (lung cancer) diseases associated with smoking in an examination of the evidence.

Always the open-minded skeptic, you want to review the evidence base related to these questions:

1. Does cigarette smoking really cause heart disease or lung cancer?
2. Does quitting smoking reduce the risk of these diseases?
3. Are smoking cessation programs effective?

Question 1: Does cigarette smoking really cause heart disease or lung cancer?

A review of the published evidence shows a strong and consistent association between smoking and lung cancer (tenfold increase in risk) and a moderate and consistent association with heart disease (two–threefold risk). Furthermore, prospective observational studies have established causal temporality by showing that smoking preceded the onset of disease. The same studies have shown that the duration and intensity (packs per day) of cigarette smoking is positively associated with the risk of developing lung cancer or heart disease. Laboratory studies on cigarette smoke and experiments involving short-term smoking by human volunteers have demonstrated multiple biological mechanisms that plausibly explain a causal link between smoking and these diseases (U.S. Dept. of Health and Human Services [USDHHS] 1989; U.S. Preventive Services Task Force 1996; Ockene and Miller 1997). Most of the criteria for causality are fulfilled, but there are two gaps: (1) cigarette smoking is neither the sole specific cause of lung cancer or heart disease, nor does it always lead to either disease (contrast this with the HIV virus and AIDS); and (2) although animal experiments have partially confirmed the causal link, there are not (and never will be) well-controlled human experiments confirming that smoking causes these diseases.

Question 2: Does quitting smoking reduce the risk of lung cancer or heart disease?

Once again, observational studies show a strong and consistent association between smoking cessation and dramatic reductions in the risk of lung cancer and heart disease that almost reach the magnitude of increased risk associated with smoking in the first place. The temporality criterion is fulfilled as prospective observational studies consistently show that ex-smokers develop lung cancer or heart disease at lower rates than those who continue to smoke. Biological plausibility related to quitting is fulfilled by laboratory studies of cigarette smoke combined with observational studies of biochemical, cellular, and physiological changes in humans who quit smoking (USDHHS 1989; U.S. Preventive Services Task Force 1996; Ockene and Miller 1997). In this case, intensity of the exposure (quitting) is not applicable, but the relative risks of lung cancer and heart disease, compared to those for continuing smokers, keep falling for 5 to 15 years after quitting. The shortfalls in proving causality are, again; (1) smoking cessation does not specifically guarantee prevention of these diseases, nor is it the only thing that protects against them; and (2) there are not (and will probably never be) well-controlled experiments of the long-term health effects of actual smoking cessation. There is, however, limited experimental evidence that shows long-term beneficial health effects of smoking cessation programs (U.S. Preventive Services Task Force 1996; Ockene and Miller 1997).

Question 3: Are smoking cessation programs effective? (i.e., Do smoking cessation programs cause smokers to quit?)

In this case, there is more experimental confirmation than observational evidence. Based on multiple controlled experiments in which smokers were randomly assigned to receive a smoking cessation program versus no special treatment, there has been a *consistent*, though usually modest, effect of smoking cessation programs on quitting rates after one year. Temporality is not an issue in these experimental data (only current smokers were exposed to the interventions). Most of these programs used either individual or group counseling; some used only brief individual advice from a physician; some combined nicotine replacement therapy or other drug therapy with advice or counseling. Intensity and duration of the program were not clearly associated with success rates, but a dose-response effect of nicotine replacement was observed. Biological plausibility was fulfilled based on animal and human experiments on nicotine addiction. Specificity of effect is lacking in this evidence base, and strength of association is, at best, moderate. Smoking cessation programs do not always cause people to quit, and many people quit without a program. In fact, programs without nicotine replacement or other medication increase quit rates by about 6 percent above the "background" rate of 3 percent to 5 percent, and those incorporating nicotine replacement and/or other medication accomplish 12-month abstinence rates of 15 percent to 35 percent (U.S. Preventive Services Task Force 1996; Jorenby et al. 1999).

For each question, you must weigh the evidence toward an answer. Do the strengths of the evidence base for each question outweigh the shortfalls enough for you to answer each in the affirmative and move on from the decision whether to provide the service to how to provide it?

Suppose you conclude that the evidence is sufficient to answer "yes" to each of your three questions about smoking. Your work is not yet completed, because you have to consider potential confounding factors that could limit the application of these findings to the people covered under your health plan. Did the smokers included in these studies have important similarities or differences compared with your health plan enrollees? Factors such as general health, age, education, motivation, employment, and social support might be important in terms of the health effects of smoking and the effectiveness of smoking cessation programs. Also, were the study circumstances surrounding the smoking cessation programs significantly different than they would be for your enrollees? Where were the programs offered? What prompted people to use the programs? In short, decision makers must bear in mind that a body of high-quality evidence that adequately fulfills criteria for causality is not necessarily applicable to all individuals or all groups. In practice, thoughtful consideration should be employed to decide if the evidence base applies to the people, setting, and circumstances under your scrutiny.

The Clinical Encounter

In order to better understand how physicians use (or could use) clinical epidemiology, let us examine what happens when a patient visits the physician. First, consider common types of questions that patients bring with them:

- What is wrong with me?
- What are my options now? What would I experience with each option?
- Can I get rid of this illness? If so, what do I have to go through, and how long will it take?
- I know what I need . . . can I convince the doctor to prescribe it?
- How am I doing with my chronic problems?
- How can I stay as healthy as possible for as long as possible?

Next, consider the same questions as they are posed by the physician:

- What is this patient's diagnosis?
- What are the treatment options?
- What is the prognosis (including potential adverse effects) for this individual for each treatment option (including no treatment)?
- Has the patient been educated according to the available pertinent medical evidence?
- Are the current and future effects of this patient's chronic problems being minimized?
- What should be done to maximize this person's health, and to prevent disability and disease for as long as possible?

Let us also consider potential areas of synergy and conflict for the physician in terms of providing the best medical care to each individual as opposed to promoting the best possible care for an entire patient population:

- What, if anything, should limit the amount of medical resources used for any *one* of my patients?
- What should my staff and I do to have the most positive impact on *all* of my patients?

These questions translate to issues of diagnosis, treatment, prevention, and cost-effectiveness, all of which can be informed by the use of clinical epidemiology by the physician. Conversely, the physician can approach them through reliance on experience, tradition, or intuition, or all three, with little attention to clinical epidemiology. The availability of reliable clinical evidence will often determine the physician's approach to any given problem, but knowledge of, and comfort with, clinical epidemiology is obviously critical. We will use two hypothetical primary care physicians to illustrate the ends of the spectrum between barely using clinical epidemiology (Dr. Lore) versus heavy reliance on it (Dr. Skeptic).

Diagnosis

Case Study: Bob Brown is a 50-year-old insurance salesman who comes to the doctor complaining of chest pain that usually occurs in the middle of the night, lasts for about an hour and goes away. These symptoms have been present for eight to ten months and are gradually worsening. Mr. Brown reports general good health and takes no medicine; he almost never goes to the doctor. He quit smoking ten years ago. His father had a heart attack at age 65. His physical exam is normal except that he is 30 pounds overweight and his blood pressure is mildly elevated. His total serum cholesterol level is moderately high. His resting electrocardiogram (EKG) is normal. Dr. Lore and Dr. Skeptic go through the same steps in pursuing a diagnosis, as they:

1. make a mental list of plausible diagnoses based on their education and experience;
2. think about the consequences of missing any given diagnosis or of pursuing treatment for the wrong diagnosis; and
3. decide what tests to get that will aid them in making the correct diagnosis.

Based on experience, they both rank three plausible diagnoses for his chest pain: (1) gastro-esophageal reflux disease (GERD or "heartburn"), (2) coronary heart disease (angina), and (3) chest wall pain. They agree that the pain is not typical for coronary disease, and the normal physical exam argues against chest wall pain.

Dr. Lore recalls his cardiology teachers' admonitions—never miss a case of coronary disease because you may next see the patient in the morgue—and he more vividly remembers his past patients with this atypical sort of chest pain who ended up having coronary disease than those who had something else. Dr. Lore tells Mr. Brown that he should have a heart catheterization procedure (dye injected through a long tube threaded into the heart) as soon as possible, and immediately refers him for this test. He tells the patient that if the catheterization is normal, he should have some tests done on his throat (esophagus) and stomach to determine if he has GERD.

Mr. Brown's heart catheterization is indeed normal. Dr. Lore refers Mr. Brown for a fiber-optic exam of his stomach and esophagus (endoscopy), plus 24-hour monitoring for acid in the esophagus. GERD is the diagnosis. Also noting that Mr. Brown's blood pressure is still high, Dr. Lore adds the diagnosis of hypertension.

Dr. Skeptic has a different approach as he thinks about the evidence base that can help him rank the probabilities of the three hypothesized diagnoses, help gauge the short- and long-term risks of misdiagnosis, and help him weigh the accuracy of diagnostic tests against their risks and costs. His experience and the results of observational studies on the incidence, prevalence, and natural history of the diagnoses in question tell him that:

1. In this type of practice setting, about 15 percent of patients who gave a history of chest pain unrelated to exercise had coronary disease, 19 percent had GERD, and 36 percent had chest wall pain (Klinkman, Stevens, and Gorenflow 1994).
2. About 4 percent of men this age in the general population have heart-related chest pain (angina), and about 3 percent report new-onset angina each year (American Heart Association 1999).
3. Based on his heart disease risk factors, this patient has about a 1.4 percent per year risk (i.e., 14 percent over the next ten years) of having a heart attack (MI), and there are effective treatments to prevent MI (Wilson et al. 1998).
4. Based on studies of men referred for exercise treadmill testing, Mr. Brown's chance of having coronary disease of sufficient severity to require bypass surgery or other invasive treatment is 10–15 percent (Pryor et al. 1991).
5. GERD is common and uncomfortable but not very dangerous; it can rarely lead to esophageal cancer after being present with uncontrolled symptoms for many years (exact risk unknown). Treatment often requires long-term use of prescription medicines to control symptoms, but treatment may not reduce the risk of cancer (DeVault and Castell 1995; Lagergren et al. 1999).
6. Chest wall pain with no obvious etiology based on history and physical exam poses no significant health risk and it usually resolves on its own, but it can be treated with a short course of an over-the-counter analgesic such as aspirin.

Dr. Skeptic also concludes that coronary heart disease would be the most important diagnosis to avoid missing. However, the evidence suggests that Mr. Brown has less than a 15 percent chance of having coronary disease and that the risk of a fatal or nonfatal MI occurring within the next few weeks is very low. Given that the pain is unlikely to be from his chest wall (based on physical exam), it is more likely that Mr. Brown has symptomatic GERD, which is treatable but usually not dangerous. Therefore, Dr. Skeptic feels that there is time to carefully consider the next diagnostic steps.

Studies on the risks and accuracy of potentially useful tests reveal that:

1. The risk of a serious complication from heart catheterization is about ten times higher than the risk from an exercise treadmill test (Scanlon et al. 1999; American Heart Association 1997).

2. Comparing the accuracy of exercise testing to heart catheterization (as the gold standard) for the detection of clinically significant coronary disease: with a pre-test probability of 15 percent, the negative predictive value of treadmill testing is 90–95 percent (that of heart catheterization is 100% by definition). By the same calculus, the positive predictive value of exercise testing is about 35 percent (American Heart Association 1997). (The concepts of sensitivity and specificity, and of positive and negative predictive value, are discussed in Chapter 2.)

3. Heart catheterization costs about 20 times as much as exercise-testing (American Heart Association 1997).

4. Fiber-optic exam of the stomach and monitoring the esophagus for acid reflux are useful for patients with suspected GERD who do not respond to therapy, but they are less cost-effective than an empirical trial of anti-reflux medication (DeVault and Castell 1995; Lagergren et al. 1999; Fass et al. 1998; Sonnenberg, Delco, and El-Serag 1998).

A positive exercise test will still lead to a heart catheterization, but for this patient the odds strongly favor a negative (normal) exercise test as the outcome. Therefore, Dr. Skeptic concludes that the modest gain in accuracy at ruling out significant coronary disease by starting with heart catheterization does not outweigh its risks and costs. Dr. Skeptic schedules an exercise test instead. If it is normal, he will explain the options of further testing for GERD versus a trial of medication to the patient.

Mr. Brown completes the exercise treadmill test with no sign of coronary disease, but his resting blood pressure is still elevated, and it goes up with exercise much more than normal. Based on all of this information, Dr. Skeptic recommends a two-week trial of medication for GERD. This results in almost complete resolution of Mr. Brown's chest pain symptoms.

Dr. Lore and Dr. Skeptic each arrived at the probable diagnosis of GERD by different paths. Dr. Lore's path was more risky and expensive than Dr. Skeptic's. They also both diagnosed hypertension. Our attention now turns to treatment.

Treatment

Gastro-Esophageal Reflux Disease: Dr. Lore prescribes an anti-GERD medication that has been used with some success for many years, as is his habit in these cases. His experience with a newer, more expensive medication is still limited so he tends to avoid prescribing it.

In contrast, Dr. Skeptic again thinks about the *evidence base* regarding medications for GERD. He considers the old medicine but reviews the evidence comparing the old medicine to the new one (DeVault and Castell 1995; Skoutakis, Joe, and Hara 1995; Thomson et al. 1998; Revicki et al. 1999; Lundell 1994). Because of the new drug's pharmacology, biological plausibility supports the idea that it may better control GERD. In fact, there is consistent evidence from several head-to-head randomized comparisons of the old versus the new medicine, showing that the new medicine controls symptoms better. However, the newer medication costs about four times as much. The comparison literature includes cost-effectiveness studies favoring the new medication (Skoutakis, Joe, and Hara 1995; Thomson et al. 1998). Finally, Dr. Skeptic notes that the newer medication now has more than seven years of reported studies about its efficacy and safety, and he is satisfied that it has a very low risk of serious side effects (Lundell 1994). From the evidence available to him, Dr. Skeptic concludes that the newer medication should be prescribed.

Hypertension: Both doctors have also diagnosed hypertension in Mr. Brown. From basic medical knowledge and experience, they both know that hypertension increases the risk of heart attack and stroke and that the standard of care is to treat hypertension with medication along with advice to cut down on salt, exercise more, and lose weight. Currently, more than 75 different drugs for the treatment of hypertension are available on the U.S. market. Dr. Lore likes to prescribe a newer antihypertensive medication (we'll call it Newpress) because it is heavily advertised to keep blood pressure down with a low incidence of side effects, and his favorite cardiologist has touted Newpress as a great drug. Like many newer drugs for high blood pressure, it costs five to ten times as much as older, off-patent antihypertensives. Dr. Lore tells Mr. Brown that he is at high risk for heart attack, stroke, and kidney failure because of his high blood pressure. He prescribes Newpress and explains that such medication will probably be required for the rest of Mr. Brown's life. Mr. Brown reluctantly accepts this fate, which Dr. Lore tells him he surely must if he wants to avoid a heart attack, stroke, or kidney failure.

Dr. Skeptic is gratified that for hypertension treatment, there is an extensive body of evidence that can guide his treatment recommendations for Mr. Brown. He considers the following:

1. Based on multiple observational studies and clinical trials involving thousands of patients with high blood pressure, Dr. Skeptic can estimate Mr. Brown's combined risk of heart attack or stroke to be 10 percent to 15 percent over the next ten years. Treating his hypertension can be expected to reduce this risk by about one-fifth (Pearce et al. 1998). His risk of kidney failure in the next ten years is less than .3 percent (Klag et al. 1996), and treatment has not been proven to push that risk even lower (Jaimes, Galceran, and Raij 1996).

2. Reducing salt intake, avoiding alcohol, exercising, and losing weight may lower Mr. Brown's blood pressure to the high-normal range, but probably will not get it down to a level at which it poses no risk ("The Sixth Report" 1997).

3. Two types of older, inexpensive antihypertensive drugs (thiazides and beta-blockers) have long been proven to prevent heart attacks and strokes without serious side effects ("The Sixth Report" 1997), but only two newer drugs (not Newpress) have yet been adequately tested in this manner (Staessen et al. 1997; Hansson et al. 1999).

4. When compared directly with each other in RCTs, the six major types of antihypertensive drugs share similar rates of side effects (Newton et al. 1993). Newpress belongs to one of those types, but Newpress has never been directly compared in controlled clinical trials with other antihypertensives. In placebo-controlled trials involving several hundred people over a three-month period, Newpress did a good job keeping blood pressure down with few side effects.

Based on this information, Dr. Skeptic advises Mr. Brown that it is acceptably safe to spend a few months trying to get his blood pressure under control through changes in lifestyle, but that he may still need antihypertensive medication. The current evidence strongly favors the drugs known as thiazides and beta-blockers because they have been proven to favorably affect real health outcomes (not just lower blood pressure). Therefore, Dr. Skeptic will prescribe one of these proven drugs if Mr. Brown's blood pressure is still elevated after a few months of trying lifestyle modifications. He will see Mr. Brown every few weeks, adjusting the treatment regimen until his blood pressure is controlled without unacceptable side-effects.

Prevention

Rational efforts to prevent disease and disability are rooted solidly in clinical epidemiology. In fact, preventive practices not supported by clinical epidemiologic evidence may be quite dangerous or costly, or both. Physicians, patients, and healthcare managers interested in prevention are presented with an almost endless array of possibilities. Time and money resources are always limited. How should they be allocated to the myriad health maladies that could possibly be prevented? Experience and tradition have led in the past to numerous practices of questionable value, such as obtaining multiple "routine" tests, including chest x-rays, extensive blood test profiles, electrocardiograms, spine x-rays, and urine tests on all adults. Results of some of these screening tests can lead to more invasive or expensive tests and treatments with little or no demonstrable benefit to patients.

Over the past 15 years, clinical epidemiology has been applied to define more rational preventive practices (U.S. Preventive Services Task Force 1996). Epidemiology is critical to our understanding of the prevalence of any disease, its natural history, and thus the burden of suffering from it. It is also used to elucidate the etiology of diseases and, therefore, their risk factors. Finally, clinical epidemiology is used to evaluate the effect of preventive interventions. For any health problem and potential preventive strategy, the following questions should be posed:

1. Is the burden of suffering sufficient to justify the preventive effort under consideration?
2. How good is the evidence to support the potential effectiveness of early intervention?
3. How practical is the preventive strategy for use with the targeted population in the targeted setting?

As discussed in Chapter 2, prevention can be conceptualized to occur on three levels:

- **Primary prevention** aims to keep disease or injury from ever occurring—for example, using condoms to prevent infections that cause cervical cancer.
- **Secondary prevention** aims to stop disease before it becomes symptomatic—for example, using Pap smears to detect cervical cancer at early, asymptomatic stages that are highly curable.
- **Tertiary prevention** refers to medical treatments used to limit the disability caused by symptomatic or advanced disease—for example, performing a hysterectomy for invasive cervical cancer in an attempt to save the patient's life.

Most primary prevention occurs without much physician involvement; it relies mainly on personal health practices, public health initiatives, laws, and governmental actions. Highway design, water treatment, pesticide use, work safety programs, and food handling/preparation all involve primary prevention. Physicians' practices usually involve secondary and tertiary prevention, although they often advise their patients on lifestyle issues pertinent to primary prevention. Because one health problem can lead to another, the distinctions between the three levels of prevention can blur. For instance, treatment of high blood pressure can be thought of as secondary prevention of hypertension or primary prevention of stroke. With that caveat in mind, we concentrate here on secondary prevention, noting that tertiary prevention can be thought of as treatment of symptomatic disease.

In clinical practice, secondary prevention usually starts with screening for a disease or its modifiable risk factors (or precursors). The disease should meet the foregoing criteria listed in terms of commonness, severity, effectiveness of early intervention, and practicality of the screening test. Since screening for the presence of a disease does nothing by itself to prevent illness or death, screening must be linked to effective and acceptable treatment or to limitation of the spread of the disease to others. The setting, population, and availability of post-screening medical services are all key factors. For example, using chest radiography to screen for lung cancer among homeless adults in America cannot be recommended because (1) there are major obstacles to the delivery of that screening service in that setting; (2) by the time lung cancer is visible on a screening chest x-ray, it is usually no more curable than when it becomes symptomatic (U.S. Preventive Services Task Force 1996); and (3) even if early detection were helpful, the needed post-screening services are often not available to that population.

Case Study: Bob Brown's adventures with chest pain have prompted him to become quite concerned about his overall health. He tells his doctor that he wants to get completely "checked out" to be sure that there are no other health problems he needs to worry about.

Dr. Lore and Dr. Skeptic are still on the case in their parallel universes. Recognizing Bob's new-found anxiety about his health, Dr. Lore recommends a full "executive health evaluation," amounting to a comprehensive battery of screening tests. In addition to the physical exam and tests already done, this includes blood and urine tests to screen for anemia, kidney disease, liver disease, thyroid trouble, diabetes, and prostate cancer. It also includes a chest x-ray to screen for lung cancer, emphysema, and tuberculosis. Spine x-rays are scheduled to screen for arthritis and osteoporosis. An examination of the colon with a six-foot flexible scope is scheduled to screen for colon cancer. Everything comes back normal except that there are a few blood cells in the urine, the prostate blood test (PSA) is at the 98th percentile for his age, his cholesterol levels are still elevated, and his serum calcium level is 2 percent over the upper limit of normal. Dr. Lore orders a parathyroid blood test because of the slightly high calcium level, special kidney x-rays with intravenous dye injected because of the blood cells in the urine. In addition, he refers Bob to a urologist for a prostate biopsy and to have a scope passed into his bladder to look for bladder cancer.

Bob complies with all test recommendations. His health fears escalate as he anxiously awaits each round of results. To his relief, the results of each subsequent test and examination are normal, but a nagging fear that he has cancer remains. He actually feels less healthy than before he got his checkup.

Dr. Lore next addresses Mr. Brown's high cholesterol levels. He advises him that high cholesterol increases the risk of heart attack, that diet can help some, but that he should take cholesterol-lowering medicine indefinitely to really get the levels down. He tells him that both his experience and published studies have shown that the medicine he prescribes does a good job of lowering cholesterol levels, and he prescribes his favorite anti-cholesterol medicine. Dr. Lore does not address whether lowering cholesterol with medicine is likely to actually prevent a heart attack.

Dr. Skeptic has a different approach to secondary prevention. He questions which screening tests really do more good than harm, which ones are worth the resources spent on them, and what needs to be done to make a firm diagnosis in response to a suggestive screening test result. He recognizes that the "normal" range for many tests is defined by the values seen in 95 percent of those tested. Therefore, the "normal" range typically excludes the 5 percent of people who happen to be at the ends of the spectrum, most of whom have no health problem related to the test result. Therefore, "chasing down" the significance of test results that are just outside the normal range in asymptomatic people often leads to discomfort, anxiety, and expense without improving or protecting health. For some tests, abnormal results in asymptomatic people indicate a high enough risk of a related and treatable disease to warrant further investigation. So Dr. Skeptic applies rational criteria in his choice of screening tests. For any potential screening strategy, he looks for high-quality, patient-oriented evidence that helps fulfill the criteria for effective screening and prevention discussed at the beginning of this section. He finds this evidence in the form of observational epidemiologic studies and in controlled clinical trials. For 50-year-old men, the available evidence argues against using blood tests to screen for nonspecific metabolic problems, anemia, kidney disease, liver disease, or thyroid disease. It also argues against the urine test, chest x-ray, and spine x-rays ordered by Dr. Lore. The evidence is mixed on the value of the PSA prostate test and on colon cancer screening, and better studies are needed to resolve these controversies. The only screening tests in this scenario that are well supported by patient-oriented evidence are the blood sugar and blood cholesterol tests (U.S. Preventive Services Task Force 1996).

Dr. Skeptic focuses on Mr. Brown's cholesterol test results. The fact that the evidence supports such screening means that effective and acceptable treatment of high cholesterol is available. But first, before making a diagnosis of high cholesterol, Dr. Skeptic recommends confirmation of the high cholesterol levels by repeat testing. Thus confirmed, he moves on to treatment. In Dr. Skeptic's view, "effective treatment" means one that should preserve or improve health, not simply lower the cholesterol level on a blood test. Weighing the potential risks and costs against the benefits of preventive treatments prescribed to asymptomatic people is of paramount importance. Dr. Skeptic's review of the available evidence shows that:

1. There is consistent, high-quality evidence that lowering serum cholesterol prevents coronary disease (Shepherd et al. 1995; Sacks et al. 1996; Downs et al. 1998); the evidence suggests that it also prevents stroke (Hebert et al. 1997).
2. Dietary advice/counseling leads to, on average, a 3–6 percent reduction in total and LDL cholesterol levels (Tang et al. 1998).
3. The most effective cholesterol-lowering drugs ("statins") lower total and LDL cholesterol by 20 to 50 percent. In the major studies looking at heart attacks in middle-aged men, these drugs lowered cholesterol by an average of 30 percent and reduced the rate of heart attack by about 40 percent without serious side effects (Shepherd et al. 1995; Sacks et al. 1996; Downs et al. 1998). These studies lasted about five years. Long-term safety and efficacy of this type of medication has not been proven. But this type of drug has been marketed in

the United States for over ten years, and with appropriate monitoring and avoidance of risky drug combinations, major safety concerns have not come to light.

4. As already mentioned, Bob Brown's risk of heart attack is about 14 percent over the next ten years. Given his normal exercise test, his risk may be lower.

5. Every one percent drop in total cholesterol level results in a one percent to two percent drop in a person's risk of heart attack (Shepherd et al. 1995; Sacks et al. 1996; Downs et al. 1998; Wilson et al. 1998). Thus, a 30 percent reduction in Bob's total cholesterol level, accomplished with medication that must be continued indefinitely, would lower his ten-year risk from about 14 percent down to about 8 percent. Low-fat dieting alone can be expected (at best) to bring Bob's ten-year risk down to 13 percent. Combined control of his hypertension and high cholesterol would lower his ten-year risk to about 6 percent.

6. The cost of the type of cholesterol-lowering medicine proven to prevent heart attacks is $35 to $100 per month. Related to other preventive treatments, this is considered to be cost-effective (Huse et al. 1998).

Presented with this information about preventing heart attack by controlling high cholesterol, Bob opts for trying a low-fat diet first. If that does not lower his cholesterol enough, he wants to try the medicine. This approach is fine with Dr. Skeptic, given the short-term and long-term absolute risks calculated from the epidemiologic evidence.

Cost-Effectiveness and the Number-Needed-to-Treat

The cost-effectiveness of healthcare services for prevention and treatment of disease is being given increasing attention. This is not surprising: our options for spending healthcare resources are growing much faster than the resources themselves. The importance of cost-effectiveness in medical decision making has been implied in the foregoing case studies, but it has not been formally addressed. Excellent overviews of cost-effectiveness analysis in medicine have been recently published (Drummond et al. 1993; Russell et al. 1996). The monetary costs to prevent one illness, disability, or death can be compared across treatment options, conditions, or outcomes. Such figures are sometimes reported as a dollar amount spent per year of life saved. Standards do not yet exist for what constitutes minimal cost-effectiveness, but many accepted screening and treatment regimens cost from $10,000 to $100,000 per year of life saved. Although practicing physicians probably envision complex economic models of cost-effectiveness only rarely, they are becoming more sophisticated about the costs to achieve a desired clinical outcome. **Cost-effectiveness** is usually expressed as the cost to prevent one unwanted outcome, or the cost per year of life saved, if applicable.

A relatively simple concept that is growing in use among physicians is the **Number-Needed-to-Treat (NNT)**. The NNT, multiplied by the unit cost of a procedure or prescription, can help physicians compare the cost-effectiveness of medical options. Mathematically, the NNT is the inverse of the **Risk Difference (RD)** (Laupacis, Sackett, and Roberts 1988). The RD is the difference between the rate of outcomes in a group receiving a certain service or treatment and the rate among those receiving a comparative treatment (or no treatment). For example, if the rate of heart attack among those receiving a new treatment is 20 per 1,000 patients, and the rate of those receiving standard treatment is 30 per 1,000, the RD will be ten heart attacks per 1,000 patients, or 10/1,000. The NNT would thus be 1,000/10, which means that 100 patients would need to get the new treatment in order to prevent one heart attack. When addressing chronic disease, the NNT is often expressed in person-years of treatment. An NNT of 100 person-years could mean that 100 people have to be treated for one year, or ten people for ten years, and so on. The actual underlying pathophysiology and clinical database must be understood to appropriately understand any NNT that includes a time factor.

Case Study: Mr. Brown has a younger sister, Mary O'Connell, who is 33 years old. Mr. Brown asks her to see his doctor to have her cholesterol checked.

Drs. Lore and Skeptic both find her to be generally healthy with no known cardiovascular risk factors except that her father has heart disease. They each opt to check her serum cholesterol levels, which turn out to be just like her older brother's. Dr. Lore gives her the same advice that he gave her brother and prescribes his favorite anti-cholesterol medicine, which costs $65 per month.

Dr. Skeptic was prepared to prescribe cholesterol-lowering medicine to her brother, but he thinks about potential differences in efficacy (and cost-effectiveness) for this treatment between these two siblings. First, he notes that women of Mrs. O'Connell's age were not included in the clinical trials that demonstrated that such medication reduces heart attack rates. But he decides to give such treatment the benefit of doubt, in the assumption that the medicine will have the same positive effect in young women that it shows in middle-aged men. Based on that assumption, Dr. Skeptic looks at the NNT. He finds that for a woman with Mrs. O'Connell's heart attack risk profile, the five-year NNT would be about 1,000 (Wilson et al. 1998; Robson 1997). That is, to prevent one heart attack using the best type of cholesterol medicine available, one would have to treat 1,000 women like Mrs. O'Connell for five years. At $35 to $100 per month for medicine, the drug cost alone would be $2 million to $6 million to prevent one heart attack. That does not include the costs of blood tests and doctor visits for follow-up. By contrast, the five-year NNT for her brother was approximately 35 (Shepherd et al. 1995; Downs et al. 1998), with an associated medication cost to prevent one heart attack of about $74,000 to $210,000. Major differences in cost-effectiveness, attributable to differences in risk, are revealed by this simple calculation. The excessive cost to those who pool their funds for healthcare, plus the lack of proof that this medicine actually works in women in their thirties, leads Dr. Skeptic to advise against medication at this juncture.

The Future

The growing evidence base for best clinical practices, especially pertaining to preventive services, has not begun to achieve its potential to improve the quality and cost-effectiveness of medical care. This is not from lack of interest or a dull market response to these concepts. For example, effective preventive services such as disease screening, immunizations, and clinical counseling are not performed as often as either patients or their physicians desire (Woo et al. 1985). One can think of a variety of reasons for this, but probably the most important is the lack of appropriate information systems to facilitate the incorporation of the current and growing evidence base into practice (Scutchfield 1992). Our Dr. Skeptic is an example of somewhat wishful thinking about a primary care physician who regularly applies clinical epidemiology in the examination room. He has overcome significant barriers to accomplish this. Without sophisticated information systems, most physicians, at best, are able to have a good grasp of the evidence base related to only a portion of the medical care they provide. The problem of "keeping up" with a constantly evolving and growing body of pertinent medical knowledge is roughly proportional to the breadth of health problems that a given physician deals with. This magnifies the challenge for primary care practitioners. Added to that is the significant problem of remembering—and finding the time during patient visits—to provide comprehensive, evidence-based preventive services to people who do not specifically request them during their visits to the physician.

Most visits to primary care physicians last 10 to 20 minutes. How can the physician assess the patient's needs, desires, and preferences, then apply the latest patient-oriented evidence to treatment and prevention? In general, the current approach is twofold: (1) pursue independent study/reading outside of patient care time to try to keep up with the evidence base, and (2) use multiple visits with a patient over time to provide evidence-based, tailored treatments together with comprehensive preventive services. This approach is problematic. Its success depends on a constant high level of personal discipline by busy physicians. It is also expensive because of multiple patient visits, and requires a lot of energy spent by office staff, physicians, and patients to keep prevention and treatment services optimal for each patient. The economic necessity of serving large volumes of patients each day discourages setting aside special time to make high-quality, evidence-based practice a high priority.

Healthcare managers can play a major role in solving this dilemma, because the answer seems to lie in sophisticated medical office management systems and medical informatics. In terms of office management, a team approach to consistently providing a high level of patient-oriented, evidence-based care is critical. This requires buy-in and active participation by all personnel, from the receptionists to the medical director. Improved methods of patient education, patient empowerment, and doctor-patient communication—all of which increase physicians' time-efficiency—require attention. Practical approaches to continuous quality improvement, motivated by tangible and intangible rewards for all involved, are integral to success.

Medical informatics holds great promise for letting physicians bring a growing and ever-changing evidence base to the point of care. This means providing the clinician with rapid access to high-quality information that is directly applicable to medical decision making for the individual patient during the visit. For example, if Dr. Lore had had such a system when he considered Bob Brown's possible diagnosis of GERD, a few keystrokes could have gained him access to all of the key evidence needed to conclude that the most cost-effective approach would be an empirical trial of a certain type of medication. He would not have felt a need to order uncomfortable and expensive tests followed by less effective medicine.

Appropriate information systems will also include computerized tracking and reminder systems that will improve the timely delivery of proven preventive services, often forgotten because they address healthcare without the motivation of symptoms to be alleviated. For example, Dr. Lore would have routinely seen a list of the screening and preventive services shown to be worthwhile for a man of Mr. Brown's age (as the computer automatically accessed demographic information entered when Mr. Brown registered as a new patient in the practice). Furthermore, the system could automatically notify this individual patient by mail of any preventive services that are past due, accompanied by instructions on how to get them done. Likewise, receptionists and nurses can be prompted to remind the patient to ask the doctor about certain services when the patient shows up for any visit. Appropriate billing, keyed to supporting documentation, will be automated, as will health plan formulary and referral restriction notifications, at the point of care. Finally, these information systems will decrease the time that physicians spend on finding and processing clinical information about individual patients, such as consultation and test reports. Such clinical information systems are in operation in many healthcare facilities across the country, with a growing competitive market for them. However, few (if any) yet have the ability to bring the latest high-quality evidence to the point of care, and many are too cumbersome to achieve their desired outcomes of improved quality at reduced long-term cost.

Optimal medical informatics and systems management remain as great challenges, but powerful economic forces will continue to push their development. Patients, physicians, employers, and insurers will all exert increasing pressures on the marketplace to deliver the most cost-effective, high-quality healthcare obtainable. Those who fail to respond to the explosion of information available to these parties as they select health plans, providers, and practice settings will likely disappear from the healthcare industry. Healthcare managers will have a major role to play in this arena. Their success will depend on their abilities to keep the quality of medical care and its associated outcomes of primary importance as they work to maximize revenue and control costs. Healthcare managers and their families will have to depend on the healthcare system that they help to build.

References

American Heart Association 1999. *Heart and Stroke Statistical Update.* [On-line]. www. amhrt.org/statistics/index.html.

American Heart Association Task Force on Practice Guidelines (Committee on Exercise Testing). 1997. *ACC/AHA Guidelines for Exercise Testing.* [On-line]. www.amhrt. org/scientific/statements.

Davignon J., G. Roederer, M. Montigny, M. R. Hayden, M. Tan, P. W. Connelly, R. Hegele, R. McPherson, P. J. Lupien, and C. Gagne. 1994. "Comparative Efficacy and Safety of Pravastatin, Nicotinic Acid and the Two Combined in Patients with Hypercholesterolemia." *American Journal of Cardiology* 73 (5): 339–45.

DeVault, K. R., and D. O. Castell. 1995. "Guidelines for the Diagnosis and Treatment of Gastroesophageal Reflux Disease." *Archives of Internal Medicine* 155 (20): 2165–73.

Downs, J. R., M. Clearfield, S. Weis, E. Whitney, D. R. Shapiro, P. A. Beere, A. Langendorfer, E. A. Stein, W. Kruyer, and A. M. Gotto, Jr. 1998. "Primary Prevention of Acute Coronary Events with Lovastatin in Men and Women with Average Cholesterol Levels." *Journal of the American Medical Association* 279 (20): 1615–22.

Drummond, M., A. Brandt, B. Luce, and J. Rovira. 1993. "Standardizing Methodologies for Economic Evaluation in Health Care." *International Journal of Technology Assessment in Healthcare* 9 (1): 26–36.

Ebell, M. H., H. C. Barry, D. C. Slawson, and A. F. Shaughnessy. 1999. "Finding POEMS in the Medical Literature." *Journal of Family Practice* 48 (5): 350–55.

Evans, A. S. 1978. "Causation and Disease: A Chronological Journey." *American Journal of Epidemiology* 108 (4): 248–58.

Fass, R., M. B. Fennerty, J. J. Ofman, I. M. Gralnek, C. Johnson, E. Camargo, and R. E. Sampliner. 1998. "The Clinical and Economic Value of a Short Course of Omeprazole in Patients with Noncardiac Chest Pain." *Gastroenterology* 115 (1): 42–49.

Ferrario, C. M. 1990. "Importance of the Renin-Angiotensin-Aldosterone System (RAS) in the Physiology and Pathology of Hypertension." *Drugs* 39 (2): 1–8.

Hansson, L., L. H. Lindholm, L. Niskanen, J. Lanke, T. Hedner, A. Niklason, K. Luomanmaki, B. Dahlof, U. deFaire, C. Morlin, B. E. Karlberg, P. O. Wester, and J. E. Bjorck. 1999. "Effect of Angiotensin-Converting-Enzyme Inhibition Compared with Conventional Therapy on Cardiovascular Morbidity and Mortality in Hypertension: the Captopril Prevention Project (CAPP) Randomised Trial." *Lancet* 353 (9153): 611–16.

Hebert, P. R., M. Gaziano, K. S. Chan, and C. H. Hennekens. 1997. "Cholesterol Lowering with Statin Drugs, Risk of Stroke, and Total Mortality." *Journal of the American Medical Association* 278 (4): 313–21.

Huse, D. M., M. W. Russell, J. D. Miller, D. F. Kraemer, R. B. D'Agostino, R. C. Ellison, and S. C. Hartz. 1998. "Cost-Effectiveness of Statins." *American Journal of Cardiology* 82 (11): 1357–63.

Jaimes, E., J. Galceran, and L. Raij. 1996. "End-Stage Renal Disease: Why Aren't Improvements in Hypertension Treatment Reducing the Risk? Current Opinion." *Cardiology* 11 (5): 471–76.

Jorenby, D. E., S. J. Leischow, M. A. Nides, S. I. Rennard, J. A. Johnston, A. R. Hughes, S. S. Smith, M. L. Muramoto, D. M. Daughton, K. Doan, M. C. Fiore, and

T. B. Baker. 1999. "A Controlled Trial of Sustained-Release Bupropion, a Nicotine Patch, or Both for Smoking Cessation." *The New England Journal of Medicine* 340 (9): 685–91.

Klag, M. J., P. K. Whelton, B. L. Randall, J. D. Neaton, F. L. Brancati, C. E. Ford, N. B. Shulman, and J. Stamler. 1996. "Blood Pressure and End-Stage Renal Disease in Men." *The New England Journal of Medicine* 334 (1): 13–18.

Klinkman, M. S., D. Stevens, and D. W. Gorenflow. 1994. "Episodes of Care for Chest Pain: A Preliminary Report from MIRNET." *Journal of Family Practice* 38 (4): 345–52.

Lagergren, J., R. Berstrom, A. Lindgren, and O. Nyren. 1999. "Symptomatic Gastroe-sophageal Reflux as a Risk Factor for Esophageal Adenocarcinoma." *The New England Journal of Medicine* 340 (11): 825–31.

Laupacis, A., D. L. Sackett, and R. S. Roberts. 1988. "An Assessment of Clinically Useful Measures of the Consequences of Treatment." *The New England Journal of Medicine* 381 (20): 1728–33.

Lundell, L. 1994. "Long-Term Treatment of Gastro-esophageal Reflux Disease with Omeprazole." *Scandinavian Journal of Gastroenterology* 201 (Supplement): 74–78.

Nawrocki, J. W., S. R. Weiss, M. H. Davidson, D. L. Sprecher, S. L. Schwartz, P. J. Lupien, P. H. Jones, H. E. Haber, and D. M. Black. 1995. "Reduction of LDL Cholesterol by 25% to 60% in Patients with Primary Hypercholesterolemia by Atorvastatin, a New HMG-CoA Reductase Inhibitor." *Arteriosclerosis, Thrombosis, and Vascular Biology* 15 (5): 678–82.

Neaton, J. D., R. H. Grimm, Jr., R. J. Prineas, J. Stamler, G. A. Grandits, P. J. Elmer, J. A. Cutler, J. M. Flack, J. A. Schoenberger, and R. McDonald. 1993. "Treatment of Mild Hypertension Study: Final Results." *Journal of the American Medical Association* 270 (6): 713–24.

Ockene, I. S., and N. H. Miller. 1997. "Cigarette Smoking, Cardiovascular Disease, and Stroke." *Circulation* 96 (9): 3243–47.

Pearce, K. A., C. D. Furberg, B. M. Psaty, and J. Kirk. 1998. "Cost-Minimization and the Number Needed to Treat in Uncomplicated Hypertension." *American Journal of Health* 11 (6): 618–29.

Pryor, D. B., L. Shaw, F. E. Harrell, K. L. Lee, M. A. Hlatky, D. B. Mark, L. H. Muhlbaier, and R. M. Califf. 1991. "Estimating the Likelihood of Severe Coronary Artery Disease." *American Journal of Medicine* 90 (5): 553–62.

Revicki, D. A., S. Sorensen, P. N. Maton, and R. C. Orlando. 1999. "Health-Related Quality of Life Outcomes of Omeprazole Versus Ranitidine in Poorly Responsive Symptomatic Gastroesophageal Reflux Disease." *Digestive Diseases* 16 (5): 284–91.

Robson J. 1997. "Information Needed to Decide About Cardiovascular Treatment in Primary Care." *British Medical Journal* 314: 277.

Russell, L. B., M. R. Gold, J. E. Siegel, N. Daniels, and M. C. Weinstein. 1996. "The Role of Cost-Effectiveness Analysis in Health and Medicine." *Journal of the American Medical Association* 276 (14): 1172–77.

Sacket D. L., W. Richardson, W. Rosenberg, and B. Haynes. 1997. *Evidence-Based Medicine: How to Practice and Teach EBM.* New York: Churchill Livingstone.

Sacks, F. M., M. A. Pfeffer, L. A. Moye, J. L. Rouleau, J. D. Rutherford, T. G. Cole, L. Brown, J. W. Warnica, J. M. Arnold, C. C. Wun, B. R. Davis, and E. Braunwald. 1996. "The Effect of Pravastatin on Coronary Events After Myocardial Infarction in Patients with Average Cholesterol Levels." *The New England Journal of Medicine* 335 (14): 1001–1009.

Scanlon, P. J., D. P. Faxon, A. Audet, B. Carabello, G. J. Dehmer, K. A. Eagle, R. D. Legako, D. F. Leon, J. A. Murray, S. E. Nissen, C. J. Pepine, R. M. Watson, J. L. Ritchie, R. J. Gibbons, M. D. Cheitlin, T. J. Gardner, A. Garson, Jr., R. O. Russell, Jr., T. J. Ryan, and S. C. Smith, Jr. 1999. "ACC/AHA Guidelines for Coronary Angiography: Executive Summary and Recommendations." *Circulation* 99 (17): 2345–57.

Scutchfield, F. D. 1992. "Clinical Preventive Services: The Patient and the Physician." *Clinical Chemistry* 38 (Supplement): 1547–51.

Shaughnessy, A. F., D. C. Slawson, and L. Becker. 1998. "Clinical Jazz: Harmonizing Clinical Experience and Evidence-Based Medicine." *Journal of Family Practice* 47 (6): 425–28.

Shepherd, J., S. M. Cobbe, I. Ford, C. G. Isles, A. R. Lorimer, P. W. MacFarlane, J. H. McKillop, and C. J. Packard. 1995. "Prevention of Coronary Heart Disease with Pravastatin in Men with Hypercholesterolemia." *The New England Journal of Medicine* 333 (20): 1301–307.

"The Sixth Report of the Joint National Committee on Prevention, Detection, Evaluation, and Treatment of High Blood Pressure." 1997. *Archives of Internal Medicine* 157 (21): 2413–46.

Skoutakis, V. A., R. H. Joe, and D. S. Hara. 1995. "Comparative Role of Omeprazole in the Treatment of Gastroesophageal Reflux Disease." *Annals of Pharmacotherapy* 29 (12): 1252–62.

Slawson, D. C., A. F. Shaughnessy, and J. H. Bennett. 1994. "Becoming a Medical Information Master: Feeling Good About Not Knowing Everything." *Journal of Family Practice* 38 (5): 505–13.

Sonnenberg, A., F. Delco, and H. B. El-Serag. 1998. "Empirical Therapy Versus Diagnostic Tests in Gastroesophageal Reflux Disease: A Medical Decision Analysis." *Digestive Diseases and Sciences* 43 (5): 1001–1008.

Staessen, J. A., R. Fagard, L. Thijs, H. Celis, G. G. Arabidze, W. H. Birkenhager, C. J. Bulpitt, P. W. deLeeuw, C. T. Dollery, A. E. Fletcher, F. Forette, G. Leonetti, C. Nachev, E. T. O'Brien, J. Rosenfeld, J. L. Rodicio, J. Tuomilehto, and A. Zanchetti. 1997. "Randomised Double-Blind Comparison of Placebo and Active Treatment for Older Patients with Isolated Systolic Hypertension." *Lancet* 350 (9080): 757–64.

Tang, J. L., J. M. Armitage, T. Lancaster, C. A. Silagy, G. H. Fowler, and A. W. Neil. 1998. "Systematic Review of Dietary Intervention Trials to Lower Blood Total Cholesterol in Free-Living Subjects." *British Medical Journal* 316 (7139): 1213–20.

Thomson, A. B., N. Chiba, D. Armstrong, G. Tougas, and R. H. Hunt. 1998. "The Second Canadian Gastroesophageal Reflux Disease Consensus: Moving Forward to New Concepts." *Canadian Journal of Gastroenterology* 12 (8): 551–56.

U.S. Department of Health and Human Services. *Reducing the Health Consequences of Smoking: 25 years of Progress: A Report of the Surgeon General*. 1989. Pub. No. DHHS (CDC) 89-8411. Rockville, MD. Department of Health and Human Services.

U.S. Preventive Services Task Force. 1996. *Guide to Clinical Preventive Services, 2nd ed.* Baltimore, MD: Williams & Wilkins.

Wilson, P. W. F., R. B. D'Agostino, D. Levy, A. M. Belanger, H. Silbershatz, and W. B. Kannel. 1998. "Prediction of Coronary Heart Disease Using Risk Factor Categories." *Circulation* 97 (18): 1837–47.

Woo, B., B. Woo, E. F. Cook, M. Weisberg, and L. Goldman. 1985. "Screening Procedures in the Asymptomatic Adult: Comparison of Physicians' Recommmendations, Patient's Desires, Published Guidelines, and Actual Practice." *Journal of the American Medical Association* 254 (11): 1480–84.

Integrative Decision Making and Managerial Epidemiology

F. Douglas Scutchfield, Steven T. Fleming, and Thomas C. Tucker

T he underlying premise of this text is that healthcare managers should embrace the tools of epidemiology and cultivate an epidemiologic perspective
with which to practice their craft. Earlier, we articulated the fundamental
concepts and principles of epidemiology and described several different kinds of
epidemiologic studies, taking care to acknowledge the flaws, biases, and cautions
associated with each. Next, we considered the basic functions of a manager and
described ways in which each of these roles might be enhanced through the use
of epidemiologic data and the development of a population-based, outcomes-
oriented viewpoint. For some of the managerial roles the connection was intuitive
and easy to see; with other functions the connection was less obvious. Clearly, the
planning function requires needs assessment, which must be based on morbidity
and mortality data. Staffing can be improved by recognizing shifts in disease that
require new or different types of skills. Likewise, the assessment of quality and
the surveillance of outcomes, all within the purview of the controlling function,
must rely on the principles and practices of epidemiology. Moreover, financial
managers must adopt a population-based perspective on morbidity and risk as they
function within a healthcare industry that is moving ever more to capitation. The
relevance of epidemiology would seem less evident, at first glance, in the directing
and organizing functions. However, we have postulated that epidemiology can
be applied to all functions of the manager, and this epidemiologic perspective
becomes evident, perhaps, in its view of the epidemiologic role as more than a
set of tools but less than a philosophy. In short, managerial epidemiology is a
perspective, a mindset, a way of thinking that can inform, elucidate, and perhaps
integrate all functions of a manager.

Integrated Decision Making

Healthcare managers make decisions and solve problems every day. It is an essential part of the job description. In theory, at least, one could classify each
decision as one that pertains to a specific function. For example, the decision to
move from a functional to a matrix model would be considered an organizing
decision. In fact, many decisions are interrelated, and thus an integrated model
of decision making would need to consider the "interfunctional" impact of each
decision. Rakich, Longest, and Darr (1992) recognize these interdependencies in

Figure 13.1, which is adapted from their text. Please note that we have included the financing function as part of the controlling function, as is typically done. Our discussion of the relevance of epidemiology to financial management was discussed in a separate chapter (11), however, because of the increased importance of epidemiology in a capitated environment. According to Figure 13.1, not only does decision making occur within each of these functions, but the decisions are often interrelated. Planning decisions may suggest new product lines that could affect the organizational design, staffing, and controlling activities.

Figure 13.1 also illustrates the premise that an epidemiologic perspective can inform decision making within each role. Consider the notion that this kind of perspective (and maybe others, such as an ethical perspective) could serve an integrative purpose and facilitate interfunctional considerations in each decision. The idea here is that an epidemiologic perspective would become a "practice style," if you will, for managers. Suppose, for example, that the measurement of disease burden is but one part of this practice style. Further, assume that a particular planning decision has to be made, for example, conversion of a 30-bed acute care wing to skilled nursing. Clearly, the manager will need to assess the need for long-term care within the population served. The practice style will dictate that disease burden be measured in this instance. This seems reasonable given the typical process of needs assessment. However, this same practice style will motivate the manager to evaluate the effect of this decision, in terms of disease burden, on other functions such as the controlling function. The manager may want to evaluate the impact of the move to skilled nursing on quality assurance activities, for instance.

Problem Solving and Epidemiology

Rakich and colleagues (1992) argue that managers are engaged in the business of problem solving, which involves both problem analysis and decision making.

FIGURE 13.1
Managerial
Functions and
Epidemiology

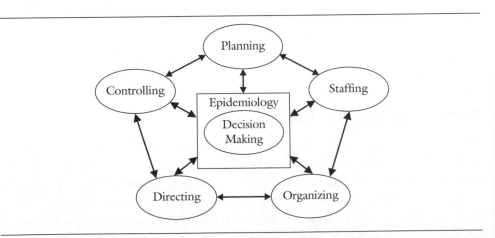

Source: Adapted from Rakich, J. S., B. B. Longest, and K. Darr. 1992. *Managing Health Services Organizations, 3rd ed.* Baltimore, MD: Health Professions Press, Inc.

Further, they argue that a number of conditions may initiate a problem solving activity: these include opportunities, crises, deviations, and improvement. With opportunities the manager must be proactive as he or she decides how to exploit new technologies, services, or product lines. Crises are events or circumstances that force managers into a reactive mode of decision making. Deviations from the expected, in terms of outcomes or performance, may also give rise to problem solving, as would normal improvement activities, such as those that occur with continuous quality improvement. The recognition of each of these four conditions may depend on epidemiologic measures. For example, smoking cessation and weight reduction programs create opportunities for problem solving, because epidemiologic studies have established each as a risk factor of disease and one can measure the prevalence of each risk in an insured population. Crises may be defined, in fact, by epidemiologic measures—an influenza outbreak or a dramatic increase in surgical mortality, for instance. Deviations from expected outcomes may be epidemiologically based as well, as was the case when some hospitals evaluated their poor performance with the short-lived Health Care Financing Administration (HCFA) mortality index (Fleming, Hicks, and Bailey 1995). Certainly, quality improvement activities involve the basic epidemiologic principle of surveillance.

Figure 13.2 modifies the problem-solving model of Rakich and colleagues (1992) to include junctures at which epidemiologic measurement may be particularly relevant. A problem must first be recognized and defined (stage 1) before it can be addressed by the manager. Each of the four kinds of conditions just described (opportunities, crises, deviations, and improvement) may initiate problem solving in this recognition stage. Problem recognition may be derived from epidemiologic measurement: a sharp increase in nosocomial infections, for instance. Problem definition, on the other hand, moves beyond signs and symptoms

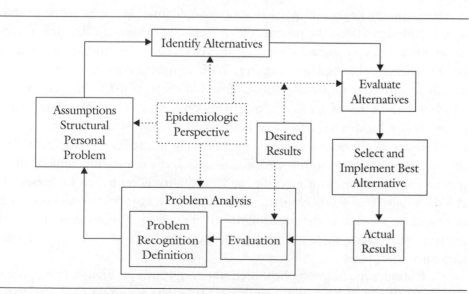

FIGURE 13.2

Epidemiology and the Problem-Solving Process

Source: Adapted from Rakich, J. S., B. B. Longest, and K. Darr. 1992. *Managing Health Services Organizations, 3rd ed.* Baltimore, MD: Health Professions Press, Inc.

to root causes. A problem may be recognized based on epidemiologic measures, such as morbidity or mortality, but defined in terms of administrative, rather than clinical, root causes. The diagnosis of cancer at a late rather than early stage may be recognized as a problem by cause-specific mortality rates, but defined in terms of insufficient insurance coverage for screening or a lack of outreach programs.

Once a problem is recognized and defined, and before alternatives can be identified, a set of assumptions need to be articulated (stage 2) based on the context of the problem (structural), the personal biases of the manager, and the problem itself (Rakich, Longest, and Darr 1992). Epidemiologic measures should be part of the context of many problems in healthcare settings. How does the problem relate to morbidity and mortality? Are there exposures and risk factors that the problem affects? Personal assumptions may include such important considerations as tolerance for risk (Rakich, Longest, and Darr 1992) and the degree to which the manager has cultivated an epidemiologic perspective. Are healthy populations and disease management important assumptions to take into consideration when the manager makes other decisions?

The problem-solving process also includes the identification, evaluation, and selection of alternatives (stages 3, 4, and 5). Clearly, epidemiology can inform the decision maker in each of these stages, as would the health services research literature. The identification stage consists of generating alternative solutions to the problem, through a number of creative activities such as brainstorming and focus groups (Spiegel and Hyman 1994). An epidemiologic perspective may be applied to any of these activities to the extent that participants in the process recognize the relevance of such a viewpoint. The evaluation stage involves setting criteria on which to evaluate the various alternatives. A number of tools may be helpful here, such as cost-benefit analysis, cost-effectiveness analysis, cost-utility analysis, decision trees, payoff matrices, and so on. With most of these methods, the manager will need to employ epidemiologic data if the problem and/or solution affects the patient. For example, with cost-effectiveness analysis, programs are often compared in terms of lives saved; thus, mortality rates would be the critical epidemiologic measure. With cost-utility analysis, programs are usually compared in terms of quality-adjusted life-years (QALY), the weighting of which is derived from the effect of morbidity on quality of life. The measurement of morbidity burden becomes key here. With decision trees, one must assign probabilities to alternative courses of action. The identification and description of exposures (both protective and malicious), and the measurement of the effect of these exposures on mortality and morbidity is central to the practice of epidemiology. This is probabilistic, which is to say that incidence and prevalence rates can be viewed as the probabilities of disease in a population. It may be necessary to include these probabilities in decision trees when one is evaluating alternative programs.

Consider the following hypothetical example of a problem-solving process. Patriot Healthcare is a 120,000-member HMO in the New York City area. Patriot has a large risk contract with the state of New York to provide comprehensive services to the Medicaid population. Patriot has been monitoring hospitalization rates and has determined that Medicaid mothers have a disproportionate share of low-birthweight newborns (problem recognition). Although these results are not necessarily surprising in a fee-for-service environment, there is some cause for concern in that the HMO must bear the full cost of these expensive hospital episodes. The senior staff defined the problem as an educational, rather than access issue relating to the understanding by Medicaid mothers of the importance of prenatal care (problem definition). The social work and nursing directors held four focus groups in different parts of the city, during which time they referred to a number of epidemiologic studies linking prenatal care with newborn birth weight. Several alternative programs were suggested (alternative identification), two of which involved educational outreach programs. These programs were evaluated using cost-effectiveness analysis (alternative evaluation) based on several studies that had examined similar programs. The key epidemiologic measures used in the evaluation were five kinds of mortality rates: infant, neonatal, post-neonatal, perinatal, and maternal. The program chosen was the one with the largest projected impact on these rates per dollar spent (alternative selection). The actual results of program implementation were measured and evaluated at some future date.

Back to the Future

Armed with the new tools of epidemiology we now have acquired, let us return to the case study from the first chapter to see if our new information might be helpful to our mythical managed care executive, Mr. Jones. As you might imagine, epidemiology will not cure his autocratic management style or improve his relations with his employees. But it might improve his capacity to make decisions and solve problems. As you recall, Mr. Jones runs Group Health East, an HMO with 100,000 covered lives. He has two large medical groups with which he contracts, as well as 500 individual physicians in the community. The HMO is affiliated with two major hospitals in the Boston area.

Many believe that enrolled members of a managed care organization form an excellent denominator for epidemiology purposes. They represent a delineated "at risk" population, from whom one can establish morbidity and mortality rates using the total number of members, or covered lives, as the denominator. This also suggests that managed care organizations, properly run, not only can influence the acute care of the members for whom they are responsible, but also can assume responsibility for the health of the enrolled population. The ability to use epidemiology tools with this group can effectively improve the decision-making process, particularly if an enlightened leadership is focused on improving population health and not just on the "bottom line." We discussed this paradigm shift, from a reactive medical care system that treats illness to a proactive one concerned with maintaining health status, in the chapter on financial management (Chapter 11).

FIGURE 13.3

Matrix
Organizational
Design

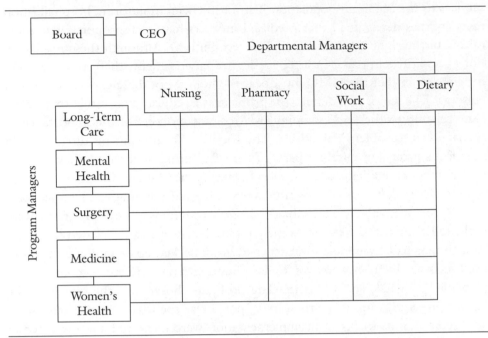

Source: Baker, G. R., L. Narine, and P. Leatt. 1994. "Organizational Designs for Health Care." In *The AUPHA Manual of Health Services Management*, edited by R. J. Taylor and S. B. Taylor. Gaithersburg, MD: Aspen Publishers, Inc.

As you recollect, Mr. Jones needed to make some decisions regarding the move to a matrix model organization for GHE; Figure 13.3 illustrates a matrix organization model, with product lines on one axis, and functional departments on the other. The first set of decisions involves the choice of product lines that should be arrayed along one axis of the matrix organization. Clearly, the disease burden of the subscribers is one area that could be used to make that decision. A review of diagnosis-related groups (DRGs) would provide insight into the morbidity burden associated with hospital episodes. The frequency of diagnoses and/or procedures could be evaluated in the ambulatory setting with the commonly used physician coding scheme (CPT, or current procedure terminology). Using these two coding formats, Jones could develop rates of hospitalization by specific condition, or rates of ambulatory care encounters by CPT code. Those conditions with the highest rates in either or both settings should be evaluated as candidates for separate product lines.

Because Mr. Jones is an epidemiologically-informed manager, he is concerned about the health of the entire population "at risk," which in this case includes the enrolled members of Group Health East. Because of this concern, Jones should collect and evaluate risk factor data on his subscribers (e.g., smoking, obesity) to identify potential areas that might result in improved population health. Risk factor intervention programs could well improve the financial health of GHE as well. Group Health East may want to complete a behavioral risk factor study on its subscribers in order to make decisions about which programs need to be developed by that managed care organization. Clearly, the target should be those risk factors that can be modified through changes in behavior. These behavioral modification programs (e.g., smoking cessation) may be separate product lines or parts of other product lines. For example, smoking cessation could be a "stand-alone" product line or part of a chronic obstructive pulmonary disease (COPD) and emphysema line.

Jones may also want to make decisions about product lines based on the cost of care for various kinds of morbidity and on the extent to which the enrolled population either has, or is at risk of developing, those conditions. Note that with this focus on the high-cost conditions, Jones would need to know the prevalence of disease and the prevalence of risk factors that may lead to disease. The DRG and CPT codes could be used to develop rates. It may be more difficult to associate a specific cost with each code, especially in a managed care environment, although Jones could borrow the Medicare "prices" assigned to DRGs and CPT codes and assume a fee-for-service environment for the sake of prioritizing product lines.

Finally, Jones may want to know the time, place, and person descriptors of the enrolled population with regard to morbidity. Some product lines may be age-specific (juvenile diabetes and Alzheimer's disease, for example). Others may be focused on specific settings or places in which the enrolled population either lives or works. For example, lead screening and abatement might be important in older neighborhoods or if a factory that makes batteries is a major employee group covered.

A number of staffing decisions also need to be made. These include the uncertainty about how the new matrix model will affect GHE staffing patterns, particularly with respect to the generalist/specialist mix, as well as the concerns of the nurse practitioners in the satellite clinics. Jones uses the morbidity data from the product-line analysis (see the preceding paragraph) to project the number of enrolled members who can be expected in each product line. He assumes an optimistic and pessimistic scenario with regard to demand increases from market segmentation. Further, he uses industry benchmarks to predict the number of generalists and specialists needed to treat each product line, assuming that productivity remains constant. For the satellite clinics he collects weekly workload statistics by clinic for each practitioner and analyzes these data to determine any statistically significant increase in patient load. He compares each quarter to the previous quarter, and each week to the same week one year ago in this analysis. A statistically significant increase in workload that persists over time would argue for increased staffing in this area.

After making some progress with the change in organizational design and staffing, Jones moves ahead to directing issues. As you recall, the governing board charged Mr. Jones with looking at an incentive system that would reward outcomes. He begins to review the literature on outcomes and is amazed at some of the material he finds, for example, work in New York and Pennsylvania on coronary artery bypass surgery. Using risk adjustment and other epidemiologic tools, they have provided information to consumers, providers, and plans on expected and actual mortality associated with that procedure. Mr. Jones recalls the discussion in Chapter 9 on this same issue. Furthermore, the board has been encouraging Mr. Jones to consider applying for accreditation by the National Committee on Quality Assurance (NCQA). As Jones looks into that process he realizes that a couple of outcome measures might be in order. Specifically, the NCQA expects health plans to examine quality by reporting results to the Health Plans Employers Information and Data Set (HEDIS). In his examination of the measures that comprise HEDIS, he realizes that they are good outcome indicators, and that many are drawn from a planning document that he had seen before, specifically *Healthy People 2000*. He recalls the previous problem, that of product lines in a matrix organization, and realizes that a behavioral risk factor survey of enrolled members might also provide information about baseline levels of several of the key HEDIS measures for his population.

Mr. Jones realizes that he needs to know other outcome variables and baseline variables in the population. Two commonly used outcome measures, for example, are the Short Form-36, developed as the result of the RAND Medical Outcomes Study. This enables individuals to classify their health status on general, mental, and physical scales. He also learns that an important quality for outcome measures is that of patient satisfaction. After careful consideration he decides to take several interim steps. First, he decides to incorporate a quality indicator in the decision about how much (if any) of the 20 percent "withhold" to return to each physician; further, he determines that the quality indicator should be tied to the HEDIS measures and to patient satisfaction. Second, with that in mind, he proposes to conduct a patient satisfaction survey and to undertake a behavioral risk factor survey of his enrollees. Third, he is persuaded of the need to know the health status of his plan members, and does a random sample survey using the SF-36.

Mr. Jones is convinced that the withhold incentive system will work better with quality indicator(s), but he is appropriately concerned about hospitalization costs consuming most of the "withhold" cache in recent years. This has caused considerable discord among physician providers who contend that they are being penalized for provided high-quality care, albeit in a hospital setting. Fortunately, Jones is aware of a promising solution to the problem. The chief financial officer (CFO) has acquired hospital case-mix information on GHE enrollees for the past several years. Several of the diagnoses that have prompted admissions are for "ambulatory-sensitive conditions" (ASC), such as asthma, diabetes, and congestive heart failure. These conditions typically should not result in hospitalization if effective primary care is provided. Thus, any hospital episode related to these conditions is considered a "preventable" or "avoidable" hospitalization.

Ambulatory-sensitive conditions can be categorized into one of three areas. Some conditions are totally preventable, such as hospitalization for an immunizable disease, such as measles. Other conditions should not typically require hospitalization if primary care is sought early enough, for example cellulitis or community-acquired pneumonia. The third group would include chronic diseases, which if tightly controlled, should not require hospitalizations, such as asthma, diabetes, or congestive heart failure. Mr. Jones needs to ponder the burden of diseases like these in the enrolled population, and the financial cost to GHE for these conditions. Although epidemiology is not critical to the consideration of the latter, it certainly is to the former.

Mr. Jones decides to implement a surveillance system with several high-cost and high-frequency ACSs. The purpose of such a monitoring system would be to determine if any potential targets exist for intervention to decrease hospital costs. The strategy is to collect the information from the surveillance system to describe ACSs and "preventable hospitalizations" in terms of the epidemiologic concepts of time, place, and person. The problem of preventable hospitalization may occur during a particular time of year, within certain neighborhoods of the city, or among specific population groups. The cause of this problem may relate to access to care, cultural barriers, or other factors, only some of which may be corrected by an organization intervention such as an outreach program.

Finally, Mr. Jones turns to the issue of setting capitation rates. He is pleased with the previous decisions that he has made with regard to product line and quality of care. These decisions have put in place a mechanism to collect the data needed to determine capitation rates. Specifically, the SF-36 should give him information about the health of his population and about ways in which he might go about determining whether his enrollees are sicker than the normal population. If he can convince employers that GHE members are sicker, on average, than other insured people in the area, he might be able to argue for higher capitation rates. Mr. Jones realizes that the behavioral risk factor data can also be an important part of that discussion, particularly if the members of his plan have a worse risk factor prevalence than is seen across the state. He decides to examine the attributable morbidity associated with several major risk factors in order to evaluate the extent to which such morbidity is responsible for a major portion of the per member per month fee. He realizes that if he can bring these risk factors under control through education, outreach, or other programmatic improvements, the potential will exist to increase profitability, particularly if he can use the data that he has gathered in rate negotiations.

As the result of learning more about epidemiological reasoning, Mr. Jones has begun to improve his decision-making and problem-solving capability. The case study illustrates a principle that we suggested at the beginning of this chapter: that epidemiology can be a very useful tool in all of the managerial functions. Moreover, it is apparent that epidemiology tools can frequently be used simultaneously in several managerial functions, that the epidemiology perspective can influence a manager's practice style in very positive ways, and that epidemiology can function as an integrative approach to management decision making. The use of the epidemiologic method and the epidemiology perspective can improve management—but more important, if the manager is committed to the goal of improving population health, it is a vitally important skill to have.

References

Baker, G. R., L. Narine, and P. Leatt. 1994. "Organizational Designs for Health Care." In *The AUPHA Manual of Health Services Management*, edited by R. J. Taylor and S. B. Taylor. Gaithersburg, MD: Aspen Publishers, Inc.

Fleming S. T., L. Hicks, and R. C. Bailey. 1995. "Interpreting the Health Care Financing Administration Mortality Statistics." *Medical Care* 33 (2): 186–201.

Rakich, J. S., B. B. Longest, and K. Darr. 1992. *Managing Health Services Organizations, 3rd ed.* Baltimore, MD: Health Professions Press, Inc.

Spiegel, A. D., and H. H. Hyman. 1994. *Strategic Health Planning: Methods and Techniques Applied to Marketing and Management.* Norwood, NJ: Ablex Publishing Corporation.

Acronyms

AAPCC	adjusted average per capita cost
AIDS	aquired immune deficiency syndrome
AMI	acute myocardial infarction
APEX/PH	Assessment Protocol for Excellence in Public Health
APHA	American Public Health Association
ASC	ambulatory care-sensitive conditions
BPH	benign prostate hypertrophy
BMI	body mass index
BRFS	Behavioral Risk Factor Survey
CABG	coronary bypass graft surgery
CD	cardiovascular disease
CDC	Center for Disease Control and Preventio
CFO	chief financial officer
CHD	coronary heart disease
COPD	chronic obstructive pulmonary disease
CPT	current procedure terminology
CQI	continuous quality improvement
DRG	diagnosis-related group
EKG	electrocardiogram
EMR	expected mortality rate
EPA	Environmental Protection Agency
ES	effect size
ESRD	end-stage renal disease
ETS	environmental tobacco smoke
FFS	fee-for-service
GERD	gastro-esophageal reflux disease
GMENAC	Graduate Medical Education National Advisory Committee
HCFA	Health Care Financing Administration
HEDIS	Health Plan Employer Data and Information System

HIV	human immunodeficiency virus
HSA	Health System Agencies
IPA	individual practice associations
IS	information system
MCO	managed care organization
MDE	maximum dollar expenditure
MI	myocardial infarction
NCQA	National Committee on Quality Assurance
NHIS	National Health Interview Survey
NNT	number-needed-to-treat
NPV	negative predictive value
OMR	observed mortality rate
OR	odds ratio
OSHA	Occupational Safety and Health Administration
PATCH	Planned Approach to Community Health
PDSA	plan, do, study, act
PMPM	per-member-per-month
PPH	primary pulmonary hypertension
PPV	positive predictive value
PSA	prostate specific antigen
PTCA	percutaneous transluminal coronary angioplasty
QALY	quality-adjusted life-years
QI	quality improvement
RAMO	risk adjustment monitoring of outcome
RAMR	risk-adjusted mortality rate
RBRVS	resource-based relative value scale
RCT	randomized clinical trial / randomized controlled trials
RD	risk difference
RR	relative risk
SMR	standard mortality ratio
SPC	statistical process control
SWOT	strengths/weaknesses/opportunities/threats
TQM	total quality management
UCL	upper confidence limit
UV	ultraviolet

Index

About the Authors

STEVEN T. FLEMING, PH.D. is an associate professor of health services management at the University of Kentucky. He is a faculty associate in the UK Center for Health Services Management and Research with joint faculty appointments in the Martin School of Public Policy and Administration and the Kentucky School of Public Health. He earned a master of applied economics, and a Ph.D. in health services organization and policy, both at the University of Michigan, and an M.P.A. from the University of Hartford. He teaches courses in epidemiology, managerial epidemiology, and community and institutional health planning. Prior to coming to Kentucky, Dr. Fleming taught at the University of Missouri in Columbia. His research interests include cancer epidemiology, quality measurement and risk-adjustment, and using claims data for epidemiological and health services research.

F. DOUGLAS SCUTCHFIELD, M.D. is the Peter P. Bosomworth Professor of health services research and policy and professor of preventive medicine and environmental health at the University of Kentucky. He is director of the Division of Health Services Management and is also acting associate dean for public health in the College of Medicine, and director of the Kentucky School of Public Health. He holds an M.D. from the University of Kentucky. His major areas of research are public health practice and administration, managed care, and preventive services, all areas in which he has published widely. He is editor of the *Journal of Preventive Medicine* and of several textbooks in public health.

THOMAS C. TUCKER, M.P.H. is an associate professor of health services management at the University of Kentucky with a joint appointment in the School of Public Health. He is the deputy associate director for cancer control and the senior director for cancer surveillance at the University of Kentucky Markey Cancer Center. Professor Tucker is also the current president of the North American Association of Central Cancer Registries (NAACCR). He holds an M.P.H. from the University of Michigan. He teaches courses in both epidemiology and health services management. His major research interests include cancer epidemiology, social factors associated with differing patterns of cancer care, and geographic variations in the burden of cancer

KEITH E. BOLES, PH.D. is an associate professor of health services finance in the Department of Health Management and Informatics at the University of Missouri in Columbia. His doctorate in economics was earned at the University of Arizona, with a master's in economics from Florida Atlantic University. His major area of research is in risk evaluation and management in a managed care environment.

JOEL M. LEE, DR.P.H. is a professor and director of undergraduate studies in the Division of Health Services Management with the University of Kentucky College of Allied Health Professions. He is also the director of the Doctor of Public Health program in the Kentucky School of Public Health and a faculty associate with the Center for Health Services Management and Research. Dr. Lee has a master's of public health in health services administration and a doctorate of public health in health services organization from the University of Texas School of Public Health. Dr. Lee's interests are in the areas of managed care, health services management, strategic planning and marketing.

JOHN N. LEWIS, M.D., M.P.H. is the corporate medical director for Health Care Excel, Incorporated, where his current work is in the epidemiology of quality improvement in healthcare. He holds an M.D. degree from Johns Hopkins University and an M.P.H. from Harvard University. He is certified by the American Board of Internal Medicine. His major areas of work have been in government public health practice and administration at the federal, state, and local levels, epidemiologic studies, and preventive medicine. His publications reflect these areas of work.

KEVIN C. LOMAX, M.H.A.C. is a doctoral student in the Ph.D. program in gerontology at the University of Kentucky. His research interests include pension income equality and international comparative aging. He is currently working with the Luxembourg Income Study and conducted research in Europe. He earned a master's degree in health administration and a graduate certificate in gerontology at the University of South Carolina.

KEVIN A. PEARCE, MD, M.P.H. is the Michael Rankin Professor of Family Medicine at the University of Kentucky College of Medicine. He is a faculty associate in the UK Center for Health Services Management and Research and holds a joint faculty appointment in the Department of Preventive Medicine and Environmental Health. He received his M.D. from the University of Florida College of Medicine and completed his residency in family practice at the Medical College of Virginia / Fairfax Hospital. He earned his M.P.H. degree in epidemiology at the University of Minnesota School of Public Health. Dr. Pearce practices family medicine while pursuing his interests in medical education, practice-based research, clinical epidemiology, and evidence-based medicine. His research focuses on hypertension, diabetes, and the prevention of cardiovascular disease.

MARY KAY RAYENS, PH.D. is the associate director of the Biostatistics Consulting Unit in the University of Kentucky Chandler Medical Center and is a research assistant professor in the colleges of nursing and medicine at the University of Kentucky. She earned a doctorate in statistics from the University of Kentucky. Her research interests include the design and analysis of longitudinal studies, both for clinical trials and surveys.

LYLE B. SNIDER, PH.D. is the research director of the University of Kentucky Center for Rural Health in Hazard with an appointment as assistant professor of health services management at the University of Kentucky. He is a faculty associate at the UK Center for Health Services Management and Research and the University's Appalachian Center. He earned a Ph.D. in health policy and administration at the University of North Carolina. Prior to coming to Kentucky, Dr. Snider served as a public health nursing manager and nurse practitioner in rural North Carolina and Alabama. His research interests include rural healthcare systems, the health professions workforce in underserved areas, and access to care.